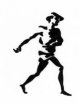

MAKING IT BIG

A Guide to Health,
Success and Beauty
For the Woman
Size 16 and Over

By
Jean DuCoffe
Sherry Suib Cohen

with photographs by Phyllis Cuington

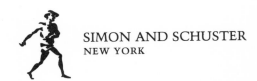

SIMON AND SCHUSTER
NEW YORK

Published by Simon and Schuster
A Division of Gulf & Western Corporation
Simon & Schuster Building
Rockefeller Center
1230 Avenue of the Americas
New York, New York 10020

SIMON AND SCHUSTER and colophon are trademarks of Simon & Schuster
Designed by Irving Perkins
Manufactured in the United States of America
Printed and bound by Fairfield Graphics
1 2 3 4 5 6 7 8 9 10

Library of Congress Cataloging in Publication Data
DuCoffe, Jean.
   Making it big.

   1. Beauty, Personal.   2. Women—Health and hygiene.   3. Obesity.   4. Women—
Conduct of life.
I. Cohen, Sherry Suib, joint author.   II. Title.
RA778.D88   646.7'2   80-13257
ISBN 0-671-25097-3

All photographs are by Phyllis Cuington, with the following exceptions: page 30,
photograph of Linda Huntington by Dan Demetriad; pages 52–53, photographs of Bevy
Chase and Lillian Nilsen by Howard Findlestein; page 69, photograph of Jeffrey Bruce by
Marc Raboy; pages 76 and 339, contrasting shots of E. Anne Denning by Marc Raboy; page
123, photograph of Kenneth by Peter McDaniels; page 156, photograph of Phyllis Cuington
and Madaline Sparks by Terry Weir; page 277, photograph of Allmilmo Corporation
kitchen courtesy of Hayes-William, Inc.; page 284, photograph of Laurette Arnel by Hans
Van Nes; page 314, photograph by Terry Weir; page 326, photograph of Armelia McQueen
by Martha Swope; page 332, photograph of Armelia McQueen and Ken Page courtesy of
Bill Evans/Howard Atlee; page 335, photograph of Linda Kline by Janet Charles; page 342,
photograph of Phyllis Cuington by Terry Weir; page 350, photograph of Rosilyn Overton
by Cameron Block; page 359, photograph of Suzanne Britt Jordan by *The News &
Observer, The Raleigh Times.*

Special thanks to our lovely models, Barbara Barten (who appears on pages 32, 51, 121, 140
and 314), Barbara Betza (pages 81, 82, 111, 113, 135, 138 and 210), Karen Bly (page 130),
Marsha Bonine (pages 93 and 172), Phyllis Cuington (pages 156 and 314), Debbi Freireich
(pages 129, 161, 166, 167, 169, 172, 174 and 222), Linda Huntington (page 30), Mary
Pequese (pages 161 and 172), Madaline Sparks (pages 57, 59, 60 62, 63, 65, 66, 67, 68, 101,
134, 156, 161, 166, 167, 187, 257, 302 and 383), Trish Weyenberg (page 238) and Esther
Yerry (pages 20 and 224).

There are thanks to be given . . .

To Ann Bramson, stellar editor at Simon and Schuster, and her supportive assistant, Jan Hershkowitz.

To William Fabrey and Lisbeth Fisher of *The National Association to Aid Fat Americans,* who have pointed the way for us and for countless numbers of big women.

To Marsha Bonine, a gorgeous, big-of-body and bigger-of-heart woman who helped in more ways than she knows.

To Gloria King and the Other Dimensions Model Agency at 393 Seventh Avenue, New York, NY 10001, who supplied many of the models and much of the support for this book.

To the professional models who appear in many of the photographs, in particular Barbara Barten, Marsha Bonine, Debbi Freireich, Linda Huntington, Madaline Sparks, Esther Yerry, Trish Weyenberg, Mary Peguese and Barbara Betza.

To our photographer, Phyllis Cuington, big, beautiful and on her way to becoming a female Avedon, who also appears in many of the photographs.

To our literary agent, Connie Clausen, for first seeing just how popular and how beautiful big was getting.

To Adam and Jennifer Cohen and Jane Suib for ideas and patience.

To Arthur Lewis who gave Jean her first job in the fashion world with the magic words "Promise me you won't diet."

And to the hundreds of big and wonderful women who spent hours answering questions, delving into their own psyches and testing the many suggestions made in these pages.

*This book is dedicated
to our supportive husbands
Roland and Larry
with love and admiration*

Contents

	Introduction: The Henry Kissinger Story	11
I	Fashion	21
II	Putting On Your Best Face	50
III	Bathing and Beauty	80
IV	The Skin Game	100
V	Hairlines	121
VI	Teeth and Mouth	140
VII	Big, Beautiful and Fit!	155
VIII	Invent Yourself: An Encounter Group	175
IX	Life Situations	187
X	How to Get a Job	209
XI	Travel	237
XII	Sex and Sensuality	257
XIII	An Organized Life	270
XIV	The Big Woman and Her Home	282
XV	Relax	301
XVI	How to Develop a Great Social Life	315
XVII	Women Who Have Made It Big	325
XVIII	Straight Talk for the Teenager	363
XIX	Facts and Myths/Truth and Lies	382
	Appendix: Large-Size Stores	413

Introduction: The Henry Kissinger Story

What has Henry Kissinger got to do with a book on big women? Plenty. What happened with Henry and my friend Marilyn is exactly the point of the book.

They were at a very glamorous party. Marilyn couldn't believe her eyes when she saw Kissinger in one corner of the living room holding forth in front of a circle of admirers on subjects like China, Nixon, Happy Rockefeller. What a terrific opportunity to hear the secrets and gossip of the century!

Marilyn hovered at the outside of the intimate circle trying to soak up Henry's pearls, but she couldn't concentrate. It seems she was on a diet, you see, probably the thousandth diet of her life, and she was obsessed with *not eating food.* Naturally, all she could think of was food. Kissinger talked away but Marilyn's attention was absolutely riveted on a dish of chocolates that sat on a corner table. Was the one with the squiggly line a cherry or a creme caramel? Was the square one butter crunch?

She was torn. She was ravening to listen to the fascinating man, but on the other hand—well, *was* it a caramel? Maybe a coconut.

"At that point," said Marilyn, as she told me the story, "I decided. Diets and food were taking over the quality of my life. I reached over, took the chocolate with the squiggle—*good,* it was a caramel—and got back to Henry Kissinger and the rest of my life."

Someone once asked Shelley Winters what she thought about

nudity and she answered, "I think it is disgusting, shameful and damaging to all things American. But if I were twenty-two with a great body it would be artistic, tasteful, patriotic and a progressive religious experience."

Funny words, but a little sad, too. Winters, like so many of us large women, gives herself the ultimate putdown. What she is saying, in essence, is "I am too heavy to be an attractive woman."

Wrong, Shelley. You could be sensational looking. Who ever decreed that anyone over size 10 can't have a great body? Can't be dynamite-looking? In fact, if Shelley Winters gave herself one-tenth as much time in preparation and in anticipation of being lovely as her skinny counterparts do, she'd be a knockout.

I was raised on the theory that all good children had a lamb chop and a baked potato for lunch. My mother was a rebel but in those days it was called a flapper. I grew up hearing her say, "Be thin so you'll be popular," but at the same time she'd slip me an extra baked potato because I looked peaked. So I was destined to be big. And rounded. And happy. The three are not exclusive. It used to be, I admit, that my idea of happy was not hearing my crotch seams split. Not now. I got smart. If *your* big moment is fitting into the size 12, look hard at yourself. Just because you don't fit into the 12, you still can fit into the social situation. Or the most stunning 42 you can find. People are noticed for their appearance and not for their size. And I, for one, spend quite a lot of time making sure my appearance is dynamic. Why wouldn't I? My mind isn't encased in fat, even if my hipbones are.

Where do you place value anyway? In Israel, where the fuller figured woman is desirable, a man wanted to give Roland, my husband, thirty camels in an even exchange for me. Roland said nothing doing. That's love.

When my mother went to the store looking for a dress and the salesperson asked her size, she used to mutter, "Size fourteen— with the zipper open." That was my mother. *I'm* not in the least embarrassed to ask for size 42.

Men may admire the skinny chicks in their impetuous days, but they end up marrying many of the heavy ones. Why? There's more comfort in a woman with a little cushion of flesh. Fat people are uppers, despite the rumors you've heard to the contrary. They like you even if you have pimples or are broke. They will cry in your beer with you. They will take you in when you're down and out because they have plenty of room. They don't smile tersely, they grin. They're nice. Give a thin person a coffee break and she'll jog around the block. Give a fat person a coffee break and she'll share a cupcake with you. And on top of all that, a fat person with her fashion consciousness raised is a great-looking person. Why wouldn't men want to marry one? Wouldn't you?

A big woman, let's say the word now, even a *fat* woman, can be beautiful. She can throw her weight around and start showing consumer interest in chic fashion, makeup tricks and life-styles not designed to hide her weight but to enhance it. And as soon as the designers and the stores start getting the message that there are some thirty-odd million women size 16 and over out there who *want* to look terrific and who will buy their products, their profits will multiply beyond their wildest dreams.

I do not expect to enjoy an early dotage, resting on my pounds of security. I will use every bit of practical advice I can glean on how to move through my years with the look and the manner of an exciting and attractive woman. And I'll share that advice with you in the following pages.

To begin with, *larger women are spending too much time trying to fit into small images and small dresses.* It's just not worth it. Apologizing for pounds just doesn't pay off.

Recently I sat near a woman at a buffet dinner party who asked her table companion what he did for a living.

"I'm a diet doctor," he answered, looking balefully down at her marvelously stacked plate.

"Um, this plate is for me *and* my husband," the woman stammered apologetically.

"And where is your husband?" asked the doctor.

"In Albany," she replied.

Enough. The time to accept ourselves has come. The time to do important things is now. The time to have fun and look wonderful is today—not when you've lost twenty pounds.

The world is waiting for sanity to return, anyway. The skinny, nervous people who are forever rubbing their bony hands together and saying, "No whipped cream, cholesterol clogs, you know," are boring. Gaunt females turn surly and hard at a young age because they've never learned the value of a hot fudge sundae *with* whipped cream for easing tensions.

What will this book do?

To begin with, it will *not* give you any diets. You already know more about diets than anyone else. If you wanted to, you could *write* the definitive diet book without even trying. You have been struggling with diets for most of your life and you have probably lost and gained and lost and regained at least 278,000 pounds over the years. And you're not exactly a phenomenon in American life. According to the U.S. Food and Drug Administration, nearly 33⅓ percent of *all* Americans are overweight. One-third of America! For persons over forty, the Health Insurance Institute says the figure jumps to a startling 35 percent. As many as 40 percent of all school-age children are overweight and nearly 85 percent of those children will *remain* fat as adults. So don't talk about diets or expect me to. They simply don't do what they're supposed to do.

I've only found one diet that ever worked. A wise old doctor gave it to me. This is it: *If it tastes good—spit it out.* Would you live your live that way? Not me.

This book will not even tell you to eat *less.* If you were hit by a two-ton truck, would the doctor tell you to bleed less? One is about as easy as the other to accomplish. When you *stop* forbidding yourself so many foods, they will lose their insane attraction anyway. A midnight salami sandwich simply doesn't have erotic allure if you know you can have it anytime you wish. Who's going to remember in a hundred years that you didn't have that piece of cake in 1980? Not *one* person will say, "Oh, terrific you, you didn't have that spumoni in the spring of 1980."

Rest assured this book will not tell you how much you should weigh, according to some antediluvian insurance-company weight chart. No book, relative, best friend, group or even doctor has the right to tell you how much you should weigh, except in the case of the severely obese who have trouble walking. If you feel good, if your blood pressure and sugar levels are acceptable, then the only person you should answer to is yourself. If any woman feels reasonably comfortable with her weight, physically and psychologically, then she should learn to live with it. Even if she doesn't actually love it, she should like it *and* herself.

Don't expect the book to tell you that you look best in black dresses. I could wear black from head to toe and *no one* is going to say, "There goes a thin woman!" So why not wear the electric colors, the prints, the styles that are uppers for me? Only two things count in fashion: (1) is it in good taste? and (2) does it fit?

On the other hand, you won't read in this book that it's terrific to be *really* enormous. No one can honestly say you look or feel your best when you can't bend down to retrieve the car keys. But most larger-than-life women don't fit that category. They are sound and very round and feminine and they have the potential of being stunning. Radiant. Chic. Relaxed. Women of accomplishment.

Okay. What this book will do is to show about 30 million (yes there are that many of us out there) heavy American women how to choose and wear the most flattering clothes, hairstyles, makeup and accessories. It will show you how to deal with special problems in the bath, in furniture stores, in the career world, in the bedroom. It will give personalized tips from famous authorities on how to oil, paint and adorn the body bountiful.

There will be material on how to prepare natural cosmetics from the kitchen that are as effective as any expensive commercially prepared products. There will be chapters on how to live well for teenagers, travelers, and partygoers. There will be many nasty myths on fatness medically exploded, and there will be tips on how to deal with everything from sexual embarrassment to getting into a car gracefully. In fact, this book will cover everything. It is the definitive guide on how to become more alive, stunning, sexy and secure if you are size 16 and over. You don't have to fit into size 9 to be a valuable person.

In order to write the book, my co-author interviewed literally thousands of big women. She asked two questions of all of them: (1) If you were *writing* this book, what do you think would be your most important chapter? and (2) If you were *reading* this book, what would you like to find out?

Boy, did the answers range. Many women talked about pride: "I'd like to find out how to develop pride even though I'm fat." Some said they were most interested in sex because it "is as important to a heavy woman as it is to Raquel Welch."

Many big women had similar experiences. For instance, when

we began this book, we had no plans to discuss dental problems. But over 80 percent of the women we spoke with had gum problems. People who eat a lot, we found out, do. Another common concern was social situations—how to get in and out of them gracefully.

So this, first and foremost, is a *practical* book. It will not lecture you about weight, but it will tell you how to live well in body and in mind.

I have spent too many years watching rotten, skinny women put away tons of food that never show on them. There is no way possible I can compete in *that* rat race. The only person who *has* to live with me is *me,* and if I spend too much time trying to change me, I'll have no time left to live.

Listen—I'll tell you a secret. What if you have thighs that a Hungarian family could eat from for a week? Do you have to love them? The answer is no. But decide right now—what *should* make you burn with passion, inside, are important causes that usually have to do with character and not thighs.

Best of all, you don't have to feel guilty if you munch a Hershey Bar when you read this book. Life is too short to take pounds or Hershey Bars seriously.

So, flaunt it! I do, every day of my life!

I am five foot ten, size 42 and a good-looking woman. Everyone says so. That's how I know. When I wake up in the morning, I could hug the world. Being practical, I hug only Roland.

Roland. When I told my mother I was going to marry this elegant and intellectual creature, she said, "Shut up and drink your milk." I did. Drank my milk and married Roland. And I've been deliciously happy and, quite incidentally, very large ever since.

I have everything. Romance, two nice kids and, I've been told, style. A classic and graceful presence. And you know what? I wouldn't change it for all the skinny bones in the world poking out of my cheeks and hips and God knows where else. I hold with the guy who said, "A skinny dame has no more secrets than a goldfish." *I* have lots of beauty secrets which I will share, here. I have lots of everything, actually. The only thing I don't have is a wasp waist. So, big deal, I don't have a wasp waist. I have goodness in my life, and I've got glamour. I have *chosen* my style and it is large and as good as I can make it. I have chosen to reject guilt and starvation. Guilt and starvation never won medals for being fun. And life, my friends, is a fashionable ball!

Of course, you can choose to dance the way many of your friends do. You can waltz with morbid obsessions about calories and diets; you can have your jaws wired; eat Ayds instead of grapes and cancel your subscription to *Vogue.* Or you can reestablish priorities. Everyone has a turning point, a decision time in the fork of life. For me, the fork of life led to an old commercial loft building. I was in my ashamed-of-being-heavy stage, it was 1968, I was dieting up and down, off and on, yo-yo fashion, and I was miserable. Getting thin was a twenty-four-hour job and it looked as if I would have the job for the first sixty-five years of my life.

I was in that particular, grimy loft building the day of my turning point because that's where the local chapter of Weight Watchers was meeting. Another embarrassing, aggravating session lay ahead. Grimsville. Walking up the steep flight of stairs, I carefully noted that *Weight Watchers* was on my left. On my right was an art studio.

I went to the right—and I've been going to the right ever since. Famous Amos cookies taste better than Valium. You pays your money and you makes your choice. And I chose freedom to be what I am. Which, incidentally, is terrific, as I mentioned a few paragraphs back.

Look, I won't kid you. I work at it. But so does Cheryl Tiegs. She wants to look thin and terrific. I want to look big and terrific.

And there are certain responsibilities. Let's face it, my crowd doesn't go braless. And if we wear large bird prints to the art opening, we look as if we're migrating.

But we live in a new world where choice counts. You can choose to start living and stop wasting time trying to fit into someone else's shoes, let alone slacks. The big woman can be beautiful—make no mistake about it. Roland thinks so. Also columnist Pete Hamill, who wrote, "If someone would walk into the offices of a fashion magazine and explain to those people that most American men like women lush and ripe, along the lines of Rubens, not Aubrey Beardsley, it would be fine."

If one-third of the nation's population is overweight, over *whose* weight are we? While we're not the majority, we sure as hell aren't a minority.

These are days of liberation. Very few people will accept rejection from the world anymore because they are a certain color or of a certain religion or racial body or sex. Why should we accept rejection because of our size?

For too many years we've been putting ourselves down, *agreeing* with the people who said we were unhappy or ugly if we were fat. Well, many of those same people are changing their minds because it's fashionable now to be individual. Take Dr. Theodore Isaac Rubin. In his last book, the mercurial Dr. Rubin said all kinds of unflattering things about large women. In his brand-new book he at least has the humility to announce that "Some of my insights and opinions have changed radically. . . . I now take issue with my previous views. . . . Ordinarily overweight people are no sicker, psychologically or physically, than thin people."

Thanks Dr. Rubin, but I could have told you that.

Look—it's easier to be thinner. The world, as it is laid out now, especially in the department stores, makes it easier to buy skinny clothes, sit in skinny furniture.

Very few of us would be telling the truth if we said we *chose* our largeness. If I tried to pawn off that propaganda in this book, you'd close it in distrust.

But the fact remains that most of us can't choose. We are what we are.

Maybe what we are is only about ten or fifteen pounds fatter than what we've been programed to believe is "right" for us. Maybe we're more than a hundred pounds higher than that weight. It makes very little difference because if you *feel* ugly or ungainly at ten or a hundred pounds extra, this book will tell you how to break free of that feeling.

Because, what have we been doing? We've been fighting a dreadful, losing battle and sacrificing our charm, sense of humor, intelligence and self-respect at the altar of *skinny worship* instead of working to make ourselves the most marvelous big women in the world.

Dumb.

We have been demeaning our really ripe and lovely bodies while we've made a cult out of Weight Watchers and a goddess out of Jean Neiditch.

Enough. Fini to all that.

The truth of truths is that *we too* are divine-looking when we make the effort to dress attractively, think positively, expand our horizons and our consciousness. And if we are having more trouble than it's worth being thin, and if being thin isn't being *us*, then let us be big and beautiful.

I'm going to show you how to be even more beautiful than you are. I'm going to show you how to be sensual, be feminine, be desirable and be fat, all at the same time. The most lethal bigotry of all, prejudice against pounds, can be banished. Guilt and self-consciousness can also go the way of all flesh. I can show you all these things because it's my job to show big women a new way of fashion and thinking. All over the country, I spend my days narrating fashion and living shows which feature heavy women showing other heavy women the way to look wonderful and live marvelously. It is my business and my life to teach high fashion and to spread the word that big can be a beautiful option for anyone. If you cannot be at one of my shows, read this book. It's all here.

A man who talks my language is Dr. Paul Scholten, former president of the San Francisco Medical Society. He says, "We can allow ourselves to be plump and contented, rather than neurotic over a few pounds. The time has come to stop the war against fat and admit people can be fat and healthy."

Sure there are many overweight, unhappy women who spend their days and their nights fighting their fat. But there are also many overweight, happy women who have learned to use their voluptuousness, their curves, to enhance their lives. They are drinking in their lives, not counting out their calories.

If you are reading this book, you are already sick of trying to fit into someone else's tiny molds. You are weary of yo-yo diets which never work and which ruin your health anyway. You are ready to accept yourself. You are ready to relax and grow lovely.

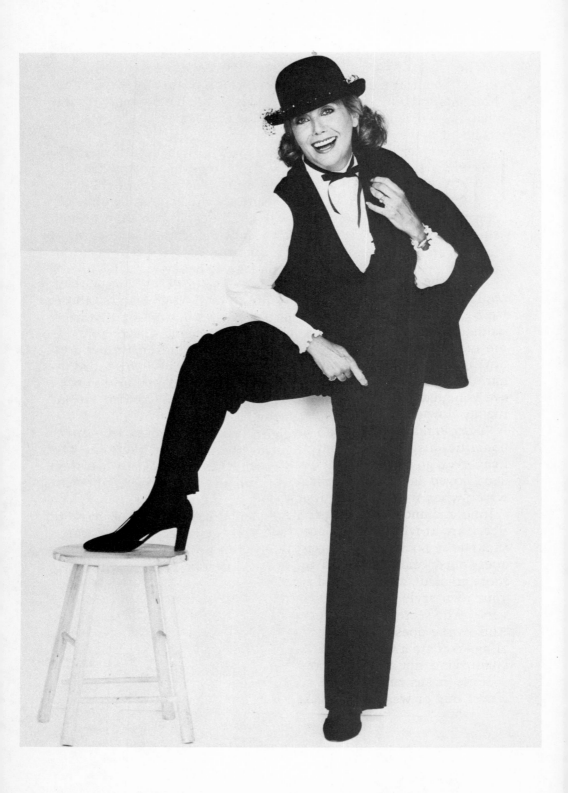

I Fashion

Of all the problems the large-size woman has, buying clothes seems to be the worst. I know a heavy woman who cried herself to sleep after every shopping trip because she felt so ungainly. This woman is truly beautiful, a successful lawyer, a well-married mother of three, and everything in her life was lovely—except for buying clothes. The day that she came to a fashion show I was narrating was, she said, the best day of her life. She waited until everyone had left, then with moist eyes she thanked me for showing her how and where and for what to shop.

"Do you really think I can stop the endless trips to the maternity boutiques just to find something that will fit? Do you really think I can even go to the beach?" asked this woman. Respected, confident, loved in every other part of her life, she was an insecure wreck when it came to fashion.

Inner radiance is the first thing. You can drape yourself in golden fleece and it will look like acetate if you don't know, really know, that you're terrific. All the traditional concepts of beauty are being questioned, and in order to get on with the business of making a more graceful, stunning and appealing you, it is imperative to find your own style. Almost anything is "in" if done with dash and verve. The secret is panache—confidence in your great big dazzle. And dazzle doesn't mean flashy, tawdry stuff. Quiet chic is dazzling. You are a Cadillac on a superhighway of Toyotas; a split of champagne, not a shot of Scotch.

Some basic rules: avoid *silliness* and court understatement. Never buy or wear anything just because it's in. Styles rarely are designed exclusively for the big woman and your choices must conform to your individual body needs. For instance, if you're a teenager and your pals are running around in short T-shirts and tight jeans, don't try to become a carbon copy of them. You can't! If you top *your* jeans with a stunning shirt that comes down to your thighs instead of to your belly button, you're doing what's right for *you*. Your whole appearance can be upgraded with one small change. It's hard to fight the fashion edicts, I know, but when you stop being one of a million sheep and start being one in a million people, you're on your way to high style! Take off the dumb turquoise polyester pants and the mad floral print. Burn the lime chiffon tent. No one is making you dress that way just because you're very large. Read the fashion magazines and watch the television screen to see what the rich and the famous and the daring and the intellectual are wearing. Then develop your own style and never settle for the Omar the Tentmaker special again. Luckily, style has begun to break through the size barriers and if you look you will find your size in the high-fashion departments of the Macy's, Bambergers, Bloomingdale's, Lord & Taylor's, and A & S's of the world. Even Lane Bryant and the small specialty shops that cater exclusively to the large-sized woman have raised their consciousness and have begun to think chic as well as coverage. Storm the stores in your area. If they don't have your size in fashionable clothes, demand to see the manager and ask the reason why. If you don't make your needs and wishes known, nobody will know you've come out of the tent.

Pantyhose manufacturers know what I mean. When pantyhose were invented, a million women sent up a cheer that you could hear in Dakar. Why not? Pantyhose are comfortable, you don't have to suffer the bite of the girdle or the sag of the garter belt, and they look great. They were as important an invention to fashion as Saran-Wrap was to leftovers. *But they came only in little-girl sizes.* Until the larger sizes got mad. They requested and demanded and petitioned for "queen-sized" pantyhose so much that finally the designers and the store owners got the picture: it would be economically to their advantage to make large-sized pantyhose. So they did. And they got rich. Every discount drugstore carries them today. Everyone said the pantyhose designers were brilliant. They were: they listened to the consumer. There are 30 million or so large-sized women out there. We *are* the consumer. We can make the designers rich and ourselves stunning if we only let the stores know we're here. Ready to spend.

I know it's hard. After all, haven't you been putting off shopping all your life because you hate the humiliation of trying on shapeless and too-small clothing in postage-stamp-sized dressing rooms? Totie Fields once said, "When they yell 'take it off,' I say, 'the hell I will. It took me four hours to get it on.' " But determine, from this moment on, that they won't keep you in the kitchen when you want to go to the opera. Make them aware that you'll buy plenty if plenty is available. And another thing: don't let any twit of a store manager intimidate you into thinking you're unhealthy or weak because you're fat.

Isn't it strange—at any Calvin Klein or Halston fashion show, the girls that waft across the stage are obviously suffering from malnutrition. Would it occur to anyone to say to them, "Do you realize it's not healthy for you to be so thin?" Why then is everyone worried about the health of the large-sized woman? One thing's for sure: you will surely stay looking younger than the cadaver models. Flesh is sensuous and softening: bones are harsh and biting.

Okay: you're big and you're beautiful. How do we make you even more terrific looking? Not thinner. *More* terrific. These ways. First:

Size

Every heavy woman must stand herself in front of a full-length mirror one day and do a kinky, a sedate, a sexy or a cultured strip. Her preference for a strip type is unimportant, but *everything* must come off. Even pantyhose. And then she must look at herself hard. And say, *I can be fitted. I look fine. I just have to know what to look for.* Sometimes we manage to avoid seeing the very areas we should be concentrating on. We twist our bodies to avoid the abdomen, the wide waist. If you think you're one who fools herself in a mirror, go to a photographer or a best friend and have a series of photos snapped from every angle. Study them: make a very honest appraisal of your good points and your bad points. It's no time to moan or berate yourself. Rather, decide how you can emphasize the good and deemphasize the bad—the next time you go shopping.

You're probably not even as overweight as you think. For years you've been hiding, crouching, humping your shoulders, letting your back sway and your rear drop and, in a million other ways, making your weight flop in all the worst places.

Is your body fat but tolerably firm? Are you *meant* to be large? Does intelligence gleam from your eyes and sensuality from your mouth? Is your skin alive with good health? You're the one this book is for, baby. You have the potential of Eve. Or any woman on this earth.

There is *no* excuse for *ever* using a giant safety pin to hold a size-16 skirt together when you really need a size 20. That's a gross and sloppy self-putdown. There is *no* excuse for ever wearing a dress that's too short or one which hikes up in the back when you bend over. Almost every emaciated buyer and skinny saleswoman makes the same mistake in trying to provide the large woman with a good fit. They simply do not know the difference between a half size and a large size.

Now hear this: *A woman who is five foot five and under can wear a classic half size.* A half size is high-waisted and has a higher bust dart. It is made for the junior-type woman who has lost her waistline. Half sizes start as low as 12½ and 14½ and are designed to fit a size-14 woman who has slipped her hourglass figure. Half sizes go up to 24½ for the woman who has slipped her whole clock. Now, *if a woman is five foot five and over, she belongs in a large size* with a lower waistline and a longer hem. If I were to go into the most expensive department store around and pick out a $500 half-sized dress, I would look like L'il Abner because I'm five foot ten and the dress would fall no lower than mid-thigh on me. If I were to buy a half-sized pantsuit, forget it. All you'd see is ankles. A long-sleeved half size is short-sleeved on me. If you ignore height when you buy, you'll walk around looking as if someone had thrown your clothes in the hot wash and they had shrunk beyond redemption.

Most large-sized women buy the wrong size. Even if you were a size 10 you'd look dopey in a size-6 Bill Blass blazer. (Bill Blass, incidentally, is one of the few designers left who absolutely refuses to design for the heavy woman, on the grounds that [he thinks] she can *never* look good. Remember that fact when he changes his mind for economic reasons, and boycott him.) If the large numbers on the sizes dismay you, pretend they're a bunch of hieroglyphics. Just get what fits and forget sizes. I have a friend who is the head of a model agency for large-size models. She told me that she was interviewing one gorgeous big woman who, when asked her size, said, "Oh, I can get into a sixteen." How unfortunate. She simply could not accept the image of big is beautiful even when she was supremely qualified to be a perfect example of the best of big. And try to find out what your *real* size is: many specialty shops have gotten into the habit of labeling larger-sized clothes according to their own system. One such store I know has only clothes from sizes 1 to 7. They say their large women love asking for the tiny sizes. That's fine if you *only* shop there, but such a system can make you crazy. It is also manipulative, not to mention silly. A large-size woman shouldn't have to say she's a size 2 when she's really a 42. Don't let them make you play games with your figure size. There is nothing to be ashamed of in facing reality.

If you manage to determine your true size, you must also try to learn the whimsies of the manufacturers. Some are known for cutting smaller waists, some are famous for their deeper-cut sleeves. Often, as the price goes up, the size goes down. Quality clothes usually have quality construction. A size 24½ in a cheap dress is often a 14½ in an Evan Picone.

Chances are also that you are either top-large and bottom-medium or vice versa. Who's perfect? The wonderful world of separates is for you. You can pull a look together if you stick to good. An impeccably tailored size-16 blouse sitting astride a size-20 pant can be stunning. Proportion is essential to look well-balanced. Never try to squeeze into an outfit if only the top half of it fits you. Good clothes need not be expensive if you shop the discount stores and the regular stores in off-seasons. How do you know good? Check the linings of garments. The fabric should have some body and should not be sleazy or rigid. Check plaids, prints, checks and squares to make sure the design is continued in an uninterrupted fashion at seams, sleeves and zippers. Watch for gathered or puckered spots at seams and zippers, also.

It's essential to remember *shoulder* size. When a woman puts on weight, her arms may grow, her waistline gets thicker, her bust may expand, but the one place that remains the same is her shoulders. If a large woman buys a shirt jacket that fits in the shoulders, she won't be able to button it. So what: don't button it. Whatever she does she should never, never squeeze it closed. We all know how terrific *that* looks. But if she looks for a jacket that will button, the gaping shoulders will make her a female Harpo Marx. What to do? Look for the manufacturer who has been smart enough to make dolman sleeves. And face the fact: classic, set-in shoulders are for classic size 10s.

Fat women often have large breasts. Lucky for them, but they need excellent bras to give them the lift and coverage to accent their great clothes. Here's a little-known tip: the one truly expert person in every store works in the bra department. She is almost always specially trained by brassiere companies to fit you properly. She is usually among the highest paid of all the salespeople. Never tell this woman what you *think* your size is. Let her measure you and tell *you.* She knows better, believe me. Why droop in your cashmere when you can be dynamite? Avail yourself of the experts who will neither point you to the stars nor squash you to the earth, but fit you with the best undergarments available. And surprise— the new wire construction bras are comfortable.

Know what you can realistically expect from clothes and look always for proper fit. A properly fitted garment will not show diagonal wrinkles. Follow the wrinkles to their source when you try on clothes and you will usually find the problem. The neck and lower armhole must be cut comfortably. When the arms are raised, the hemline shouldn't fly up also. Sleeve width must be full enough to cover the heaviest part of the upper arm and not bind into the flesh. If the upper part of the dress acts like a constricting brassiere to reveal rolls of flesh, it is too tight. Too tight is unforgivable. Even Dolly Parton looks crummy in skin-tight T-shirts. Too gappy is almost as bad. Baggy pants, drooping waistlines and yards of extra material evoke images of elephants. Clothing that is too tight or too loose equally exaggerates fat. Your clothes should touch you and show your sensuality, not just slide on your body like Hawaiian muumuus. Then again, they shouldn't touch you so tightly that buttons pop open, blouses pull hopelessly across breasts and skirts cup in under your bottom.

You are a big and wonderful-looking woman. Check that mirror again. Do your clothes look as if Halston had designed them after thinking about your proper size for a week? They should.

Fabric

Let's face it. Larger-size women perspire more than their skinny sisters. That dark stain spreading under the arm is not calculated to make one feel like Jackie Kennedy. Natural fibers like wool, cotton, linen, soft silks, gauze, make you perspire less than synthetics. If you really care about things like perspiration, you will not fill your wardrobe with dacron and polyester. On the other hand, if you really care about washing, ironing and cleaning bills, you will not opt for natural fibers. Determine your priorities but be honest with yourself. What is your life-style? What really counts most? Natural fibers are cooler in the summer, warmer in the winter and generally look better. Synthetics are easier. Cheap polyester hangs on the body somewhere between cement and cardboard. But there are certain polyesters that allow perspiration to come through and be absorbed by the air. Visa is one of these. It breathes. And then there are compromises. You can buy synthetics blended with silk, cotton and other natural fabrics. They are always more comfortable and prettier than the pure synthetic. And listen—no woman should consistently wear clothes that she can throw in the machine along with the shag rug and the baby's diapers. She is shortchanging herself and the people who love her no matter what her life-style is. Never be so oppressed and so grateful to have found something in your size that you will be too intimidated to ask the salesperson, "What's this made of?" You have a perfect right to ask about the fiber content of any garment. Be a judgmental shopper. Your money and your experience should buy you good and comfortable clothing.

A tip: Heavy, knobby fabrics tend to make you look larger. Woven fine fabrics cover up styling mistakes and counterattack the clinging look of synthetics.

Style

Find out what you love. Next find out what you look good in. Then find out if they're the same thing. If you like layered looks and if you note that you have a layered look when you're still undressed, you will not want to put on six extra layers. Fads are not for you. No one should be a slavish follower. For someone to wear the Annie Hall look when she is built like Annie Auditorium is just plain silly. I wouldn't wear white socks with high heels if I were four, let alone thirty-four. Someone with a very large super-structure will not want to wear a tight T-shirt with a tiger's head because the tiger will look as if it had mumps. Big prints are not to be tolerated. If a tiny size 10 wears a blouse with huge roses, it looks like a rose-printed blouse. If a size 24 wears the blouse, she looks like the whole garden. But she can wear delicate prints magnificently.

Forget the rules. If you think horizontal stripes are becoming to you, wear them. I say there are two kinds of stripes, pretty and ugly, depending on each woman. A large woman wearing ugly vertical stripes looks as if she were wearing a big cage. And she can wear colors grandly, the way colors were made to be worn. Nothing is out if it's a good-taste color. Chartreuse does not come under this category. Cherry red doesn't make anyone look fatter than before she had the cherry red on. I guarantee she won't look thin in cherry red, but she won't look thin in black, either. The point is to look terrific, not thin. A silky cherry-red blouse and a brown velvet blazer cut in the classical style will make heads turn in envy, not ridicule. Too many colors together distract from a unified look. If you're short and feel dumpy, concentrate on monochromatic (one color) styling. It will elongate you.

Certain current vogues are fine for fat women. Textured hose, for instance. You may have to look farther for them than the little skinny mini who finds her size in textured hose anywhere. But do it! If you carefully pick the styles that were made with you in mind, you won't get in trouble. Thick, long sleeves may be pretty on some of the people some of the time, but on heavy women, under a suit, they are insane. They are bulky and make you feel hot and klutzy. Sleeveless shirts were invented to be worn under jackets. On the other hand, sleeveless shirts are good for nothing else. The Venus de Milo could not wear a sleeveless shirt effectively. Neither could Twiggy, Marilyn Monroe or Jackie O. Right? You can wear plaid skirts and blazers, tweeds and angora, flowing gowns, hats, boots and whatever else you love—if you do it with taste and flare. For instance, you do not wear a plaid skirt and a tweed jacket *together.* Skirts should not have deep pleats or wide flares.

And another thing—wear what looks good on you today, not what you felt marvelous in when you were sixteen. This does not separate you from your skinny sister. She also looks silly in sixteen-year-old clothes. Which means you should both throw out the three-inch false eyelashes.

Designer clothes are available to you now and they never have been before. But don't buy just for a name. Buy for fit. On *our* fannies, names mean less than on tiny bottoms. Listen, we could have the name of the designer, the cutter, the sewer and the guy who delivered the item to the store embroidered on our bottom and still have room for more names. Say yes only if the name means fit. Gloria Vanderbilt obviously fitted her large-sized jeans on fat models; she understands *ample* not only from a coverage but from a flattery point of view.

A further word about life-style: it has everything to do with your clothing and nothing to do with your size. If you're a countrywoman all week or on weekends and go to barns, auctions and state fairs, you will wear well-cut denim and look smashing. If you wore black silk to the auction, you would look like a dodo If you're a city executive running a huge corporation, you will not wear material that clings or rustles when you walk. You will wear a dress with a matching jacket. Both denim and dress must be of good fabric, must fit and must be clean and look neat, let alone attractive.

The point is to wear clothes that fit in your environment. A large woman wearing a lovely silk pantsuit when everyone else is wearing ratty blue jeans will look fatter than she is, even if the silk pantsuit is of good quality. The "right" dress or suit isn't "right" if it's worn for an inappropriate occasion. I once saw a huge woman come into a funeral parlor in a red fox coat. Now red fox on a fat woman is pretty funny, but it's ludicrous within the environment

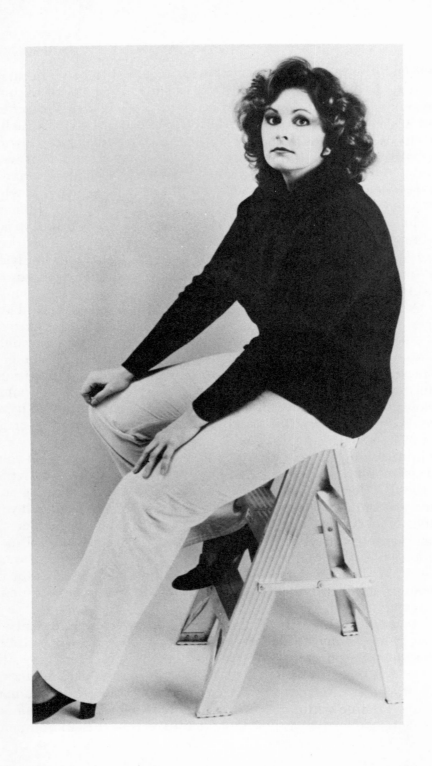

of death. It's silly. And no one's life-style dictates silly. Car coats represent a certain life-style. Car coats are an abomination to me —even long car coats that cover the hips. (*No one* should be caught dead in a car coat that doesn't cover the hips.) Still, if you spend 60 percent of your time in the car, chauffering children and grocery bags, what do you do? You wear car coats. *But you ditch them as soon as you can. You only wear them in the car.* In the supermarket, you throw them over the wagon.

Designer clothes are fine *only* if they fit *you.* Never buy just for a label that yells expensive. Gloria Vanderbilt, for instance, has introduced a large-size collection of blouses, tops and simply super jeans in her new line. The jeans are classic and give the big woman the same quality, fit and designer detailing that size 8s have come to expect from Gloria Vanderbilt. Jeans in brushed cotton, corduroy and denim, blouses in silky crepe de chine and cotton knit— they're dynamite! Pierre Cardin and Sasson have also just come out with "stout" jeans. Be selective and choosy. Don't settle for inferior cut and style. You're in the news now—have you noticed? More and more designers are following the fashion road to the big, beautiful woman. Givenchy enters the field this fall.

How do you make a style for yourself? *Be* yourself. I have always loved long scarves and I'll often put a gorgeous, dashy long scarf on a solid-color dress to give myself verve. Here's a personal fashion hint: go to your scarf drawer even before you go to your closet, and choose a dynamite scarf. Then pick out two articles of clothing for the day that duplicate or blend with two of the colors in the scarf: you can't miss being smartly turned out. I never wear short scarves that disappear into neck folds. On the other hand, I never wear overlong scarves either. Any scarf that floats too far or drags too long will eventually be floated or dragged through the food, despite Marlene Dietrich. There was a dame who wore long scarves magnificently. It just so happened there was a soft breeze always blowing her scarf out and behind her gracefully. It never fails that when I wear that length scarf, the soft breeze inevitably blows it across my lipstick. I end up choking on pure silk with these lip marks all over it.

Arlene Francis always wears a diamond heart and develops a look around it. That's *her* style. Someone else may always wear shining, pristine white next to her skin so whatever she wears, a

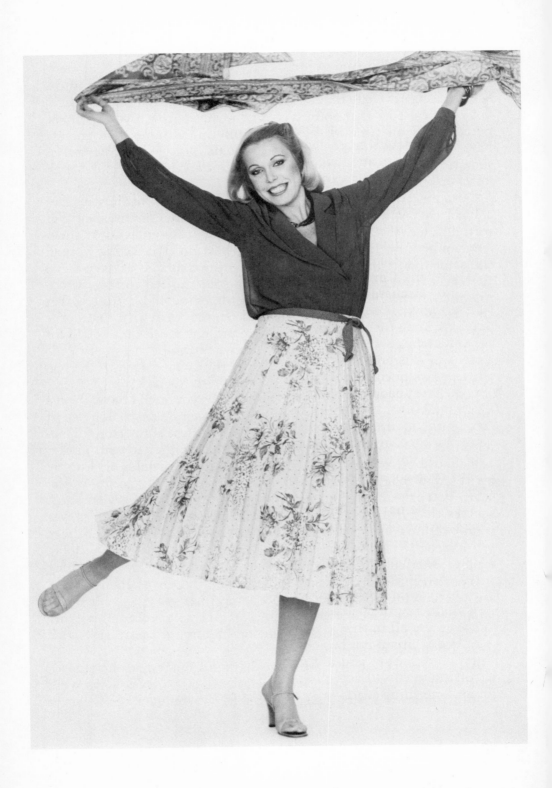

suit, dress or coat, that stunning white blouse or sweater or scarf will peek out. That's style. It is *not* style to wear little Sears Roebuck housedresses, even in your house. Their comfort may be a temptation but their repulsiveness can't be matched. Pass a mirror while wearing a zip-up-the-front job. You'll cry if you really look. Elongated looks given by long scarves, high boots that disappear under the hem, and longer lengths all look marvelous on the heavy woman. They are created for her. Her skinny sisters may steal the style but will never look as dynamic as the big woman in it.

You simply can't ignore the *presence* of the big, stylish woman. Make the most of your size. If you're overweight you do not have to look dowdy for a moment. More and more designers are jumping on the *big* fashion bandwagon. Donald Brooks is making large sizes. Pierre Cardin jeans are available up to a size-40 waist. We've already discussed the great Vanderbilt stuff. And the big bride is being acknowledged in fashions by Alfred Angelo, Francell and others. Look for line plus style as well as size!

If you are really committed to the navy-blue pantsuit, you are in trouble. It is probably not a reflection of your taste, style and feeling. It has nothing personal about it. It has been imposed on you by sadistic people. If you wear only navy-blue pantsuits, you are putting yourself down. As long as you buy only navy-blue pantsuits, the manufacturers will endlessly call, "Cut Navy!" They are guided by your pocketbook. How many pairs of navy-blue shoes have you in the closet? More than one, I bet. I don't know how navy even got started—it's just one of those dumb things. And you know what? Navy is the *worst* color to match. You can never match one navy with another, so why bother? In three shades of navy, you look as if you were hiccuping.

Another hint: If you buy a plain, inexpensive suit, go down to the main floor of the department store and splurge on the simple but elegant scarf that will *make* that suit.

I once arranged a fashion show for large-sized women that consisted solely of the manufacturer's grotty-looking raincoats. The coats were all in that shade of nondescript beige that does so little for any woman, but before the show was over, the women observers were oohing and ahhing in ecstasy over the show's models. You know why? Every plain raincoat came down the runway wearing a smashing scarf—a citron yellow, a brilliant sun orange—and it made all the difference in the world. Of course you shouldn't take spots of color that way and wind it around your *fanny* tightly: on scarves or sleeves, it's terrific!

If you're creative, you can design your own clothing. Or try someone else's patterns. For the first time, large pattern makers like Butterick and Simplicity have created a whole new market of fashionable large-size patterns. And they have cleverly modeled the fashions on large-sized models so you'll get to see how they'll really look.

Your style if you're very heavy? It can be warm and sophisticated. It can be charming and understated. *It can never be cute.* Cute is puffy sleeves and laced-up bodices and ribbons on hair bunches. Any grown woman who is not gravely ill in body or mind should not wear cute children's clothes. Avoid excesses of gathers, flounces, material, ruffles, buttons and bows. Rest assured they'll fall precisely on your worst problem area and emphasize it! You can not wear "cute" clothes when your body says Valkyrie.

Combine your own personality with your own common sense, mix in a little trial and error and close observation of the fashion magazines, and your style-conscious friends and, *voilà.* You too have style! You're a knockout!

The latest fashions interpreted in large sizes include: dresses with shirred or draped sleeves; shorter, narrow jackets, many with some type of shoulder padding; interesting belt treatments on suits and dresses; pretty prints for daytime and evening; slim, straight-legged pants; pleats as well as modified slits in skirts; shorter skirts.

If you are the mother of the bride, don't go to a company that specializes in mother-of-the-bride dresses. You will end up in something that is foam yellow, azure blue or mint green and look like a clone of 20,000 other mothers of the bride. These dresses are churned out by the thousands and all have flowing chiffon sleeves which usually get stained by the salad. The little sparkles at their necklines inevitably leave a rash. You will have total invisibility in a dress like that. You don't have to settle for it and you *never* have to buy anything you don't like. Look hard and you will find a dress in simple lace, satin, silk, velvet or matte jersey that expresses *your* style. Luxurious colors and fabrics that shout *I count!* can be had with a little extra effort. If you can't find the dress, have it made, but never compromise your potential message of elegance and beauty.

Mood Dressing

You can dress to fit your moods. If you feel authoritative one day and you happen to be fat, you can really make a statement with charcoal grays, deep maroons and tweeds. Suits, shifts and tailored blouses and skirts are for you. A successfully authoritative person will burn her mustard-yellow pantsuit and her frilly flamingo-pink shirt.

If you feel like being cuddly and you are fat, God, can you be cuddly! Warm camel-colored sweaters and pale-blue wool skirts and subtle perfumes and a quality fur coat and never, never tight, sprayed-on pants and gaping, revealing necklines. That's cuddly. If you feel intellectual and you are fat, you are a presence to be reckoned with. You can dress in earth tones of rusts and browns. You can wear denim if it's wonderfully cut and you can wear exotic clothing like Indian blouses and Guatemalan shawls if they are not too outrageous. Long blazers and reefer coats are splendid. If you feel kinky and you are fat, forget it. Kinky fat is not pretty or witty. It is one of the few areas, in the interest of good taste, which is out for you.

Neatness Counts

A word about neatness. No matter what mood you're in, it counts. Just as it did in third grade. Certainly, everyone needs one terrible, grotty-looking outfit, preferably with ice-cream stains, to wear just as a release. It makes you feel better. But only wear it in the backyard. And then only if the backyard is fenced in. The large-sized woman can tend to look disorganized if she is not careful, and there is nothing worse than a button missing or a fruit stain on her bodice to give her an unkempt look. She has to be more careful than her skinny counterpart.

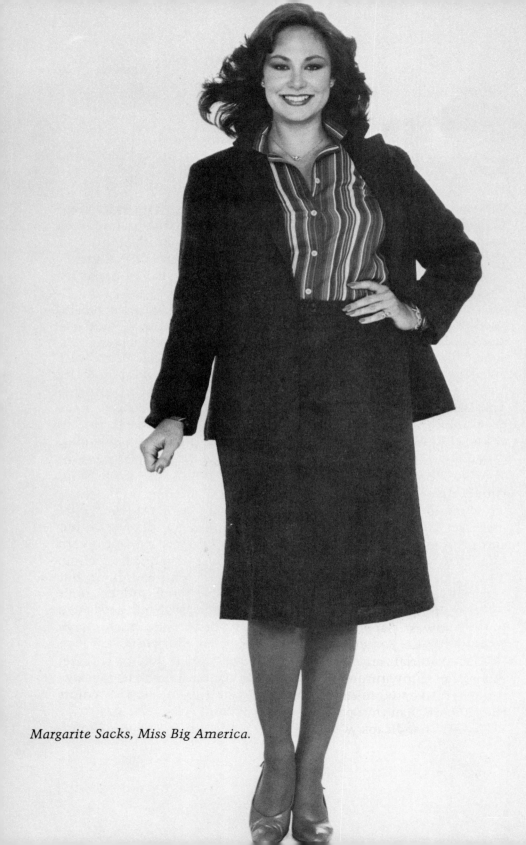

Margarite Sacks, Miss Big America.

Wise Words:

• You can be heavy and look sexy.
• You can be heavy and look sophisticated.
• You can be heavy and look casual.
• You can be heavy and look demure.

The one thing you cannot be, and still be heavy and good-looking, is *sloppy*.

• Heavy and sloppy simply do not go together.
• Heavy and sloppy look *miserable*.

So, comb your hair, iron your blouse, throw out the scuffed loafers. *Sloppy is not for us.* Or for many others, either. Well, maybe a sixteen-year-old, size-6 cheerleader.

Clothing Messages

Make no mistake. Clothing is the loudest nonverbal communication there is. Your clothes are seen before your voice is heard. Your economic status, your educational level, your profession, your state of mind, are instantly judged by your apparel. Blue-collar workers and Ivy-Leaguers communicate different emotional messages. "Glad rags" or party clothes transmit a message of fun and excitement. Mourning clothes, Sunday dress, patriotic garb like Nazi brownshirts and Green berets all communicate feeling. Take color: beige in New York says you're fashion-conscious, but beige dies as soon as you get to Paramus, New Jersey, and you can't sell beige for potatoes in Idaho. Blue, on the other hand, says class in the Midwest. Sapphire blue, robin's-egg blue, azure blue or navy blue—but blue. Forget celery and celadon in Chicago.

Take material: any material that says budget or bargain basement (like shiny, turquoise nylon) says cheap, poor, coarse. Heavy people are even more easily labeled by the material and the colors they choose than thin people.

Physical handicaps, weight, other things that make you "different," are not as significant in the first impression you make on people as clothing. First impressions of ill-fitting and sloppy or poor-taste clothing are hard to erase. The people who hold the power in today's society are the educated, the rich and the creative. They almost always look it. Stained shirts and acetate pantsuits shout *powerless* or *bad taste.*

Heavy people must be especially careful of their clothing messages. They can spell dynamic, successful, happy, tailored, gorgeous. Or they can spell tacky and insecure.

A few examples: clothes with designers' names and initials should be worn by the designers—not lovely, individual you. Leather sends a message of quality. Plastic is poor. Shirts and blouses that say things, give messages like "Mexico" or "A Woman's Place Is *Everyplace*" are okay for the marina or the beach but crummy for the theater. Little-girl bows say kittenish. Fabric that would look good as wallpaper or draperies says gauche. Coats, unlike blazers and jackets, often get buttoned. Therefore you must get a coat that fits—all over. There should not be countermovement in a coat. You and your coat must go in the same direction. Otherwise, the message to the world is, "I don't care. I don't *have* a direction."

Have It Custom-Made, Madam!

You used to be able to buy a car with a radio and an air conditioner for what you pay today for a large-size, highly styled dress. There's a better way, if you want to take the time. Maybe not really cheaper, but better and sometimes not even more expensive.

There is no village, no town in America so small it doesn't have a village dressmaker. And that dressmaker usually has, as the *backbone* of her business, the large-size woman. If you don't see what you want in the stores and you don't want to settle for something that doesn't fit and doesn't have quality—have it made! Usually the price difference between what you have custom-made and a good, lasting piece of apparel that you buy in a store is negligible. Sure, a dressmaker off the Rue de la Paix in Paris will charge a fortune, but a dressmaker off Main Street in Hohokus or even

Manhattan will not be that expensive. Use the same positive attitude that tells you it's silly to make a fetish out of *not* having the lemon meringue pie to find yourself a reasonable dressmaker.

First: Ask around, look at the Service Available section in the want ads of your newspaper, or even put your own ad in the paper stating that you are looking for a reasonably priced custom dressmaker. Check the Yellow Pages for listings under Dressmakers, Custom-made Clothes or Custom Tailoring.

Second: Look in the magazine ads for a picture of something you love: bring it when you go to see your dressmaker. Perhaps she will be one of those talented women who can make her own pattern for your size and copy the design from a picture. Perhaps she will ask you to look through the pattern books for a style and/or pattern.

Third: Now comes the best part—your dressmaker will tell you how much fabric she needs. The greatest luxury in the world is picking out one's own print and fabric for a dress, a blouse, a blazer. Most department stores have fabric departments. Ditto J.C. Penney's, Sears Roebuck, Wards, Woolworth's. Make sure you read or find out the washing instructions of the fabric you choose: there is no law requiring yard goods to be labeled in terms of washing instructions as there is for ready-made garments.

Fourth: You will probably have two to five fittings before the garment is ready to wear. And—joy of joys—it will fit! And you will feel like a million pampered dollars.

Let me give you one small example of why it's lovely to have some of your clothes made to your own ample specifications by a professional dressmaker. Take the matter of bust darts. A few years ago, *all* blouses for large-sized ladies were made with the same 18,000 unflattering bust darts. A bust dart is supposed to flatter the wearer, but tell that to the manufacturers who put the same-size dart in the same place in every large-size blouse that came off the assembly line. I hated bust darts with a passion. If I put on a blouse where the bust dart was too high, it looked as if my breast was hanging from my ears. I bought those blouses and I suffered and looked pathetic. So did 25 million other women. Then we got mad and we stopped buying so many tops, because they looked unbelievably awful. The manufacturers heard the message.

They found a way to manufacture tops without bust darts. We started buying again. And the blouse market went bananas.

Today, three and four tops are sold for every bottom sold because today's tops don't have peculiar bust darts and they look like every other blouse made for thin women. We don't stand out, we are not freaky-looking, we wear tops that fit. *Which is not to say that bust darts were retired.* On the contrary. A bust dart on a small blouse looks like a marvelous little dressmaking detail. It works! On the mass-produced blouses I mentioned, the darts looked as if they were each a yard-long slash. They were superimposed on the material and on the design, changing everything. But when a dressmaker fits a top specifically to your body, she will put a bust dart in that belongs. It belongs because it's *your* bust dart and not Morris the Marker Maker's bust dart. It is a custom detail.

Dressmakers know how to cover the bulge that is 7¾ inches off your shoulder blade. They know how to drape the material so it won't slide up on *your particular behind* as you sit down. Check it out.

And, I might add, check out making your own clothes. All over America, women who have never held a needle in their teeth for even button-sewing purposes are finding that the patterns designed for large-sized ladies make it much easier to create your own wardrobe. I've known the most militant feminists who have been delighted with a newly developed skill of dressmaking. I know a woman writer who got a bigger personal kick from a stunning caftan she made with her own writing fingers than from a $10,000 advance on a new novel.

Accessories

I detest a lot of *jewelry*—on anyone. Luckily, with the large-size woman, much of the jewelry doesn't fit. Chokers interfere with breathing, but long chains look attractive. Irregular or angular-shaped beads are great for very full faces. Large gypsy earrings should be limited to gypsies. Avoid overloads. The days of the twelve bangles and the ring on every finger are mercifully gone. Rhinestones during the day are crazy. Wide bracelets are right for heavy arms, delicate link chains are a matter of personal choice, but charm bracelets are out. No jewelry should be so tight as to squeeze the neck or arms. Pearls are perfect except with pants. Good costume jewelry is fine, but glitter like glass beads, sequins and anything with metallic thread is not fine. Thank God they got rid of rhinestone-rimmed glasses. Avoid bosom-length beads on large bosoms. Long, delicate, slim earrings increase facial length. (Make sure they're not brassy or gaudy.)

Wield accessories as if they were potent weapons. You can win any difficult fashion battle with them. Suppose all you can find in your hometown (not that I believe it for a moment) are dumb, double-knit, navy polyester pants. You don't have to end up looking dumb. Match a gorgeous pure-silk blouse with them, add a sophisticated print scarf, then a contrasting good wool jacket and, finally, a piece of real gold jewelry.

Tight *belts* are taboo; loosely fitting belts are usually acceptable, even if you do not have a waist. If you have trouble finding a belt that fits, link two or three together to get the double-belted look that is popular. And if three belts still don't fit, quell your sensitivity and improvise. But *don't* squeeze your middle, *ever.* Unless you like the sack-of-wheat look. And if you don't like belts, forget them. No law requires you to define a waistline that has disappeared.

Large *hats* are smashing on larger women. They offset your size and flatter your face. Add a stunning hat and your outfit is sensational! Too much hair is not pretty under hats. Less than swanlike necks look more graceful with wide-brimmers. See Bella Abzug. Slightly irregular brims and higher crowns do wonders for triple chins.

Shoes

Choose comfortable *shoes.* Pained expressions are not glamorous. Itty-bitty evening shoes of satin and velvet look silly on everyone. Gold and silver shoes are the pits. Your life-style should dictate shoes. If your back doesn't scream in protest, emphasize your height with high heels. They *stretch* you out. And even if your back does hurt a little, for special occasions choose high heels that flatter whatever else you have on. And compromise: wear your bedroom slippers in the car and change to the heels seconds before you get to where you're going. When I have an important function at night and I know I have to be walking around all day, I wear my flats and carry the heels in a large chic, purse (never a supermarket shopping bag, please).

Open-toe shoes are not particularly flattering to heavy legs. Shoes on heavy legs should be of one color, have an unbroken line, and should not have chunky, squared-off toes. Ankle straps call attention to stocky ankles and calves. White shoes draw the eye to the heavy leg like a flag. Suedes are great and dull-finished shoes are fine. The simple, ever-classic pump is your best bet.

What if your town doesn't have stores that stock very wide shoes, and you need them? Quietly but firmly tell the buyer: "I'm going to write to the president of the store, I'm going to speak to customer relations, I'm going to make a million phone calls—but you must not ignore the woman with the wide foot! If you service me, I'll bring in thirty wide-footed friends: I demand high style in shoes. Order shoes that will fit me!" You'll get them. Remember when everyone smoked anything on airlines? It wasn't until enough people said they resented cigar smoke in their lunch that the airlines forbade pipes and cigars. You must speak up or be ignored.

It is kind of difficult to shop for shoes by mail order, but if you *really* can't find anything to fit you, consider sending for the catalog of the Lawson Hill Leather and Shoe Company, 580 Winter Street, Waltham, MA 02254. They are specialists in hard-to-find sizes and offer a large selection of stunning leather shoes with a ten-day, no questions-asked guarantee of money return if you are not satisfied with your purchase.

No longer do *handbags* have to match shoes. Never try to hide your middle behind a pocketbook. It should be carried over the shoulder or over the arms and *to the side* of your body—never poised on the stomach.

A Special Word on Bathing Suits

Have you ever said, "Oh, God, it's July, I have to take off my coat, I guess . . ."

Well, scratch that attitude. It is true that we traditionally feel uncomfortable at beaches. But times have changed. You're allowed to live now as well as your emaciated counterpart. Ignore your mother who tells you to stay home from the beach. Joie de vivre is what counts. But know one thing: if you persist in wearing that navy-blue, skirted sack to the beach, you will not look thinner. You will only look like a large navy-blue rock on the pale sand. Beiges and lighter colors are much better because they help you to blend in with your environment instead of sticking out like a boulder. Inner bras are a must for the heavy top, and widely spaced straps detract from top-heaviness. You may be gorgeous in your massiveness, but a bikini and sometimes even a two-piece suit is back to silly again.

There *are* bikinis in size 52. I prefer not to comment on *that* look. Quiet elegance, understated dignity it's not.

There's no getting around it: the beach *is* a difficult place for large women. Even the most liberated, successful big women have confessed their discomfort in bathing suits.

But try hard to remember: you are not so visible as you think. In fact, you are pretty invisible. No one is staring at you, no one really cares. People are caught up with their own self-images and they hardly see you at all. Why should you deny yourself one of the great pleasures of life because of *imagined* side looks? If your bathing suit bulges—let it.

Try to blend in with your environment, here as elsewhere. If everyone else is wearing one-piece maillots, the navy skirt with the white piping down to your knees will stand out like a sore thumb.

Actually, *nothing* hinders *or* helps very much in a bathing suit. You're pretty much down to basics at the beach, so look as chic as you can and don't worry about camouflage. I love to swim, and you can bet I'm not staying home in August. I do, I must admit, spend a lot of money on marvelous-looking cover-ups and beach jackets, and when I come out of the water, I slip into them. But I don't worry about hiding—and you shouldn't either.

To sum up, scratch bikinis, check out the straight, good-looking one-piece maillots, stand up straight and be the great, big, beautiful doll of a bathing beauty you are meant to be.

Glasses

A word about your eyeglasses: if you need them, they're as important a fashion consideration as any suit or dress. Glasses can be stunning or silly.

Meyrowitz, one of the largest chain of opticians in the country, gives us the word through one of the chain managers: "When you buy glasses, go to a place where the selection is enormous. Your choices are severely limited at the neighborhood frame store unless your neighborhood is Broadway and 42nd Street. Designer frames are now available, but you may find that your shape face does not need an initial or a famous name decorating it."

Here are some suggestions for glasses that look great:

- Don't buy glasses that are the same shape as your face. Opposites go together. A large woman with a large, round face looks unnatural in tiny, round frames.
- Rimless glasses emphasize the roundness of the lens; round, pudgy faces look terrible in them. (Also, they are quite fragile.)
- Half-frames are disaster on chipmunk cheeks because they focus attention on the lower part of the face.
- Round faces look stunning with frames that are deep and angular or geometrically shaped. (A modified square or rectangle is particularly nice.)
- Coordinate your glasses with your skin tone, eyes and hair. The wrong color frame or lens can make you look perpetually drained or tired.
- Wear enough dark mascara to give your eyes the soft, curving depth that glasses tend to take away.
- Squarish faces shine with rounded frames.
- Long faces like wider frames.
- Oval faces can do no wrong.

Glasses should follow the natural brow line. Frames should be level with or slightly above the natural brow.

Marilyn Bernard, beauty and technical advisor to the glasses company of Univis, notes: "There is nothing more distracting than a woman who has two sets of eyebrows, one that moves and another that doesn't."

If your complexion is pink or rosy, cool greens, blues and grays are the colors that will best flatter you in lenses and frames. Pale or olive complexions do well with warm browns, rusts and plums. Amber looks well on almost everyone.

If you are farsighted and have trouble putting makeup on, Ms. Bernard suggests a makeup eyeglass frame. "Each lens folds down on the cheek so you can put makeup on the eye while looking through the lens which is not folded down."

Last glass words:

- Glasses should not feel heavy on the bridge of your nose.
- Rhinestones are definitely out. Anyone who wears rhinestone-frame glasses ought to wear fake beauty marks and an acetate rose in her hair.
- Be sure a licensed optician waits on you in the eyeglass store, not his teenage trainee.

Shopping by Mail

If you order clothes from catalogs, be sure everything is returnable.

Elnora Worder's *Designer Collection, the Large-Size Supplement* is one of the biggest catalogs on the market for the large-size customer to check out and buy the newest looks from. It concentrates on clothes from American designers like Gloria Vanderbilt and Baron Peters, among others. Dresses, coats, suits and ensembles in all the 20s sizes are included. The catalog is available at Elnora Worder Designer Collection, 200 East 36th Street, New York, NY 10016. For faster service, Ms. Worder can be reached at (212) 685-6183.

SPECIFIC DO'S AND DON'TS FOR THE LARGE WOMAN

Do Wear	Don't Wear
Elongated objects like long scarves, chains	Bulky stuff in pockets
Straight-leg pants	Kinky, silly clothes
Coat dresses	Spangles and bangles
High boots that disappear under your hemline	Foam-yellow chiffon
Longer lengths	Tight anything
Natural-fiber products like wool, cotton, linen	Shirts tucked into pants
or	Dirndl skirts
Synthetic *and* natural-fiber blends	Large, ugly prints
Fullness at front of skirts	Anything too short
Shirt jackets	Too-tight underwear (makes for odd patterns)
Blouses worn out, reaching the hip or even lower	Double-breasted anythings
V necks, scoops, square necks	Turtlenecks (not great on short, heavy necks)
Tailored suits	Baby-doll dresses
Tunic dresses	Baggy pants

Who Are We?

We're heavy housewives and corporation presidents and restaurant owners and entertainers and college students and accounts-receivable secretaries and writers and saleswomen and bankers—and we all care about how we look.

We're Puerto Rican and Irish and third-generation Americans and Italians.

We're Jewish and Protestant and Catholic and Buddhist (and maybe one or two Hari-Krishnas).

We're black and white and tan, and I know one large woman who has yo-yo dieted for so many years, the striations on her body make her look striped.

Some of us are jolly, just as they think. Some of us are testy as hell. Some are sophisticated. Some are naive. None of us, if we are fashion-conscious, is sloppy.

Twenty percent of us are under 35.

Thirty-seven percent of us work full or part time.

More of us than the skinny ones are married: 83 percent of sizes 16 to 52 are married, as opposed to 66.2 percent of sizes 4 to 14. (How do you like them apples?) The fat lady doesn't cry alone in her beer every night, as most people think. She is more likely to go discoing and dining with her adoring husband.

Twenty-five million of us wear size 16 or larger, and 8.5 million wear over size 22. (Over 30 percent of the adult female population of the United States.) Marjorie M. Reich, President of Merchandising Motivation, Inc., of New York City, did a carefully documented study of the fashionable big woman and came up with these amazing statistics, which are closely supported by fashion and sociological studies all over the country.

Why Should Anyone Listen to Us?

Because the large-size woman who is aware of her fashion sense is big business. In 1977, she spent $675 million on dresses and $420 million on slacks and jeans. In 1980/81, because of the new interest in her fashion and her immediate buying response, the big woman will come close to doubling that figure. Did you know that if 53 percent of the American women who weigh over 140 pounds spend only $200 a year on clothing, that's *5 billion* in the coffers of the fashion business world? (It has been estimated that 40 percent of these women spend almost four times as much: no small potatoes.) No wonder more and more manufacturers are waking up to the challenge of designing for this market. They have been making the same dumb, idiot, half-size dress since time immemorial and it was difficult to get them to change the pattern as long as we kept buying what they churned out. Since the big woman has awakened to her fashion potential, the selections from which she has to make choices have grown and grown. In 1955 there were only about 150 manufacturers of large sizes; in 1978 there were at least 500.

And the specialty shop for large women has been invented. The specialty shop that is chic and glamorous.

"It's not just a question of taking a junior style and making the whole thing bigger," says a salesperson at The Forgotten Woman in New York. "The big woman gains in her abdomen and her hips, but other parts of her, like her shoulders, never get any bigger. Styling for a big woman must be based on research and experience. Big women should not patronize a manufacturer who jumps into the market with a large-size line that doesn't take her special needs into consideration. That manufacturer is interested in dollars only, not good looks."

We have become a potentially powerful group with big buying power and we must be careful to use our power intelligently. Any manufacturer who courts us is in for hefty profits.

Because we are so grateful to finally have attention paid to us, we are easy dupes for quick putdowns. At least in the past, we have been. Take cute little Oscar de la Renta, who is not really so cute. He said he would never design for the large-sized woman because he was not in the upholstery business. One day, I guarantee you, Oscar will be designing for us because he will have found out that there's money in the big woman. Even if he changes his tune, I won't. *Nothing* could get me to buy an Oscar de la Renta hair ribbon. Let Oscar be forever stuck with the skeletally chic.

Take multiple sales: we are too often what has been called "multiple unit sales." I have, in the past, been so grateful to find a dress in my size that I bought the thing in mauve, plum, black and blue. That is a true self-putdown. Don't buy it unless you really love it, and then only buy one. With a little effort and time you'll find other things which fit you and which you love. Select, don't settle. The market will reflect your desires if you're buying. If you buy only navy-blue polyester, again, that's all they'll cut.

We are entitled to hard fashion news. Some manufacturers are still trying to get us into that double-breasted navy-blue spring coat with the two pockets, one for the gloves and one for the candy. The rest of the fashion-conscious country knows spring coats and gloves are out and raincoats and boots are in. No one *needs* spring coats any more. But as long as we'll buy them (and be very out of style, unknowingly), they'll cut them.

According to a study done in 1978 by The Fashion Group Inc., an organization of over 5,000 people in the chic fashion world, it was found that the large-size customer wanted, in clothing, five things, in this order of importance:

1. Good fit
2. Quality
3. Color choices
4. High-fashion design
5. Moderate price

Amazing! Before this study, designers and manufacturers thought the big woman was mostly a dowdy dame who cared about price most of all. Now, they found out, she follows the fashion pattern of any other American woman. She has the same needs, wants the same choices of fit and quality as her hungrier, leaner sisters. And, most surprising of all, *she's willing to pay for it!*

Her greatest complaint, according to the study, was that the clothing she found was too tight at the armholes, bustline and hips.

She also wasn't thrilled with the lengths of the garments found in the large-size department. Just because she's heavy doesn't mean she's tall. Sixty percent of *all* women are five foot six or shorter.

She wants to see what she'll look like in the clothes the stores offer her and she therefore is happiest when big, beautiful models show her size in the catalogs.

We have been a badly neglected group, but the message is coming across, surely though slowly. Fat power is winning.

We *will* be listened to in the fashion world because we have the taste to insist upon excellence and the money to buy what we like. We will not diet our lives away in the fruitless battle to fit into Oscar de la Renta's size 6s. Instead, we will live and eat normally.

We have $5 billion in our fists to spend on fashion. We'll spend it wisely and well.

II Putting On Your Best Face

Who did it?

Well, for one, Cleopatra loved to do it. Also Jezebel, Nefertiti, Clara Bow, Princess Pignatelli. Ophelia did it against Hamlet's wishes. Lots of others did it.

Who wouldn't?

Queen Anne wouldn't. Cotton Mather's wife, the author's daughter, Margaret Mead. Lots of others wouldn't. And didn't.

Do *what?*

Face painting, that's what. Otherwise known as makeup.

Just as fatness was *in* during the Golden Age of Greece, *out* during the Dark Ages, *in* during the Renaissance, *out* during the twentieth century—the art of making up has also seen its share of ins and outs.

The ancient Egyptians wouldn't be caught embalmed without a pot of black kohl, and Nero's Roman beauties whitened their faces with chalk and used barley powder to camouflage their classic Roman pimples. Primitives and witches painted their faces. Also Rosalyn Carter. Also Gloria Steinem. Also my mother.

Then again, it was definitely sinful for the Puritans and English-women of the sixteenth century who were subject to a law saying a woman "who seduced any one of Her Majesty's subjects by using face paint and false hair" was guilty of witchcraft. The law didn't say anything about shy young maidens pinching their cheeks to raise color, so they did a lot of that. Even the Bible comes down hard on makeup wearers: it suggests that "the assembly shall stone them . . . and burn up their houses with fire." Somewhat of an overreaction, even if it is the Bible.

King Louis XIII of France thought makeup was terrific. King Louis XIV didn't. Eleanor Roosevelt ignored it. Jackie Kennedy did not. Clearly, a controversy exists.

Suffice it to say that even in the most prudish of times, women found a way to color and moisten their faces with oils, lubricants and the color from natural berries.

How come? Simple. Makeup, subtly, cleverly used, *makes you look pretty.* It really does. Most women and particularly large-sized women don't feel good unless they think they look pretty. And no matter what anyone says, the freshest-faced virgin, the apple-cheekiest maiden, along with any sized woman, can all do with a dab of mascara, a blush of rouge—particularly if they're over thirty. And before, depending on their God-given assets.

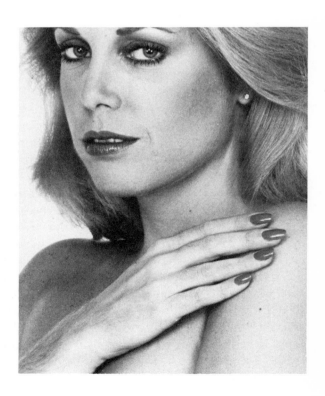

It's particularly important for us, whether apple-cheeked maidens or matrons, to learn how to apply cosmetics softly. Makeup draws attention to the face, your strongest asset. It gives you that chic, stylish, lovely look. It makes a very plain face attractive and a very pretty face irresistible. It completes a well-groomed, appealing appearance.

But, you say, your husband likes the "natural" look? Like Debbie Reynolds, Cheryl Tiegs, Pollyanna, Rebecca of Sunnybrook Farm? I guarantee you, three pounds of cleverly applied makeup could probably be scraped off any one of those faces at any given moment. Pollyanna probably wore the most, with Rebecca running a close second.

The point is that you can wear a dozen flattering colors or tints in blusher, eye liner and lipstick to the office or the den mothers' meeting and, if they are applied artfully, you could look as if you were wearing no makeup at all. You just look smashing.

Of course, when the den mothers' meeting is over and it's disco or seduction time, you can whip out your mysterious midnight-blue eye shadow, your lusty bronzer and your sparkle-plenty lip gloss and knock them all dead!

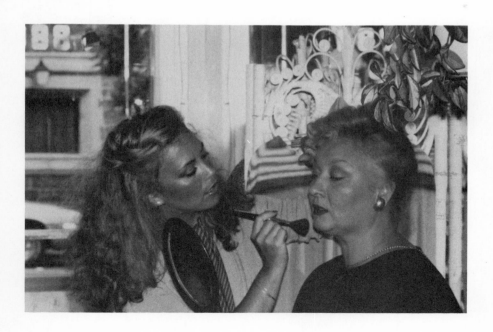

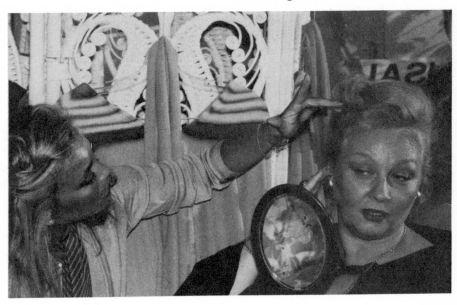

Bevy Chase, makeup artist, shows Lillian Nilsen, salesperson at The Forgotten Woman, how makeup can make you look "like you but better."

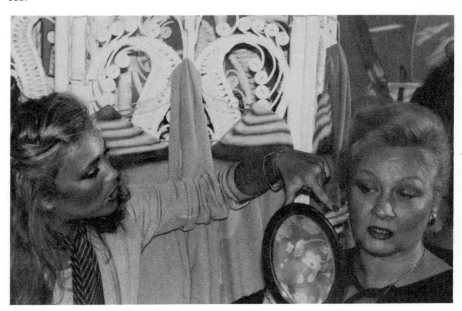

You think nothing of spending weeks looking for the skirt that is stylish without being too tight, the boots that fit over your calf, the blouse that doesn't look like a potato sack—why stop there, at the neck? Inspect your face, experiment, learn about cosmetics. As Bevy Chase, a makeup expert especially for the larger woman, says, they will make you look "like you but better."

All makeup is a combination of unlikely ingredients: fish scales, wool fibers, seaweed, ambergris, flower oils, sulfides, acids and vegetable coloring, to name a few. Generally it's all wrapped up in a tinsely package guaranteed to make you start fantasizing. But it's not fantasy. And even if you don't buy everything the Kiss and Sell Guys, better known as the cosmetics industry, push, it *is* a fact that fleshy eyes can be made to look wider and less fleshy, jowly chins can be made to disappear (almost), and cheekbones submerged in fat can be pulled out. Fat faces, bland faces, can be made into shapely faces, interesting faces.

Just because a cosmetic carries an expensive price tag doesn't mean it's good. And many of them are expensive. You can buy, for example, a lipstick cased in sterling silver from Marcella Borghese, for —are you sitting down?—$200. The refill costs $8.50 (which should give you an idea how much the actual product costs to make).

And just because a product is new doesn't make it good, either. Some of the new commercial face creams, for instance, have mineral bases that make the creams just lie there on your skin surface, never penetrating or moisturizing—as a matter of fact, drying. And the new mustache removers which burn faces and the mascaras which irritate eyes, while being new, are nuisances. On the other hand, just because a product is old and your grandmother swore by it, doesn't make it terrific. *My* great-grandmother loved leeches on her skin to freshen it up, get rid of all that dirty old blood. Blecch. Take Ovid's cure for freckle removal in A.D. 15. He pushed a neat concoction of eggs, honey, white lead, narcissus bulbs, bird excrement and other goodies. Sure. The women were dropping in *hordes* for centuries from lead poisoning from that particular freckle cream.

Good advice? *Listen* to the experts, experiment and then become your own makeup artist. It's really no mystery, once you get the hang of it. *Our* experts, Bevy Chase and Jeffrey Bruce, have perfected the art of makeup for the heavy woman. They agree on some points and disagree on others, but that's what makes the world go round. Listen then, try everything out and find out what works for *you*.

Advice from a Pro

Bevy Chase has spent much of her life as a makeup artist, training with Elizabeth Arden, Lancôme, Orlane, Nina Ricci—you name the company, she's been a professional there for a while. But the best of all, she's discovered, is making up the wonderfully eclectic big women who come to The Forgotten Woman, a dynamite and voguey dress shop that caters to the over-size-16 crowd on Manhattan's fashionable East Side. Their faces are fresh and lovely palettes which, incidentally, come in all shapes from oval to square to round. Very often, although not always, when a woman puts on weight, her face becomes fuller. Her makeup must become more specialized and geared especially to her needs. What follows are Bevy's beauty secrets culled from years of experimenting, studying and teaching. *All* the beauty tips for the large-size woman may not apply to your face if it is angular and narrow. But except for the specific advice on how to enhance and slim a round face, the beauty messages are timeless, tried and terrific for everyone.

1. START WITH A FREEBIE

It is shamefully easy to get a free makeup from a professional artist. Or two or three. Seeing how the professionals work is worth a thousand words in print on the subject. First, go to a large department store or even a drugstore. It is better to go to a place where you are not very well known so you will be more comfortable about leaving without making any purchases (if that is what you decide to do). It is easier to accept freebies from strangers than from the neighborhood crony.

Remember that the woman behind the Revlon, Estée Lauder or Max Factor counter wants primarily to sell makeup to you. Therefore she will do her best to make you look good, and most often she is quite well trained in the art of cosmetics. Approach her honestly by saying you wish to find a foundation, a blusher or a lipstick that will be right for you. Ask her to make suggestions and ask her to apply the makeup on you the correct way. That is her job. Do *not* approach a makeup artist saying, "Look, I'm not going to buy anything. I just want to learn." No one will whip out her talent and her makeup line in great joy at that overture.

Study your face while she's working and when she's finished. Only if you are transformed with wonder at what she has done to your face should you buy her products. You're allowed to say, "I'm going to walk around the store for a while to see how it feels and then, perhaps, I'll be back." Do just that. Look into mirrors as you amble and try on clothes. If you're happy with your new look, go back and buy only what you think you can use. Don't trust anyone who tries to sell you kits or more than a few items. Again, remember you are under no obligation to spend even one dime—even if the pressure is hot and heavy. Don't even feel slightly guilty: rest assured Revlon will not fold if you don't make your $10 purchase.

Hint: If you notice one of those classy makeup artists who are picking women at random from the crowd to illustrate his products, you should go over to ask if *you* can be the next guinea pig. Chances are, sad to say, you'll have to wait forever before an artist will invite a heavy woman to sit in his chair. With the country's infatuation with skinny, the artist knows he can meet with more popular approval if he chooses a slender, chic, young woman who is already great-looking in everybody's eyes and he can make her even more great-looking to sell his wares. But consider it time for a little consciousness raising: if you volunteer to be the model for the admiring crowds, you'll illustrate just how terrific a big woman can look.

Tip: If you love what the artist has done to your face but don't want to purchase anything because you're worried you might get an allergic reaction—stop worrying. Chances are, if you are going to get a reaction at all it'll probably be within the first ten minutes of wearing a product. Makeup reactions are not like chicken-pox reactions: they don't wait until next Tuesday to show up.

Getting free makeups is a super thing to do because it gives you ideas to start with.

2. SCRUTINIZE YOUR NAKED FACE—CLEAN UP YOUR ACT

Let there be light. A *good* light or it doesn't count. A mirror near the window is fine for daytime but don't depend on it. Sometimes it's cloudy out and you put enough blusher on to sink the *Queen Mary*. Fluorescent lights and makeup bulbs installed in your bathroom by a professional are fine. If you can't afford that, get yourself a simple gooseneck job with a 100-watt bulb and aim it toward your face.

Start cleaning first: use soap and water, cleansing cream, cleaning oils—whatever you swear by—but get that face down to bare essentials. Part of cleaning up is facial hair removal: if there's hair peeking from your nostrils, your ears, your chin, your upper lip, between your brows, under the smooth brow line—think hard. Do you really *love* those curls, *there?* If not, get rid of them. If you go

Start with a good look in the mirror.

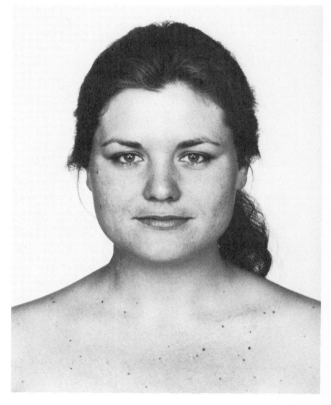

to a professional, you can have electrolysis or waxing. If you do it yourself, soft peach fuzz can be bleached with a commercial preparation like Jolen cream or removed with a depilatory. (If your skin is irritated by any preparation, apply a cold compress and then a moisturizer.) Brows can be tweezed professionally or with your own skillful hand. Nose and ear hairs can be cut with a manicuring scissors. *Never* shave, unless you want to look like Burt Lancaster. Shaving leaves stubble, kind of cute on a lover but not on you.

Tip: It's one thing for a 98-pounder to let her eyebrows and mustache grow for two weeks. It's another thing for you. You may cry *unfair, discriminatory,* but it's true. If you want to erase the image of Big Fat Slob that the rest of the country carries around, you must be meticulously neat. Neater than *anyone* else. You can be pretty no matter how heavy you are but, like it or not, it takes more vigilance and time than pretty and skinny takes. These are harsh words but true ones. Anyway, come to think of it, they're not so harsh. We're talking about twenty minutes a week, that's all, which is all it takes to use a cream depilatory or bleach and tweeze your brows.

3. MOISTURIZE?

I say *yes!* Although there is much controversy about the efficacy of moisturizers, I love them. Never confuse a moisturizer with oil. Moisturizers are water. Oil is oil. Moisturizers do not make skin oily. They penetrate the top layers of skin while oils just sit on top, clogging away. A cheap and lovely moisturizer is a drugstore-bought glycerine. Mix in a drop of honey or rosewater and you've got yourself something good which would cost five times the price if it came in a fancy bottle. Use a thin layer of any moisturizer you choose, commercial or homemade, under your foundation.

4. "EARTH'S FOUNDATION STANDS AND HEAVEN ENDURES" (A. E. Housman)

If your foundation stands, your makeup will endure (Bevy Chase). What color should you use? Heavier women almost always have a more reddish tone to their skin and a slightly uneven color quality. This is because their adrenaline pumps a little faster and their blood vessels are closer to the top of their skin, and also because their skin is stretched a little tauter, a little thinner. They are also subject to broken capillaries. Therefore, large women should almost always choose a foundation in either a light or a dark beige tint. Foundations with color washes give faces a glow which the big and the beautiful generally do not need. So peach, rose or pink foundations are not recommended. Beige tones are.

We will find that extreme heat or extreme cold works havoc on our complexions, giving an unnaturally ruddy look. A soft, beige foundation tones this down.

All our foundations must be *water-based.* Check carefully to see that yours is. Our weight creates extra perspiration. Water-based foundations don't melt off your face as an oil-based product might. A water-based foundation will not clog your pores, either. If your skin is very dry, you might blend a little liquid moisturizer into

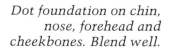

Dot foundation on chin, nose, forehead and cheekbones. Blend well.

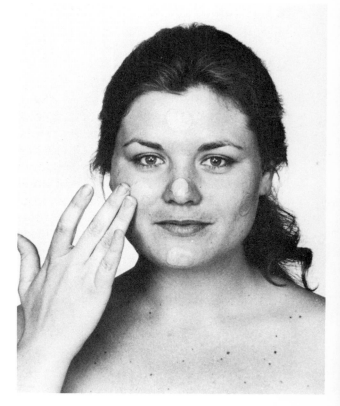

the palm of your hand with the foundation to create a more creamy consistency.

Dot the foundation on your face in five dots on your chin, nose, forehead and two cheekbones; gently blend so it forms an allover, unblotchy coverage. Check around your nostrils and under your chin to see that the foundation is not blotched. Smooth the foundation over your eyelids, lips and as far out to the hairline as you can go without painting your hair beige. Because of our tendency to perspire, we often "lose" our makeup. When you cover your lips and eyes with the foundation base, your eye shadow and lipstick will last longer.

Tip: Don't thickly cover lines or eye bags with foundation. A thick layer of foundation over anything is like an arrow pointing to the area you wish to hide. It will cake in the folds of a fleshier face. Instead of a person, you'll look like a mask. Instead, dot some under-eye cream on an eye bag before you apply the foundation. Then, blend in, *very gently.* You can also use a neutral-color erase product. The same cream or erase product can be used on lines

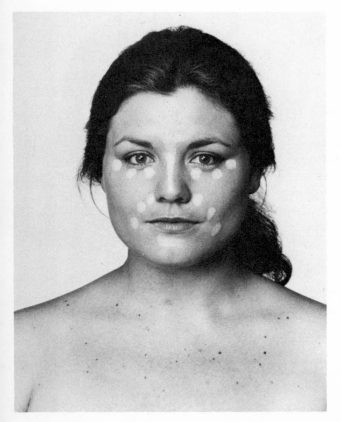

Dot highlighter under eyes, down the nose and on the crease at the sides of mouth. Blend in gently.

that waft out from the nose and lip corners or any prominent broken capillaries.

How do you know if a foundation is good? Does it feel light on your face? Does it smell sweet and not like old eggs? Does your face look naturally pretty after it's applied? Be careful with foundations which label themselves bronzers or tanners. If not blended carefully, they can make you look like a spotted leopard.

How expensive does it have to be to be good? Not very. Of course, you don't have to look long to find foundations that cost a fortune. For instance, Alexandra de Markoff puts out a product called Countess Isserlyn Creme which at last look sold for $25 for two ounces. It *advertises* that it's expensive for a certain snob appeal. According to a recent study, the Isserlyn Creme jar listed twenty ingredients, most of them garden-variety chemicals and not one of them particularly expensive. Mostly they were moisturizers, emulsifiers, color pigments and preservatives. And a whole lot of water. If you want to spend your Milk Duds money on a cream that spells itself creme, go ahead. Rest assured of one thing: it will not make you a countess.

5. CONTOUR OR CON ARTIST?

If you have high cheekbones and a natural contoured sculpture to your face, anyone who tries to sell you contour shading is a con artist. *You don't need it.* Oh, I know it's the rage, and I know you read contour-contour-contour in every magazine, but if the lines are already there, save yourself the money.

On the other hand, if you have no discernible cheekbones (and most of us with fleshy faces are in this category), contour makeup is essential. You can chop off much of the roundness of your face by using it cleverly. Contouring shadow should be used in a red/brown shade. You will probably decide to use a cream contour if you have dry skin and a powder contour if you have normal to oily skin. Cream contour is applied with the fingers and powder with a brush or a piece of cotton.

How? Like this. *Suck your cheeks in.* Find the hollow in the bone and work the contour color up from the hollow to the outer

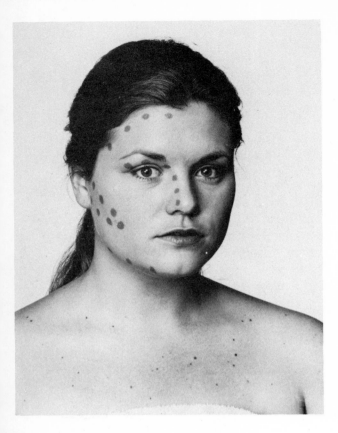

Contour makeup can chop off roundness to flatter a full face.

cheekbone. Blend the makeup up and around the outer corner of the eye, making a soft U-turn around the hairline and under the eyebrow. Then blend in a brigher color in red, peach or plum tones along the cheekbone line. (This brighter color should blend in with your lipstick color and your clothing. In other words, if you are wearing a bright red blouse, plum color on your cheekbone *won't* look terrific.)

Remember: The trick is to use the red-brown contour color *with* the brighter cheekbone color or else you will look like Zacherly's sister. Contour makes for hollows in your cheeks and slims them down. Color makes for prettiness. And again, if you already have a narrow face and high cheekbones, skip the contour stuff and only use the cheekbone color.

If your skin is black, you may find some very gray areas. Your contour shading ought to be in clear red or coral instead of the red-brown. *Very* black skins must use a very deep and dark contour color.

Blend in a brightly colored blusher along the cheekbone line.

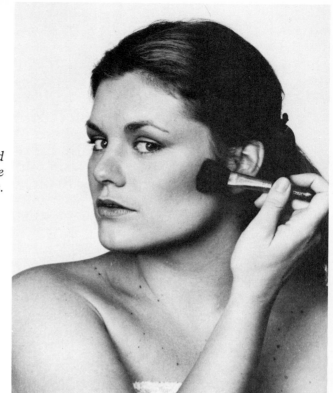

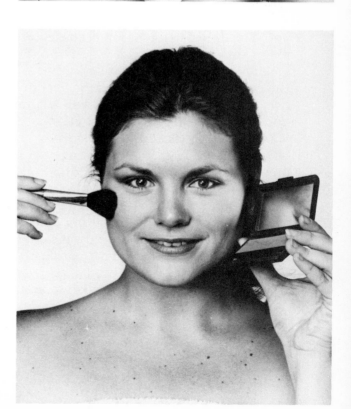

6. NOW, MORE MAGIC

Use the same red-brown contour powder or cream to camouflage that jowly hanging under your chin. With the widest brush you can find, softly paint the throat and under the jaw and blend in down the neck. If you plan to be in soft light, you can go deeper in color. Daylight calls for a more subtle color. One of Judy Garland's stage tricks was to make her neck and underchin almost black. It gave her a small, firm neck and a strong jawline. Your own jowls will recede before your very eyes.

7. EYES COLORED LIKE A WATERFLOWER . . . AND DEEPER THAN THE GREEN SEA'S GLASS (Swinburne)

Your eyes can look like lush waterflowers. They mirror your soul, not to mention the sense of humor and sensuality the big woman is blessed with. But many big women have fleshy, almost oriental eyelids—which is magnificent if you are born Oriental but not so magnificent otherwise. You have two choices for eye shadow color but no choices as to a cream- or powder-based product. You must use powder because your excess perspiration will make any cream eye shadow run into the creases around your eyes.

Your color choices: You can use a white (or any light tone) on the entire lid, blending up to the eyebrow, and then a darker shade, over the light one, on the eyelid alone. This does wonders for widening those fleshy eyelids. Or you can use just one light shade.

Eye makeup should be an accessory to what you're wearing; it does not have to match the color of your eyes. The green-as-grass dress is finely emphasized by a quiet and subtle eye shadow.

Liquid eye liner is for the big woman instead of a pencil. It is more defined, will last longer and will not smudge into fleshy eye folds. Eye liner should be in any color *but* jet black (even if your eyes are black), because it is always too harsh. Dark blue, dark gray and dark plum are effective. Black skins look gorgeous with a dark-blue eyeliner.

To apply: (Be patient. It takes practice.) With pointer finger at

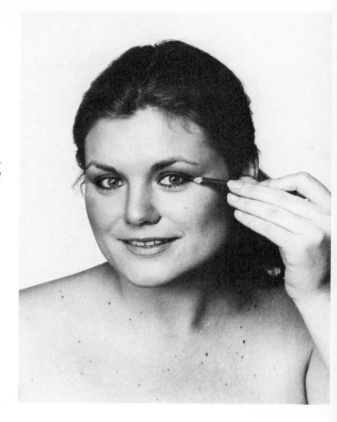

Use an eye liner pencil to add subtle color and drama to eyes.

corner of eye, stretch eye out toward ear. Line the entire eye, aiming to get as close to the lashes as possible. There should *not* be a flesh-colored space between your eye liner and your lashes when you are finished.

Time for mascara: Black. Nothing else. No matter what color your lashes are. Loads of it. On upper and lower lashes. Expensive stuff? Many Ford models I know swear by the cheapest product of all—Maybelline. Experiment to see which brand runs and which lasts the longest on you.

Tip: Mascara is a product that always tends to get thick and clumpy. Never keep any mascara for longer than six months even if there's still a lot left. It will look ghastly and clot up your lashes.

Tip: False eyelashes went out ten years ago. They are phony-looking and you can always tell.

Tip: Keep Q-tips in your purse at all times to give a quick dab to any smudge lines that develop as you go through your busy day.

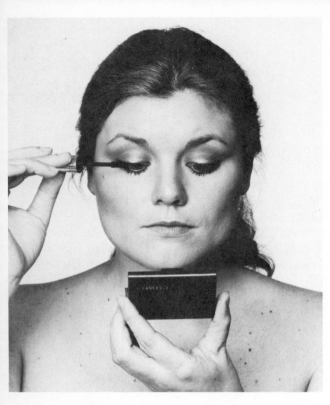

Always use black mascara —lots and lots on upper and lower lashes.

Your brows: The thinner the brow, the fatter the rest of the face looks. Your brows should be naturally full and gently arched up and out to accent your eyes. Overplucked brows sometimes *never* grow back. By gently refining the brow line, you can counteract that droopy look so many big women have around the eyes, and make your eyes soft and luminous. If your eyebrows are bushy, have a professional tweeze them at first, to get a good line. Explain to the cosmetician that you despise thin lines over your eyes. Softly *feather* in bald spots in the brow with light, tiny strokes. And never draw a Halloween straight black line across your fore-head—it will make you look like a comic-strip character. Today's brow pencils glide on in soft sands, smokes, pearl grays and taupes. Always use a very sharp pencil and follow your own brow line.

8. A PURPLE MOUTH IS THE PITS

Lips should never be purple. Or bright orange, for that matter. Lips just don't come in those colors. The lipstick should coordinate with your outfit. The older you get, the brighter your lipstick should be—no matter what the trends are. Don't listen to the *Vogue* editor if she tells forty-year-old you to put earth brown on your lips. Earth-brown lips look like dirty lips. The big woman should have a kissable, shining mouth. Would *you* want to kiss you? Or does your lipstick look so thickly smeared on, other lips could get stuck?

To avoid lipstick "bleeding," powder your mouth with translucent powder (baby powder's fine) before you apply lipstick. Those tiny lines that come with age over your lips are aggravated terribly by smoking. Outline the lips carefully, putting two dots at the top of the bow and joining each dot to the corner of the mouth. Precision is everything: the highest points of the bow should coincide

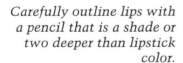

Carefully outline lips with a pencil that is a shade or two deeper than lipstick color.

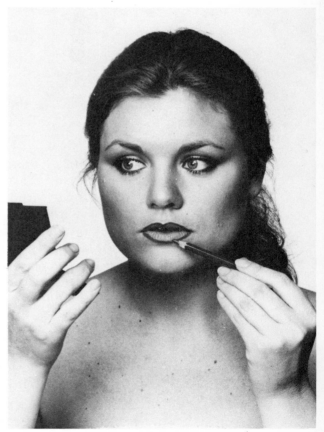

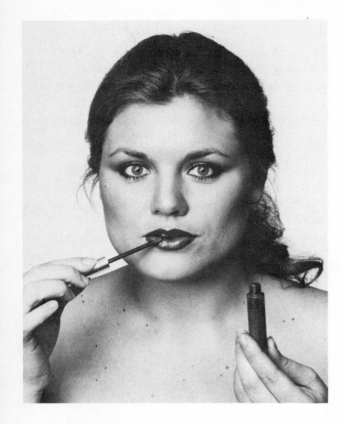

Finish off with lip gloss to make lipstick last longer and to give your lips an irresistibly kissable look!

with the center of the nostrils. Pretend you're coloring in an eight-year-old's coloring book and fill in the lips. Blend down from the outline to subtly define the mouth without a visible line showing. Top the whole thing off with a dab of sheer gloss.

Lipstick generally stays on for about five hours.

Gloss alone for lip color lasts only about an hour.

Lipstick and gloss together last about three and a half hours.

How come lipstick disappears at all? Blame eating, smoking and talking. (Not to mention kissing.)

9. NOW YOU'RE FINISHED

Except for one thing. Dip the widest brush you have into a finely milled, neutral shade of translucent powder. (Again, baby powder is fine.) Blow off the excess from the brush and lightly dust your face, throat and neck. That sets the makeup and gives a matte finish. It also tones down by at least 25 percent any overzealous makeup efforts.

A Date with an Artist

Look in the mirror. Are you gorgeous? You are.

Still it's always good, as my mother used to say, to get another opinion. In this case, the other opinion was famed makeup artist Jeffrey Bruce.

Jeffrey Bruce started off his career working for the famed New York Kenneth salon. He sharpened his skills with Estée Lauder and Revlon and today is one of the top makeup men in New York City. If you have a special date and wish to be made up by Bruce, bring a clean face and $100 to his studio. It had better be a *very*

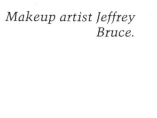

Makeup artist Jeffrey Bruce.

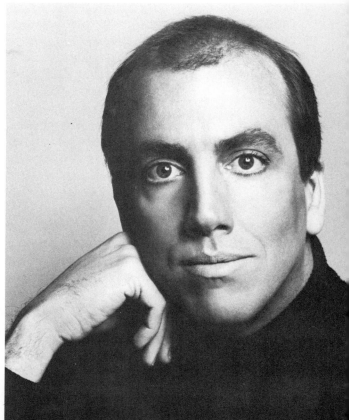

special date. Some of Bruce's clients are Eydie Gorme, Raquel Welch, the entire Kennedy galaxy of women, Ann-Margret, Cher, Dina Merrill, Kim Novak, Ursula Andress, Candice Bergen, Melba Moore, Mary Ann Mobley, Leslie Uggams and Carol Burnett. Just to name drop a few.

While I was on the road narrating another fashion show for big, terrific women, my co-author, Sherry, had Jeffrey Bruce make her up—just to see how it felt. Let her tell it:

I am a wreck. I sit in Bruce's chair, alone in a tiny, rosy-lit room staring straight into an enormous mirror ringed with round, unlit bulbs. There is nowhere to look but at myself—good, you can't see this morning's chin pimple—the rosy light masks it. I try to relax, pretend I'm Jackie waiting for the 3,000th makeup of my life. Instead of old me, having a New Experience.

Bruce comes in, all business, all action, snaps on the mirror lights and God—there it is, all right, what Bob and Ray used to call a skin blossom. He ignores the pimple, frames my face with his hands (surprisingly gentle) and lifts my head up and straight and long on my neck while he studies my features for—what? Inspiration? More skin blossoms? And then, before he even starts to work, a strange thing happens. I start to feel prettier. Maybe it's the attention, maybe it's his hands cradling my face, but something makes me look better. It is a *nurturing* experience: he is holding my cheeks, paying attention only to me, *all* his attention. He is appraising, he is expert, he is almost seductive. Look, if he's not worried about the pimple, why should I be? I sit up straighter, suck in my cheeks, open my mouth just a tiny sensuous drop and, maybe for the first time in my life, also look hard and straight on at my face. Hmmmmm. It's not so bad, after all. There *are* bones there, and contours. My sense of professionalism tells me that having a makeup is more than just a makeup; it is a definite turn-on, a pick-me-up. I feel that I should analyze it but instead I just let myself relax in an orgy of being pampered.

"Beauty should not stop at the neck," Bruce says. "Women have a tendency to buy chic boots, expensive dresses, the most stunning jewelry and then walk out of their homes with the same faces they cook dinner with. There's no need to do that. You can transform yourself—make your self gorgeous with the proper attention to makeup.

"In the first place, bigger women who have rounder faces can carry *more* makeup. Small faces shouldn't wear a lot of makeup. Are you ready? Let's start with the night before."

I'm ready.

"Cream cleanser to get off the whole day's dirt. Very important. The cleanser emulsifies the old makeup, raises the dirt out of the pores, and gets it to the top level of the skin where you can just wipe it away. Here's a trick: most women complain that they can tissue endlessly at the cleanser and removing it is still an endless process. Apply the cleanser and brush your teeth. Tweeze the stray hair from your eyebrows. Then, after about three minutes, wipe off the cleanser. It comes right off, and you finish with a washcloth drenched in warm water to remove the whole shebang."

"How come I can't use soap, as I always have?" I ask Bruce. "Good old soap?"

"The worst! Soap, especially the highly perfumed stuff, clogs pores and gives acne. Glycerine soap is even worse. It gives surface dryness and makes skin almost impossible to work with. People who have oily skin and use products which dry out the top layer of skin actually succeed only in keeping all those pimples and black-heads underneath. Ugh."

Chastened, I vow to be good.

"After your cleanser, take a freshener or an astringent (depending upon your skin type—a freshener has no alcohol, an astringent contains alcohol) and use a lot of it to remove all traces of the cleanser. Then finish off with a night-cream oil moisturizer. *Even if your skin is oily.* Moisture and *oil* are two different things. You're ready to sleep."

I feel as if I need Bruce to tell me what nightgown to choose, the pristine bride job or the old Pucci number. I am developing a dependency on him, fast. I react strongly to assertive statement-makers.

"Okay, you wake up in the morning, you don't need to spend a whole lot of time cleaning—you're clean already. Just a thin and light facial wash will do, and again, the freshener. Believe me, you'll be a lot cleaner than if you used, ugh, soap.

"You *must* use a moisturizer under your makeup. The foundation won't slide on properly unless you do. And if your dermatologist tells you that moisturizers don't work, you have to decide whom you'll listen to—him or me. But what does he know about beauty? All he sells is hope. I show people *how.*"

I immediately decide to listen to Bruce. For now, anyway. He's pretty emphatic.

"Time to drink a glass of water, one of many you should consume during the day," Bruce says. "Water flushes and purifies the system. If you're heavy, you lose a lot of water in perspiration; it shows on the face, right away. Okay. First makeup that goes on is your cream foundation in a color a half-shade lighter than your own complexion, *never* darker. Big women often have hormone imbalances and that results in facial hair. A darker foundation makes the hair and any lines on your face more obvious. Make sure you apply the foundation evenly and over your lips as well to mask the blue that many women have in their lips.

"Next comes the corrective work. Don't believe anyone who tells you to contour *under* your foundation. Ridiculous. All corrective work goes over the basic makeup. Contouring is the key word for heavy faces—not highlighting. Remember that darkness hides and lightness brings out. You don't want to highlight a full face. Look for your cheekbones."

I looked. I couldn't find them.

"There are two ways of doing it. Suck in your cheeks, go up half an inch—there are your bones, and there's where you contour. You can knock off twenty pounds by contouring. Or find that bone on the top of your cheeks—good, got it? Underneath, where there's nothing, is really muscle. *That's* the place for contouring or shading. Don't be afraid to shade heavily. Look directly into the mirror and imagine a V with the point at the ear and the two lines going out to the eye corner and under the cheekbone. Inside those lines is where you contour, with a big brush. What to use? Ask at the makeup counter for dark, rust-colored, powdered blusher. Don't forget to go straight out to the hairline with the powder. Also, shade your entire neck—just paint your entire throat (even behind the ears). That lengthens the neck and camouflages jowls. It gives a very beautiful look.

"Now comes the cream rouge. That adds color. Dot it on, above the contouring and blend. Because you perspire more, you will tend to absorb the cream rouge into your skin. How to keep it on? Take a blusher powder that's the same color as the rouge and pat it on, which in effect "sets" the rouge.

"Then, with a big, fat brush, powder with translucent, colorless powder over the whole makeup, to set that also and give a refined matte finish. I loathe a moist face. Moist makeup looks dirty because facial hair has color. Powder down quite a bit and carry a compact with you always."

Whew. I hope I can remember all this.

"Now the eyes. If you are very large, you will probably have a little ledge, or kind of an overhang over your eyes. Remember, again, lightness brings out, darkness hides. So lightness goes under your eyebrow, and darkness goes on the lid and on that ledge. Always use lightness in the form of *powdered* eye shadows. Creams coagulate on heavy women and get oily. What color lightness? Beige or pink or yellow—*never* white. White's unnatural.

"Then either a darker beige, brown or gray on the lid, crease and on the overhang. *Never green or blue, never pastels.*"

I cringe at the thought of pastels on the overhang, as I am meant to do.

"Okay. Now the mascara. Tons of mascara. First spend the price of a Maybelline curler. Do this first, as soon as you wake up in the morning, and never curl your lashes with mascara on them—unless you want to lose a few dozen. Keep building on coats of mascara, letting each coat dry before you build with another. You want to bring out the eye. You want to call attention to the mirror of the soul. Line the inside of your eye with blue crayon liner. It makes the whites look whiter. Cover up any circles under your eye with a concealer—but not Erase. That pulls the eye, it's too thick.

"Ready for the mouth?"

I was. My mouth was all aquiver.

"Powder everything except the eyes—even over the lips. Use a lip liner in a burgundy or natural brown color to give a good, neat line. Fill in your lips with a soft, natural color—and for God's sake, never use *orange* lipstick!"

Me? Orange lipstick? Are you kidding? I'd rather die.

"Gloss on the top and the bottom lip and that's the only part of your face that should be shining. *Fini!*"

I look in the mirror. Garbo, at the very least. I am a vision.

Jeffrey is not quite finished.

"I have some more tips—one-liners, if you will.

"1. Eyebrows should be seen and not heard. Understated. I loathe bushy eyebrows.

"2. If you use treatment products, don't panic if the day after you give yourself a facial, your face breaks out. Common sense should tell you that the impurities are raising out from the lower skin layer. It's what you *want* to happen.

"3. Black women generally have the most gorgeous skin in the world. They must use rouge colors in ambers and roses—colors that are softly complimentary to the skin—and not dot their cheekbones with vivid reds. They must be careful with concealers: naturally, they have to be darker in color. And again, they also must wear a foundation a half-shade lighter than their skin.

"4. Your makeup should not be dramatically different in the day and in the evening. Your face should not know what time it is. At night, just touch up with a little more contour, mascara and lip gloss—and that's all. I loathe the 'disco' look. I never do it."

I stare at the mirror. At home, I was pudgy and pimply. Here, I am someone you'd turn around to look at again—if I do say so myself.

How to reach Jeffrey or Bevy:

Jeffrey Bruce
  3330 West 56 Street
  New York, NY 10019
  (212) 757-5192

or

The Forgotten Woman
  880 Lexington Avenue
  New York, NY 10021
  (212) 535-8848

Bevy Chase
  30 East 60 Street
  New York, NY 10022
  (212) 421-7555

Treatment Products

Be careful. There is a difference between makeup products and treatment products for the face. One is supposed to make you look pretty. The other is to soothe and heal any skin problems that may be present or that may be thinking of creeping up on you.

People who treat skins with treatment products are known variously as cosmeticians, facialists and, a new one, estheticians. They were inevitable. After generations of applying layers of makeup to cover all ills, the American woman is becoming concerned with cleaning, lubricating and healing the skin itself. Although there has always been controversy as to whether the skin can be lubricated by outside creams and oils, everyone agrees that skin can be cleansed and healed.

Naturally the American woman has gone bananas about buying anything sold by people who call themselves experts. "Miracle creams" range from hundreds of dollars an ounce to 59¢ for a jar of good old cold cream. The creams are made from herbs, sheep placenta (good to retard aging—do you believe it?) seaweed, avocado and heaven knows what else. An hour's facial costs from $20 to $40 in most places. It has been known to go for $100 an hour. If you pay $100 to have a blackhead removed, you deserve sheep placenta on your face. Most medical doctors say that the treatments do little else than massage the ego. (See chapter 4, The Skin Game.) And some honest experts like the famous Georgette Klinger say, "Magic creams don't exist. There is no magic in anything. It is absolutely not necessary to pay a hundred dollars for a facial. That's just for prestige."

Bevy Chase has the following suggestions on treatment products and treatments in general:

1. Don't go to an esthetician who thinks she can do everything including midwifery. If you are being promised miracles, get suspicious.

2. A large-size woman will make very sure the table she climbs up on is absolutely sturdy. Ditto with the stool you stand on. *Ask.* Don't be shy. And don't climb on anything unless someone is near

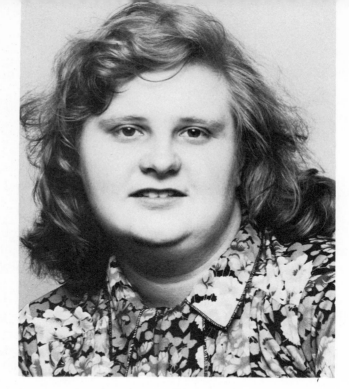

The miracle of makeup, illustrated
by contrasting shots of E. Anne Denning, Cable TV hostess. Makeup by
Jeffrey Bruce.

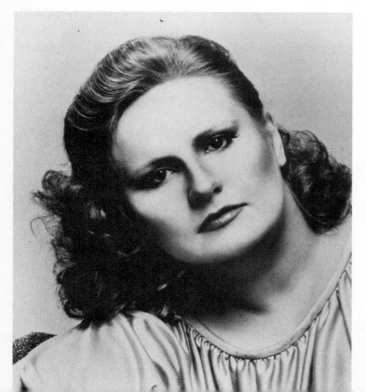

to steady you. For your $30 you are entitled to keep your bones intact.

3. Your facial should be given in a private room to ensure relaxation and comfort. You will lie back and be covered by a large quilt or towel. (Bring your own if theirs is too small and stingy.) If you are more comfortable with your blouse and bra removed, say so. Most facialists will want to work on your upper chest and neck, anyway. You will probably have a treatment to soften pores, an herbal or seaweed steam facial, a manual and deep-pore cleansing, a tightening mask, and if you request it, a makeup and skin care consultation.

4. *If it hurts, stop whoever is doing the hurting.* It's no good. You don't get extra credit for pain. Hurting is not useful for anyone but masochists. If it's really hurting, run for the water and wash whatever it is off immediately. Astringents that burn can also cause redness, irritations and, sometimes, lasting skin problems. Your skin is more sensitive than a size 10's skin because your blood vessels are closer to the surface and react quickly and fiercely to stimuli. If your facialist is Old Hammer Hands, get another facialist. No one should put *anything* on your face that burns. A severe acne condition might warrant some pain in treatment, but normal skin conditions do not, and you should not tolerate pain for a moment. If something seems to have hurt your skin, ask for some ice immediately.

5. Your cosmetician should stay with you most of the time. If she's gone for more than ten minutes, she's probably giving about three facials at the same time. You're being short-changed in attention.

Cosmetics from the Kitchen, the Grocery, the Medicine Cabinet

Here are some natural cosmetics and treatment products you can make yourself. Remember that homemade, natural products are whomped up without preservatives and some must be used immediately or kept in the refrigerator to prevent spoiling. Use your head: if the product includes mayonnaise, you *know* it's got to go in the refrigerator. I don't swear by any of these products, but I've tried them all and they're lovely. They are usually nicer smelling, more effective and certainly cheaper than anything you buy commercially prepared. Also one feels more virtuous with strawberries on her cheeks rather than triethanolamine or even propylparaben.

- Marigold petals mixed with safflower oil is said to heal acne. Can it hurt?
- Slices of cucumber, potato or carrot are a delicious psychological pick-me-up for veiny and tired eyes. Grated potato and carrot has the same cooling effect. Also cotton pads soaked in milk.
- Sliced, raw, juicy tomatoes when applied to the face seem to tighten the pores and, it is said, they equalize the skin's natural acid content. (But lie down to avoid tomato juice stains on your shoes.)
- A honey-and-almond mask draws impurities from the skin while it moisturizes.
- A beaten-egg mask does wonders to tighten and makes five minutes of lying down seem like a night's sleep.
- Mash four or five strawberries with six tablespoons of vegetable shortening and three tablespoons of witch hazel. Voilà! A delicious and effective cleanser when massaged into skin. (Be sure to remove thoroughly, and if your skin is oily, don't use at all.)
- Plain yogurt cleanses marvelously. Ditto sour cream. They're also cooling on a hot day.
- A healthy skin or scalp gives forth a mild acid which protects against infection. When you bathe or use astringent cleansers, you remove some of that acid shield. A vinegar concoction restores the acid. Try one pint of pure cider vinegar mixed with one pint of hot water. Complete the potion with half a teaspoon of rose geranium and half a teaspoon of any kind of oil. Apply to face or scalp with cotton. (And thank Gaylord Hauser for the tip!)
- Big women often have sensitive skin. If soaps and detergents make you break out, try a wheat-germ mask: one tablespoon of wheat-germ flour, one tablespoon of yogurt and mix till

smooth. Apply and relax on your bed for a while. When mask is dry (fifteen to twenty minutes), remove with warm water and follow with a cold-water rinse. Great!

- You want to know delicious? Sensual? (Only for you women without oily skin, I'm afraid.) Take a tip from Tutankhamun and Cleopatra and the rest of the smart money crowd and give yourself a rich oil rub now and then. It's definitely worth it. But watch your sheets and/or couch. Oil seems to rub off bodies onto furniture. Baby oil is good but you can experiment with your own combinations. Try this one for openers: two tablespoons of sesame oil, two tablespoons of wheat-germ oil, one tablespoon of avocado oil and a tablespoon or two of any essential perfume oil. Stir. Makes about a half a cup.
- Mayonnaise conditioner and cleanser: add a few drops of lemon or lime juice (which are astringents) to some plain old mayonnaise. It softens and cleanses practically better than anything.
- Crisco makes a neat cleanser also.
- Many people swear that liquid capsules of Vitamin E, when broken open and patted on the face, tend to tighten and smooth away weariness lines. (If it burns, remove it immediately.)
- Blackhead chaser: concoct a mixture of one tablespoon of epsom salts and three drops of iodine in half a cup of very hot water. Soak absorbent cotton in mixture and hold over blackhead area. Do it again and again. Blackheads, you will find, are softened and will squeeze out gently. Never squeeze hard: if you have to do that, the blackheads are simply not ready to come out and you can injure delicate skin tissue.
- Warm tea bags are luscious for puffy, pink, tired eyes.

Remember: Acids in any preparation may cause irritation, so think and test before you use oranges, lemons, limes and any citrus juices.

Peaches and cream on the face do not necessarily produce peaches-and-cream complexions. Ditto yogurt. Ditto mayonnaise. They're fun, they feel and taste good. They smell nice. *Sometimes,* they do nice things for your skin. As Georgette Klinger says, "There are no miracles."

III Bathing and Beauty

In the beginning was gaminess. Nobody thought it was terrific to be clean. In third-century Rome the people bathed, all right, but there was an ulterior purpose. Because nudity was equated with lewdness, the lusty pleasure-seekers cavorted in the public baths but mostly for sinful debauchery rather than sanitation. In France, Marie Antoinette also held that nakedness was a sin and she took her occasional bath wrapped in a white flannel nightshirt. Queen Isabella of Spain boasted that she would only have three baths in her life, one when she was born, one when she was married and one when she died. In sharp contrast was Queen Elizabeth the First of England, a regular cleanliness fanatic who announced that she bathed once a month "whether it was needed or not." Liz even went for a brisk rubdown with wine after her monthly cleanup and insisted that her marvelous complexion stemmed from that bathing ritual. The masses had to content themselves with milk, which was cheaper. France's Louis IV put one of the two bathtubs that existed in all of his country in the royal garden to be used as a fountain—it shouldn't be a total waste.

Somewhere the odors must have started getting grim, because Henry IV of England established the Order of the Tub to convince his noblemen to wash. It didn't work. In Paris, they invented perfume to cover up body odor for the few who were offended by the national rankness, but most Frenchmen still believed that sweaty was sexy, as did Baudelaire who telegraphed his ample mistress, "*Ne lave pas: j'arrive demain*" (Don't take a bath—I'm coming home tomorrow).

Things weren't much better here. The American Colonies

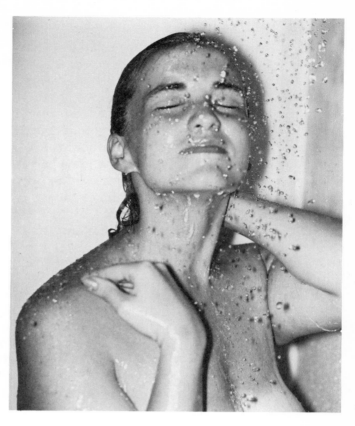

thought baths were silly and even dangerous. You could go to jail in Philadelphia if you took more than one bath a month. And there was no bathtub in the White House until 1850 when Mrs. Millard Fillmore said enough is enough. Just as Jackie made pillbox hats popular, Abigail Fillmore made body odor scandalous. The first deodorant, Mum, was invented in 1888. Phew! Phinally! Muslims and Hindus have always bathed for ritual purposes, as do Orthodox Jews. In medieval monasteries one bathed for cleansing and penance; never, God forbid, for enjoyment.

And now, here we are in spic and span America. Being clean is a national trait, a patriotic hobby and, for some mothers, a life's work.

Some of us take showers. They're okay. No worry about slipping or pulling more than 120 pounds out of a bathtub. And hot showers happen to be perfect for bursitis if one directs a hot stream to the affected part for about five minutes. It is more fun to shower with a large-sized woman. Showers probably clean better than baths because the spray loosens up the grime and you don't have to sit in any water that has become less than pure. Start at the top with a shower, washing from the face down, so no dirty water falls on parts that have already been cleansed. Soap-on-a-rope is a good bet to avoid those torturous bend-downs to retrieve the soap; just hang it on any available hook when you don't need it for the moment. The shower nozzle attachments are great for playing around with a friend and for giving yourself a heady and pulsating water massage. Sure, showers get you wet and clean and can perk you up.

But for an experience, a happening, almost a theater piece—take a bath. A bath can relax or stimulate and it can influence moods. A little music, a candle on the toilet seat and you have a setting that's comparable to a Roman-bath orgy. Besides making you smell sweet, a bath can be a sensual experience that's almost as good as making love or eating Raisinets.

Large women should take serious baths. Which means they should determine their needs and plan their baths accordingly. No frivolous dip-in-the water jobs for us. We must consider whether we want to be healed, cleansed, tranquilized, awakened or sexually

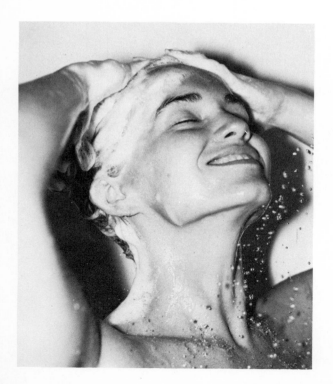

When you take a shower, start at the top.

stimulated. In terms of healing: extra weight and self-doubt are often related to each other and each of them is related to excess perspiration. Sweat means heat rashes, odor, sometimes more serious skin infections. Baths are palliative *and* curative. Changing the temperature, the consistency, the length of the bath, opens up a horde of other interesting possibilities. The action of the water on your skin carries sparkle and rejuvenation to your senses as well as it sparks blood circulation. Baths can make you pretty, sleepy, romantic or perky. What follows are some suggestions for making the amply endowed woman a true bathing beauty: comfortable and graceful in a plethora of baths.

The first thing to consider is that fat floats. Put a pound of butter in your bathtub and the butter will float like a cork. The fat in your body is no different. And while our skinny sisters sink to the bottom of the tub, all skin and bones dead weight against the hard enamel, poor kids, we can *luxuriate* in our weightlessness. Our arms, our legs, our breasts float sensually and relaxed in pleasurable water abandon. Baths were made for heavy women. Unfortunately, that does not always hold true for bathtubs. If you're thrifty, you can save up your pennies to buy a wonderfully large tub. A simple white-enamel job that is six feet long and three feet wide (a foot longer and wider than standard) can be ordered from any plumbing supply house for about $530. Then, of course, you have to make your own best deal with the plumber for installation. If you're *really* thrifty and have lots saved, you can consider buying either a whirlpool bath or a sauna, both of which do wonders for circulation, skin and frame of mind. Approximate prices for those run from $1,500 to $3,500.

Another national phenomenon, begun in California and now sweeping the country, is the redwood hot-tub Jacuzzi. Women with circulation problems from weight, women with bad backs, injured ankles, swollen legs, chronic headaches, seem to have found the panacea of panaceas in this hot-water tub which can be placed outside and used in the snow as well as in the balmy days of summer. Placed indoors, it becomes an addiction. Hanging out in a tub of hot water alone, or with pals, naked or bathing-suited, while the rest of the world rushes madly by, is the ultimate in pleasure. Those with high blood pressure or diabetes should check with their doctors before investing. No one should stay in so long that she feels as if her bones were melting. And never, never mix alcohol and drugs while soaking in a very hot tub. The combination can be, and has been, fatal.

Port-A-Spa is another wonderful water thing to look into. Its $2,495 price tag is stiff, but this portable supertub cures stiff necks, backs, fingers—you name it. It can be plugged into any household electric outlet. Sixty-eight powerful jets transform 200 gallons of hot water into millions of soothing bubbles.

If you cannot afford the luxury items, you can still make your own bathtub such an instrument of pleasure and health that size can be overlooked.

Sometimes your bountiful self can throw you off balance. It's a good idea for anyone, but especially for large-sized people, to have an expert install (very securely please) a holding rail in the tub area as a worthwhile precaution. Slippery tubs, temporary imbalances and stumbling can be compensated for if you have a firm grip on a bar as you enter or leave a bath. Never trust tile soap dishes affixed to the wall. They are invariably malicious creatures which just wait for you to grab them and then break off from the wall just as you trust them the most. For the challenges sometimes presented by getting into the tub, a sturdy chair, preferably with rubber-tipped legs (available in any orthopedic supply store), is a panacea. Place the chair as close to the tub as it will go, sit down on it and swing your legs over the edge of the tub, placing both feet flat on the tub floor. Slowly stand and then, with one hand holding the guard rail, gently lower yourself down. To get out, hold rail, stand, sit down on your chair, swing legs over the edge of the tub and then down to the floor for a safe and easy exit.

If you have only hard water where you live, it pays to invest in a commercial water softener. Not only does it save the soap, but it encourages a richer lather and rinses much more effectively.

When preparing the bath, be careful with extremes of temperature. Although you may love a boiling hot bath, too-hot water can shock the system and dry and wrinkle the skin prematurely. Too-cold water can create other problems by constricting blood vessels. Persons with heart problems and older people should check with their doctors about water temperatures. Also remember that natural ingredients recommended for baths, like lemon or grapefruit, may be irritating to some skins because of their acid content.

Soaps

Is one the same as the other? Yes and no. They all clean. And basically, the American woman decides by scent, color, transparency or wrapper which soap she cannot live without. There are subtle differences.

Transparent or glycerine soap has a higher vegetable fat content and thus is more expensive, but it is doubtful that these soaps are truly less drying than the milled or regular soap.

Milled soap is what you see in the supermarket. It's the most common and is generally very good. (Cashmere Bouquet and Camay are two examples.)

Superfatted soaps contain an excess of fatty material and usually deposit a thin coat of oil on the skin surface. They are good for very dry, scaling skin. (Dove and Basis are two of the many superfatted soaps.)

Deodorant soap usually carries a perfume to mask perspiration odors and/or an antibacterial agent that inhibits the growth of odor-causing bacteria. (Dial is one brand of deodorant soap.)

Multimilled or French soaps give a foamy lather and make you smell like candy, but are usually superexpensive.

When ordinary soap causes irritation, use a soap substitute. We large women have enough trouble from heat rashes to have to worry about soap rashes also. The substitutes have less alkali than regular soap: some of the brand names are Lindora, Aveeno, Lowilla and Basis.

Special soaps for special problems: If you have extraordinarily oily skin, you will do well with Ivory soap and the acne soaps like Acnaveen and Sastid which contain ingredients to dry out and cause peeling.

NOTE: Very dark-skinned people should stay clear of the agent resorcinol, found in some of these soaps. It can stain and blotch your skin. If you have extraordinarily dry skin, you will do well with soaps like Dove and imitation soaps like Oilatum and Lowilla. Don't use deodorant soaps or any sulfur and tar soaps, which are irritating to the skin.

There are so many hard-to-reach parts when you are over size 16. Easy solution: Who said those nice long back brushes are just for backs? Use them on feet, knees, backs of necks—anyplace you can't reach.

Okay, are you ready? Here are your bath choices. Notice that a lot of these ingredients come from the kitchen, which is nice because it keeps you close to the food.

Therapeutic Baths

The sulfur bath. You've heard about mineral-sulfur baths all your life. Presidents and beautiful people make pilgrimages to get to these watering holes because, legend has it, the baths seem to ease the nagging aches of arthritis, gout and rheumatic complaints. Some people think they're good for pimples. Some people think they're better than Valium. Well, good news. You don't have to go farther than your own bathroom. Ask your friendly druggist for a prepackaged mineral-spring-type sulfur bath and you are on your way to making a spa out of your own friendly tub. Let the water run at body temperature and empty the package of bath powder into the running water. As you slothfully relax in the water, gradually increase the water temperature. The grinding aches and the tiredness just seem to evaporate and your skin will feel like rose petals. Because the heated water has a sauna effect on your skin, use a good penetrating moisture cream on the opened pores right after the tub, or even while you're in it.

The colloidal bath. Women with bountiful poundage tend to suffer from heat rashes, hives and other mild skin inflammations. Colloids, which do not blend into the water but hang suspended in tiny soothing particles, have deliciously soothing effects on these skin problems and sometimes the benefits last for many hours. Oatmeal is a colloid. (If you hate oatmeal, don't try bran. It won't work.) After breakfast, squeeze some of the leftover guck into a few thicknesses of cheesecloth and swirl it around in your tepid bath water until a creamy material oozes into the water, reminding you of a science fiction movie. That's good, not bad. Cornstarch is also a colloid: mix some with mineral oil into a liquid paste, add to bath water and you have relief from dry or eczema skin. Linit, a commercial preparation, is another effective colloid bath.

The tar-baby bath. Skin problems like psoriasis, eczema and rosacea (a disease of the oil glands that looks like acne) respond nicely to a solution of coal tar (available in your drugstore) in your tub. No, you won't stick to the enamel. (Balnetar is one brand.)

The epsom-salt bath. Super for reducing pain and swelling caused by sprains, twists and pulls. It will also tone up your muscles. Also, if you remember, your mother used to give you epsom-salt baths. Can it hurt?

The ocean-dip bath. Take home some ocean from the beach in your cute tin pail or go to any fish restaurant or drugstore and buy some natural sea salt to turn your bath into an invigorating ocean dip. Feels like Atlantic City without the roulette wheel. Sea salt is antiseptic and deodorizing for those with heavy perspiration problems. It is said to be a balm to many rheumatic complaints. Use more than you need—three cupfuls, at least, in the tub and then some extra to rub onto your body. It scrapes away dead and dry skin cells because it has a mildly abrasive effect—if you don't use it as a medieval torture weapon and rub until your skin is raw.

The open-air bath. Day and night our bodies schlep their clothes around. Except for the few brief moments when we undress—just to dress again in nightclothes—we are covered. Think of it: breasts, buttocks, that have never seen the light of day—or even the dark of night, for very long. Billions of pores that are never exposed to fresh air!

Try sleeping in the raw: it's great, and freeing! You can't imagine how liberated and refreshed you'll feel in the morning. If possible, during warm days, find a place you can strip in the fresh air for even a short while. An open-air bath is cleansing to the soul!

The sitz bath. Sitz means sit in German, and that's all you do: sit. In only about four or five inches of water. Good is a steaming-hot sitz bath, which relieves painful hemorrhoids, common as the cold in large women. Also painful periods. Also bladder inflammations and vaginal irritations. Sit in the hot water for about fifteen minutes with your knees bent and your feet flat on the tub to get the good of the water where it counts.

Rose-vinegar bath. Nice for oily skin because vinegar is an astringent. It also tends to do lovely things with your complexion, making you rosy as a babe. Always put a nice scent in the vinegar so you don't smell pickled.

Mix one half pint of vinegar with one teaspoon of rose geranium oil (or one teaspoon oil of cloves). Mix with half a tubful of warm water and soak for twenty minutes.

The apple-cider-vinegar bath. In a recent letter to *The New York Times,* Dr. Herbert N. Smith writes, "For years I've been pouring one cup of apple cider vinegar in my bathtub and after three-quarters of an hour of happy immersion, I rise out of the tub totally relaxed, tremendously refreshed and full of ginger—and I am eighty-nine years old."

Beauty Baths

The lemonade lulu. One cup of fresh lemon juice (the bottled kind smells evil) in a hot-water bath reduces skin oiliness and makes you taste tart and terrific. Because lemon is a mild acid, when used as a rinse after shampooing, it rubs away soap scum and makes hair look brighter and shinier.

The bubble-oil bath. Tubs of fun and nourishment for the psyche. Oil softens dry skin and winter itch, which is worse than crotch itch. It also forms a nice protective film all over your body and makes you very squeezable. Bubbles make you feel all frothy and champagney and extravagant. The combination is mind-boggling. You can buy a prepared bubble-oil mixture, but I prefer making it myself from kitchen stuff because it's cheaper and gives me a chance to experiment with exotic combinations. To make it yourself, put a little sesame oil (peanut or corn oil is also lovely) in a bowl. Add two tablespoons of a liquid shampoo. Then add about a teaspoon of your favorite perfume or any other essential oil aroma, like oil of geraniums or roses or coconut or musk, and beat the whole thing up in a blender on *low* speed or with an electric mixer or, even better, with an egg beater. It will keep indefinitely in a closed bottle. (If you have sensitive skin, you can skip the perfumes.) Bubble baths should be mixed well with the water before immersing your body to prevent the slight chance of a urinary tract infection. If you think bubbles are for kids, a few tablespoons of Alpha Keri oil, or baby or olive oil, in the water will hydrate the skin.

Tip: for the thigh burn that is so prevalent and caused by skin rubbing against skin as you walk, firmly massage some of the pure oil into your thighs. Be particularly careful when getting out of the tub after using bath oil because the tub becomes peeled-grape slippery.

The milk bath. Although there's very little value in milk baths unless you drink them, they're still fun and they feel glamorous. The American actress Anna Held swore that they were responsible for her legendary smooth skin. Put a cup of powdered skim milk and a cup of laundry starch into a muslin or cheesecloth pouch. Swish the pouch around in a warm, not hot, tub until the water is milky white. You can pour a little of the homogenized stuff in for good measure. Then alternately relax and rub—with the pouch of goodies. *Rinse yourself very well* to prevent stickiness. Dry gently. You have had a movie-star bath and you should feel very gorgeous. Also organic.

Fruit-salad bath. Puree in a blender some fresh cucumbers, strawberries, or peaches and add to the bath water. It makes you smell peachy (or whatever), and some people think that it acts as a perspiration deterrent. If it feels so good on the inside, how could it not be good on the outside? I love pureed avocado in my bath. No one can tell me it's not good for skin. And it's not even fattening, this way.

Herb-and-flower potpourri bath. Mix any sweet-smelling herbs such as chamomile, lavender and rose petals with an equal mixture of Borax and orris-root powder. Create a sachet in a silk or cotton bag and tie up the pretty mixture with a ribbon. Hang the sachet from the hot-water tap so the fragrance is released as the bath water soaks the bag. What a sweet-smelling delight!

Pick-Me-Up Baths

The Perrier and water bath, please. There's a reason why the whole world is drinking this new carbonated beverage. It tickles one's tongue and the tiny little bubbles pop in millions of little points all over the mouth, making for an exhilarating effect. Try it on your body. Mixed with bath water, two bottles of Perrier imitate an invigorating massage and feel quite delicious. Seltzer works just as well, but doesn't sound as classy.

The loofah bath. For a morning wake-up bath, try coolish water and a loofah sponge, which is a slightly rough, fibrous sponge that is great for general scrubbing and light scouring. It not only sloughs off the surface dead-skin cells and imbedded grime but provides a real massage action, while making the skin tingle. Scrub your face gently, using moderate pressure and a circular motion for the flat surfaces and a horizontal or vertical motion for the contoured planes. Say goodbye to blackheads.

The Queen Elizabeth of Hungary secret bath. Robustly exquisite Queen Elizabeth concocted a bath to which she ascribed her mind-boggling beauty and enormous energy. It has a wake-up astringent quality and it is delightful. The secret ingredients were only discovered years after her death. From your kitchen, collect one ounce of fresh lemon peel and one ounce of fresh orange peel. Add an ounce of whole cloves, an ounce of dried mint leaves, an ounce of dried rosemary leaves and one pint of rosewater (get in drugstore). Also a pint of a nonsmelling alcohol like spirit of wine. Let the whole stew seep in a closed container for a couple of weeks, then strain it before using to avoid whole cloves entering your system, somewhere, as you sit in your queenly, eye-opening bath. Cucumber slices are delightfully cooling. Gently placed on tired eyelids as you soak, they really make for refreshed vision.

Lay-Me-Down Baths

A go-to-sleep bath should be tranquilizingly warm, not hot, because too hot can overstimulate and cause restlessness. This is a serious, tub-soaking, languorous time. A magazine, a munch or maybe a split of champagne (Dr. Pepper, if you're a teetotaler) to sip while you soak, spurs relaxation. Put some fresh flowers on the hamper or toilet seat and invest in one of those nice little neck-supporting bath pillows. This is also a good time for a gentle self-massage in the tub. Knead your muscles gently between the palms of both hands or the thumb and finger of one hand. Use the tips of your fingers to push, explore and unknot hidden muscles. Aid your circulation by gently exerting force in circular motions on thighs, upper arms and abdomen. Stretch, stretch, stretch your arms and legs in the warm water and twist your feet and hands at the joints in gyrating spirals. A little warm bath oil added to the water adds mood and fragrance. You might also try, in another bath, a half-cup of mineral bath crystals for a nice boost to relaxation. The important thing is to be totally selfish. After a day of running around for boss, family and the rest of the outside world, this bath, this before-sleep time, belongs wholly to you. Breathe slowly and deeply. Contemplate your navel. When you are finished, pat, never rub briskly, dry. Go straight to bed. Do not pass Go. Do not indulge in invigorating conversation.

A list of relaxing baths wouldn't be complete unless I included Harriet Hubbard Ayer's suggestions, written in 1889, in a weekly beauty column for *The New York World*. She suggests you take these baths as relaxants *and* if you have committed the "sin of dowdiness."

Aromatic Bath for Nervous Women

Sage—25 grammes
Rosmarine—30 grammes
Serpolet—40 grammes
Menthol—15 grammes
Lavender flowers—25 grammes
Make an infusion in about a quart of boiling water. Let stand until cold. Pour into bath.

AUTHOR'S NOTE: Rosmarine and serpolet are rosemary and thyme, respectively.

For a Bath of the Aristocracy

To 100 grammes of tincture of benzoin, add 40 grammes of aromatic vinegar. This quantity is for a large, full bath.

AUTHOR'S NOTE: Let's have none of you peasants taking this bath, now!

After-Bath Activity

Despite the controversy over the effectiveness of moisturizers, you *may* choose to massage every part of your body with a cream or lotion moisturizer, after bathing. Moisturizers come in a variety of guises called oils, lotions and creams. If you have an oily skin and are acne prone, do not use any oily moisturizer. Instead, use a product that chemically attracts moisture but doesn't clog pores. Aqua-care and Carmol are brand names of two such products. Moisturizers are supposed to seal in the skin's natural moisture by slowing down its evaporation into the air. Crisco is as effective as any brand-name stuff for doing this—honestly!

Special attention should be paid to the parts which support a great deal of our weight: heels and elbows. Count how many times you lean on your elbows while reading, eating and working. That makes for rough and chapped skin. Comedian Mel Brooks wasn't crazy when he said Saran-Wrap was the greatest invention of modern times. *Try this Saran-Wrap magic:* after a bath, use a pumice stone to scrape away the dried, dead skin from heels and elbows. Then put a layer of moisturizer or, better still, plain Vaseline or petrolatum on the areas. Wrap the Saran-Wrap around the elbows and heels, taping the edges onto the skin. You can even wrap a plastic food bag on each foot and cover with a pair of socks. In the morning—voilà! Your elbows and your heels have been transformed into a Gerber baby's elbows and heels—soft and cuddly. How? The wrapped skin has increased the temperature and the humidity of the skin and the moisturizer has been able to penetrate deeper and deeper and faster.

After the bath, inspect your abdomen and thigh area. Have the hundreds of useless diets over the years left stretch marks all over your body where the weight has come and gone and come again? Rub some wheat-germ oil or coconut oil or even a little melted cocoa butter gently into the area. Gradually, hopefully, the stretch marks will fade. Even if they don't, you'll smell fine.

Tip: Lemon or grapefruit juice, rubbed into after-bath elbows, smooths and lightens.

Footnotes

If you don't respect feet, you're mad. Think of the weight they carry around. Your very soul resides in your feet. They mirror your psyche. If your feet hurt, your face will show it. Forget about going

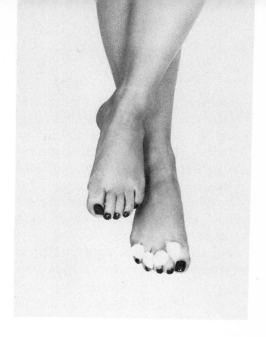

discoing and to the movies as well. If your feet are cold, twelve blankets won't warm you. Only woolen socks will. Making love does wonders for an aching back but it does borscht for tired feet. *Nothing* will taste, feel or sound good with a burning corn or hot, aching toes. In the case of big women, they're harder to reach also, which tends to make us ignore them more. A big mistake.

Fact for foot fetishists: About 70 to 80 percent of the nation's women have feet problems. Big women make up the largest group of these women because they are forever trying to fit into shoes that are too narrow for them. (*Tip: You must wear properly fitting shoes if you are to survive!*) Bunions, hammertoes, ingrown toenails and nail dystrophy, not to mention calluses, rough skin and diseases like athlete's foot, are in store for you unless you insist on a proper fit. There is probably a shoe store in your neighborhood that specializes in wide widths. If not, get in your car, plane or bus and find a store that has shoes which will fit. Buy several pairs at one time. You must. It's that important. Then consider the following directions on foot bathing and foot care.

FOOT BATHS

Fill a tub or a basin with the following concoctions to relieve sore, aching and hot feet. A five-minute foot bath in the middle of the day is worth $9 million.

Fire-and-ice foot bath. The hottest water you can stand followed by the coldest water you can stand—three minutes of each. Eureka! You can walk again. This kind of "contrast bath" is terrific!

Baking-soda foot bath. Pumice-stone dry skin off, then add one tablespoon of baking soda to lukewarm water and soak. Soothing as can be.

Saltwater foot bath. A cup of sea salt added to lukewarm water: the alkali in the salt helps remove dead skin, debris and odor sources.

All of these baths stimulate the local blood supply and aid circulation. Dry very carefully, particularly between the toes.

FOOT MASSAGE

If you simply cannot reach your feet to massage them, have someone else do it, or better than nothing, use a vibrator. Placing a chair or a stool under your feet sometimes makes the difference between reaching them and just missing. You can create a long-handled vibrator by taping the vibrator onto a thin ruler or any long stick-shape. Move the vibrator slowly in circular motions on the ball of the foot, along each toe and each tendon on the top of the foot. Pay special attention to the arch.

If you can reach your feet with your hands easily, however, there is nothing like a manual foot massage. Begin by crossing your right leg on your left knee. Lubricate your hands with cream and knead your toes, one by one, giving a twisting massage action from the tip of the toenail to the end of the toe. If you can grab your right foot with both hands, join your fingers above the instep and stroke firmly in a definite rhythm from the toes toward the heel. Then knead the calf muscles with circular finger presses. Finally, massage the sole of the foot. Cross your left leg over your right foot and repeat the process. Apply a light moisturizer with your fingertips and rub in until it disappears. You can use an aerosol powder which you spray from a distance. Or, with a large five-and-dime-store powder puff, pat the whole thing dry with cornstarch or a medicated, unperfumed powder.

Always dry feet very well to prevent athlete's foot.

THIS LITTLE PIGGY WENT TO MARKET . . .

Toenails grow at a slower rate than fingernails, but they must not be ignored. If they extend beyond the edge of your toes you may trip on them. Also you'll look like Howard Hughes in his last days. Long toenails interfere with walking and shoe comfort and may even cut into the skin of other toes. Always clip them straight across to protect and preserve the nail corners. If you round out the corners, you are opening yourself up to ingrown toenails. After cutting, file them down a bit to prevent stocking snares. You can use a pumice stone on toes, while bathing, to rub away calluses and dry skin. Toe hair is definitely not attractive. Remove it by depilation or plucking. (Well, maybe there's someone, somewhere who is turned on by toe hair, but I can't think of anybody.)

Did I tell you to change your shoes *very often?* No? Well, do. That really helps aching feet and toes.

ITCHY FOOT CURE

Sprinkle them with an antifungal powder like Stiefel Lab's Zeasorb medicated powder. Actually, this particular powder is good for fungal infections *anywhere,* except the vaginal area.

SWOLLEN ANKLE CURE

Big women are plagued with swollen ankles. If you lie, for ten minutes every night, with your feet propped higher than your head; if you remove all constricting socks and stockings during the sleeping hours; if you exercise daily by picking up pencils or marbles with your toes—the problem will be greatly relieved.

CORN AND CALLUS CURE

Don't fool around with self-treatment of corns, calluses and foot diseases that need cutting or other medical treatment. See a chiropodist, who will not be terribly expensive. Seeing a foot doctor regularly, for the big woman with her many feet problems, is no more luxurious than seeing a dentist twice a year.

SMELLY FEET CURE

Spraying newly washed pantyhose or stockings with a dry foot deodorant helps attack foot odor problems all day. If you daily powder the soles of your feet with a foot talc, they'll perspire less and smell less. Cornstarch with a powder puff works beautifully. You might also try this recipe, which military foot soldiers swear is magic for sweaty feet: Grind together one teaspoon of thymol, two tablespoons of boric acid, one and a half tablespoons of zinc oxide, almost half a cup of talc (all ingredients available at drugstore).

PRETTY FEET

It's a downer for anyone to cast their eyes down the length of a great-looking big woman and end up at her smelly, swollen, callused, boring feet. Don't stop at the hemline: give your feet a fashion once-over also. Which means a pedicure and a coat of shining, glossy color or clear nail polish. It's the perfect finishing touch to a bath.

Tip: Stuff wads of cotton in between each toe until the polish dries to prevent overlapping toes and smudging.

Shaving the Legs

If you cannot comfortably reach your legs to shave them, you can make any manual or electric razor easier to wield by taping it onto a long wooden ruler. Be very careful that your skin is wet and lathered before you use a blade. Styptic pencils are *musts* for stopping the bleeding from minor nicks. Always use cream (but never anything with alcohol) after you shave to prevent irritation. If bending down to shave is just too uncomfortable even with a razor extension, you will want to consider the luxury of having your legs waxed about once a month. It should cost from $15 to $30, or even less if you can find a private technician who will do it free lance, in her home or yours. Almost every beauty shop or department store has an expert in leg waxing. Health clubs also generally provide the service.

Snaring Sweat

We perspire more than small women. When our emotions work double time and we're falling in love, getting embarrassed or raging with fury, those old apocrine glands in the armpits start releasing smelly sweat. The eccrine glands, which work as body waste and heat thermostats as they release sweat, aren't much better, although this kind of sweat, by itself, does not produce an unpleasant odor. Still, sweat is sweat, and even the eccrine kind will not smell terrific when it mixes with the pollution, grime and other body debris you carry around.

Perspiration not only ruins composure but it tends to make you feel slightly inelegant when that dark stain under your arms begins to spread to your knees. You can, of course, wear a cotton arm shield if you don't mind being trussed up like a Christmas turkey. Also, arm shields are a little impractical with short-sleeved dresses. All those white straps look funny.

It was this very odor of the dank armpits and the moist crotch we speak of, that drove our evolutionary ancestors happily crazy. They *liked* it, but it's hard to find a sweat freak in today's market. As we've said, it's not the perspiration that generally smells, but the perspiration that blends with bacteria. And bacteria, *those* little buggers, love warm, moist, hairy hiding places like rainforests, underarms and crotches.

Aside from underarm armor, what can be done? Plenty. Lots and lots of soap and water works best. If you have a heavy problem, it can't hurt to jog into the ladies room during your coffee break for a quick wash down. And carefully find, by trial and error, the antiperspirant and deodorant on the market that works best for you. Check out the difference between the two: antiperspirant reduces and retards perspiration upon application. The more you use it, the better it works. If you use an antiperspirant, you do not need a deodorant also. A deodorant masks or perfumes body odors. That's all. You can buy a product which is a combination of both although each is essentially different. And although the ads will never tell you this, Virginia, neither is foolproof, and even if they work, they will only be effective for a limited amount of hours, at best.

No deodorant lasts for two days, no matter what they say. Impossible!

Some tips:

- If you've been exercising heavily, don't jump into a shower immediately upon stopping. Eccrine sweat glands keep working about fifteen minutes after you've stopped exercising, so wait that long before taking a cooling, cleansing shower.
- Never use antiperspirants or deodorants immediately after your shower, either. You will tend to be hot and sweaty from the air temperature and the product will be diluted by our increased perspiration. Wait at least twenty minutes.
- Watch what you eat because what you eat is what you sweat. No one is telling you to go easy on the garlic and spicy meat sauce that you dearly love, but just be aware that body odor loves it too. Asparagus seems to make people sweat—not green, but pungent.
- Don't use antiperspirant products right after you shave. It *hoits!*

PERSPIRING HANDS CURE

Although your hands, because of your pounds, are gracefully wrinkle-free, they perspire more than your cousin Jenny's (who has all those bulging veins in her skinny, dry hands). In fact, your hands always seem to be wet, particularly under stress—not great for shaking hands with the future boss. Try this: Mix one teaspoon of alum (an astringent you can buy in the drugstore) with half a cup of hot water and two tablespoons of rosewater or orange flower water (also in drugstores). Rinse your hands in this mixture and pat dry. They'll probably stay that way for quite a while—Sahara dry.

TOWEL UP

Remember your mother always told you to dry *very well* after a shower, especially *there?* She was right. Nothing makes perspiration and bacteria connect faster than slightly damp, warm areas.

DOES CLOTHING COUNT?

More than almost anything. Change your underwear twice a day, instead of twice a week (arrrrgh). Launder your clothes frequently: the most terrific-smelling person can become fetid in a gamey blouse. Loose, porous clothing and limited physical energy help control perspiration. If you're going for a job interview, don't wear a tight polyester blouse as you run around the block for energy.

CROTCH SPRAYS IN STRAWBERRY, VANILLA?

Well, they come in flavors, but don't use them anyway! They can really irritate, and they have no medical usefulness whatsoever. Burning and blisters and worse have been known to occur from crotch sprays. Don't even ask *what* worse; you wouldn't want to know.

DOUCHES ARE ALSO DOUBTFUL

Whatever entices and excites lovers, douches aren't among them. Even raspberry douches. Unless your doctor tells you to use one, douching can injure the cells in the vagina lining and actually encourage unpleasant-smelling discharges. If God had meant you to douche, you would have come with a bag and a syringe.

IV The Skin Game

Before we even start this chapter, take two minutes to complete a simple true-false test. You may feel a little silly because the answers are so obvious. *Everybody* knows that chocolate gives you pimples, right?

TRUE   FALSE

_____ _____ Chocolate gives you pimples.

_____ _____ Emotional problems are usually responsible for poor skin.

_____ _____ Dieting makes complexion and skin tone gorgeous.

_____ _____ Moles with hairs in them are potentially cancerous.

_____ _____ Cellulite disease can be cured.

_____ _____ Obese people definitely have shorter life spans because of high blood pressure.

_____ _____ A diet without fat is super for the skin.

_____ _____ Hair bleach causes cancer.

_____ _____ Wrinkle creams, used conscientiously, fade wrinkles.

_____ _____ Moisturizers are marvelous and should never be forgotten.

_____ _____ Daily bathing keeps the skin glowing and youthful.

_____ _____ True hypoallergenic makeups are deservedly expensive.

_____ _____ Smoking and drinking are not great for lungs and liver, but they never hurt the skin.

_____ _____ Vigorous facial massage is great for the circulation and keeps the skin looking youthful.

Wrong. Chocolate _doesn't_ give you pimples, according to the best medical advice. And wrong again, to the rest of the questions. _Read on and find out why._

"Bid Them Wash Their Faces" (Coriolanus)

Skin talks. It's your telephone to the world. It shouts your reactions to whatever you're thinking, feeling, doing. You can hide nothing from your skin.

Frightened? Watch the hair follicles broadcast the fact by rising to attention.

Nervous? That thin line of sweat over your upper lip announces it.

Embarrassed? Blushing proclaims the big news.

Cold? Everyone knows it because of the goose bumps pimpling your skin.

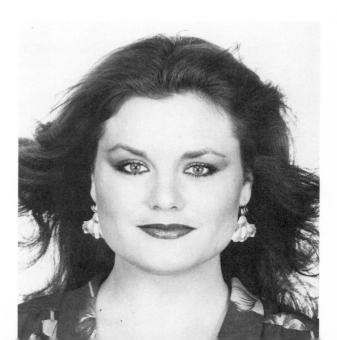

Falling in love? Your skin warms up to tell about it. Furthermore, your skin can be treated as a giant canvas on which can be painted beauty, disguises, even health.

We are ahead in the skin game. We can't compete in the wasp-waist department and we can't even come close in the narrow-calf race, but we have our pounds working for us on our face. Check out a round middle-aged face. It looks years younger because that extra plumping out tends to erase wrinkles. Look at the hands of a big woman next to those of a skinny mini. The big woman's hands are smooth, her veins and wrinkles obscured by pounds. With a minimum of care and some sound, commonsense advice, we can win any race hands down when it comes to super-looking, glowing, exquisite skin. In fact, the only thing that can seriously crimp our advantage is crash dieting—the yo-yo kind of starve and stuff, lose and gain game. It will take firm, fine, plump skin and create a sagging mess. Don't do it. If you must diet, do it very slowly.

Dr. Irving Abrahams is a dermatologist in the New York metropolitan area. He is also associated with one of the world's greatest medical institutions, Columbia Presbyterian Hospital. He was interviewed closely for this chapter. You may be very surprised at some of his answers because he does not parrot the views of the commercial cosmetic industries and even other doctors. He makes sense. The question-and-answer session which follows will give you a medical background. Then check out the information, culled from cosmeticians and other specialists, which *will* give the big woman that extra dash and verve in her skin that spells s-t-u-n-n-i-n-g.

Q. What is the biggest skin problem for large women?

A. Without question, it's intertrigo, which is what people mean when they're talking about chafing. It's an irritation and an infection of the skin folds in the groin, under the armpit, beneath the breast, on the abdomen and in other areas where it is moist and warm. The problem has to do with heat, lack of air and moisture. The heavier the woman, the more skin folds she has. The deeper these skin folds, the more moisture and heat, the better the atmosphere is for bacteria growth. The most common problem is a fungus or yeast infection called moniliasis. It looks like a red rash with pustules and it is very itchy. Now *all* women, particularly those who are diabetic, very sexually active, who take the birth control pill and who take antibiotics, are prone to this yeast infection in their bodies and they often have vaginal infections as a result. If a very thin person carries this yeast infection in her body and the weather is cool, the moniliasis is contained in her vaginal area. If a woman is fat, that particular bug gets into her skin folds and that's when she gets this red, itchy rash on her body.

Q. *What do we do about this infection?*

A. First, you dry very carefully after bathing. A hair dryer works wonderfully to dry out the hard-to-reach folds in the body. Next, dress as coolly as you can. Heavy women tend to wear old-fashioned underwear like girdles, slips and too-tight pantyhose. Occlusive garments like that don't allow skin to breathe, make you hot and moist and contribute to the problem. *Never,* never wear undergarments to bed. Think of treating a baby with diaper rash: a bare end cures the rash almost overnight. Essentially, you should apply the same principle and expose as much as possible of your body to air and dryness. If the rash persists, you may have to see your doctor for medication.

Q. *Does overeating chocolate or fatty foods create skin problems?*

A. Today's thinking says that what you eat does *not* contribute in an important way to acne. Pimples are not the property of fat overeaters, that's for sure. Chocolate, French fries, malteds and nuts simply do not give you acne. I see heavy people who eat these foods in great quantities and have perfect skins. A conscientious doctor simply cannot counsel heavy teenagers who have acne that if they stop eating chocolate and fried foods, their acne will go away. It won't. Now it is true that people who overeat these foods will gain weight. And heavy people are more likely to get heat rashes and skin problems of that sort because their body temperature is higher, as a result of their weight, than the body temperature of thin people. Heavy women wear a built-in sweater against the outside world. It's nice for warmth in the winter, but it sometimes does create rashy skin problems, indirectly.

Q. *Myth has it that women gain surplus pounds because of emotional problems. Although the weight of new evidence is clearly against this theory, do you think that emotional problems can trigger off skin diseases?*

A. I know that many skin doctors say yes, but I am not a great believer in that theory. When that kind of excuse is used casually, it probably means that the doctor doesn't know what's going on. Emotional problems can sometimes be related to eczema, but that's not a particular problem of heavy women. Of course, *if* a heavy woman has eczema which is related to allergy, the increased moisture and airlessness of her body skin folds *can* make the disease worse than it would be in a thinner woman.

Q. *Do medicated powders help to prevent intertrigo?*

A. Maybe, slightly. Powders like Mexana have ingredients that are slightly germicidal and antiseptic. Perhaps, to some small extent, they're helpful.

Q. *What does yo-yo dieting do to the skin?*

A. At a young age, it doesn't do much at all. When you're older, you do lose some of your natural elasticity, and women who lose, gain and lose weight again and again, quickly, tend to have hanging skin. Dieting like this is treacherous. It is a pity that females have been the victims of this "skinny" propaganda for so long in this society. Relaxing a diet in the wintertime and rigidly adhering to it in bathing-suit time and relaxing it again is lousy for the skin—let alone the rest of the body and psyche. Decide what weight you can realistically be, and make up your mind that you'll be that weight forever, but don't say I've got to lose so many pounds in two weeks and then suffer. It's unhealthy—all that suffering.

Q. *Everyone's talking about cellulite. Can big women hope to free themselves of "the disease of ugly cellulite," as the ads put it?*

A. Cellulite is an invented disease, which means it's not a disease at all. The anatomy of women's fat is different from men's fat. Women's subcutaneous fat is divided by fibrous tissues shaped like arches. Men's fibrous tissues are not in this arched pattern but more erratic. When a woman's skin thins, as she gets older, and as she accumulates fat, it tends to push up in fingerlike projections because it's held in that skin compartment by arch-shaped connective tissues. Men do not have this problem. It is *normal* for a woman to have that cobblestoned skin which is known as cellulite. You *can* change it by loss of weight and exercise and that is the *only* way to change it. Many so-called authorities who say they can treat the condition and dissolve these fat deposits by enzyme injections, heat packs, vibrators, massage, special ointments and electro-currents are conning the public. This is pure and simple quackery. Don't be seduced into any such treatment because there is absolutely no evidence that it works. The AMA has recently called all the attention to cellulite an "exploitation of women" and denounces any group or individual who says they can "cure" cellulite.

Q. Is it true that fat-poor diets are good for the skin?

A. There is also no evidence that this is true. Do you think that Africans and Chinese, who eat almost no fat at all, have better skins than the Swedes and Danes, whose diet is very rich in fat? They don't. Who has prettier skin than a Swedish young woman? What about Eskimos, whose diet consists greatly of whale blubber and other high-fat products? Bad skin? No! Absolutely not.

Q. Lately we've been hearing rumors that obesity is not so closely aligned to high blood pressure as we've been led to believe? Have you any ideas on the subject?

A. I do. Traditionally, high blood pressure is associated with early death and all kinds of medical problems—everybody knows that. And fat people are supposed to have higher blood pressure than thin ones. The way we measure blood pressure (putting the cuff you're familiar with around the arm) is actually a very indirect way of measuring the pressure of the blood. Sometimes (although rarely) circumstances dictate that doctors measure pressure by putting a gauge directly into the artery. In that way they get a true and accurate reading. The fatter the arm, the farther the estimator is from the blood. The sound is dulled and the reading is less true. The thinner the arm, the closer the true blood pressure is to the estimator and the more accurate the reading. Fat people who have been labeled hypertensive (having abnormally high arterial blood pressure) are probably not as hypertense as we think. As a general rule, fat arms provide for falsely high blood pressure readings.

I don't know how accurate we've been all these years when we say that fat people die earlier than thin ones. One surely sees a lot more thin old people than fat old people, but maybe that's because people tend to lose weight as they grow older. I used to think fat was a disease; I don't anymore. I certainly see many healthy fat people.

Q. Do skin specialty salons like Georgette Klinger's really help skin?

A. They do very little. Look—if a person has blackheads and she goes to a place where blackheads are removed in a sanitary way, then the place has made her look better. But most of the value lies in psychological value which is also quite important. If a person feels good, then the skin salon is a worthwhile place. But make no mistake. All the creams and steams and presses in the world won't give you a beautiful skin. Only good health does that.

Q. What erases wrinkles?

A. *Nothing*, absolutely nothing takes wrinkles away but surgery. Wrinkles are a function of aging and sun-damaged skin. All light-skinned people who are exposed to the sun will get wrinkles. Dark-skinned people get them too, but later. Look at black-skinned people who are not terribly responsive to sun rays. Eighty-year olds look as if they were forty! Women come in and show me their "old skin." I ask them, "Why isn't the skin under your arms and the skin on your buttocks 'old' skin? They're the same age as your facial skin. The reason your face skin looks seventy years old and your buttocks skin looks forty is ninety percent due to sun exposure." The threat of skin cancer from the sun is a very real danger. If women are not afraid enough of wrinkles to wear a sun-screen product when they're outside, then they should be afraid of cancer.

Q. I've heard about the sexual flush—that rush of blood to the face after orgasm. Is it good for the skin?

A. I certainly believe in sexual flushes. But they only last for a minute and benefits cannot be very strong. Any sustained flush, particularly from exercise, is nice for the skin.

Q. Are the abrasive loofah sponges as wonderful for the skin as we've been told?

A. Who gets so dirty that abrasives are necessary? Only grease monkeys. All most women today have to wash off is makeup. Loofah sponges are supposed to take off the superficial keratin which is the dead outer-skin area. I don't know why anyone, to tell you the truth, would want to do that. That's the normal protective layer of the skin. It keeps the sun and soot off you. Loofahs are a good massage and if they feel good, I suppose they can't hurt too much. Still, be careful of overuse.

Q. Will a heavy woman with a lusty appetite have worse skin than a thin person with a meager appetite?

A. No.

Q. Does tweezing hairs on moles cause cancer?

A. No. Hairy moles do not become transformed into melanoma if you tweeze them. Almost as an absolute rule, hairy moles are not cancerous. It's the ones without hair that must be watched.

Q. Can skin-bleaching creams cause skin irritations?

A. Only if you're allergic to them.

Q. What about hair bleach?

A. The evidence is very, very slim that hair bleach causes cancer, despite the recent hullaballoo. It's a possibility but a very remote one. If I were a woman and wished my hair bleached, I would continue to bleach it—at this time.

Q. Does frequent bathing keep the skin glowing?

A. For some people, older people especially, too much bathing is irritating. In the wintertime, if your skin has gotten a little thinner due to age, you tend to become rashy and wrinkled with a lot of washing. Males tolerate bathing a little better than women because their male hormones promote oiliness. Bathing four times a week is actually plenty—unless it offends your sensibilities. And it's better for your skin.

Q. Here's the big question: We have been besieged by a moisturizing madness. Every skin product, every TV show tells us to moisturize, moisturize, moisturize! We are battered by advice to dampen ourselves. What is your feeling about the subject?

A. The most astonishing thing about being a doctor is that people really believe what you're saying. A stranger comes in here and she'll do anything I say—simply because I'm a doctor. Except one thing. She will never give up her moisturizers. That's how brainwashed American women have become. Acne conditions are *always* made worse by oiliness. Anyone who has a tendency toward pimples should not use moisturizers. In the summertime, when everybody sweats more, moisturizers plug up the oil glands and cause real problems. Women are made to believe that they need a morning moisturizer, an afternoon astringent, a night cream, a removal cream, a Swiss action cream, and a hormone cream that costs $200 a shot. Insane. Most moisturizers cause blackheads and whiteheads. People who haven't washed their faces with soap and water for forty years would be aghast at someone not washing his body with soap and water for forty years. But it's the same thing, really. Women ought to get back to the soap and water, for sure.

There are certain times when a moisturizer makes sense: a freckled, blond, thin-skinned woman has delicate skin which dries out fast and she should use a moisturizer to prevent drying. Most of us, though, are definitely better off without moisturizing products. Still—back to the old adage—if it feels good, do it. The psychological value is greater than any damage done.

So much for the medical advice.

The second half of this chapter is devoted to tips, ideas, natural product recipes and good thoughts about skin. Every now and then, in your reading, you might come across the words "If you have a dry skin, stay away from . . ." Or the same if you have an oily or a normal skin. Do you know what kind of skin you have? It's about time you found out. Check the clues below:

You have an oily skin if most of your answers are yes.

Do you ever have acne?

Do you require daily shampoos because your hair is so oily?

Does your nose always shine?

Did you ever notice redness, itching or even scaling between eyebrows?

In a magnified mirror, do your skin pores seem quite enlarged?

You have a dry skin if most of your answers are yes.

Does your face sometimes feel so tight it will crack?

Does your hair need washing no more than once or twice a week?

Does your face often feel chapped and look flaky?

Do you have tiny splits in your facial skin?

Is your skin dry to the touch?

Do you have tiny, premature wrinkle lines around your mouth and eyes?

Do you rarely have blackheads or pimples?

In a magnified mirror, do you have tiny or no visible pores?

Does your skin stay red for more than a second after a pinch?

If you pinch your neck skin out, does it kind of wait a second or so before it jumps back on your neck?

You have normal skin if most of the answers are yes.

Do you hardly ever have dandruff?
Is your skin smooth?
Does your makeup stay on without getting blotchy or oily?
Do you have pimples around your menstrual period perhaps, and when you've been careless with cleansing, but rarely otherwise?
Do you tan easily?
Can you say your face rarely feels tight or itchy?

Now, down to basics—and beauty. Whatever is good for a thin woman is generally good for a heavy woman—with an important exception. We perspire a lot. Much more than any thin person. Because our body temperature is higher than a thin woman's, sometimes we sweat so much that the gland openings in our skin can't handle the volume. They become clogged. We have many problems caused by bacterial and fungus infections. I even know someone who woefully announces to anyone who will listen that she usually has "crotch rot." Argggh. It's a real problem. So it's generally not a good idea to further clog pores with excess creams, oils and heavy makeups. Occlusive (obstructing) face junk is particularly bad for heavy women. So use your judgment always.

What Do You Do for Heavy Perspiration?

Research shows us that body odors occur more during times of emotional stress. You might have noticed it doesn't take a hot kitchen to make you perspire profusely. Make sure you use an antiperspirant and not just a deodorant. (There was more on that in the last chapter.) An antiperspirant partially closes the pores and inhibits the sweat glands. Be sure to read package directions: some antiperspirants require you to use them the night before so early morning showers won't nullify their effects.

Powders work by absorbing perspiration. It's particularly effective to apply bath powder between your thighs, under your upper arms, anyplace that meets another place to prevent chafing.

When you find yourself sweating up a storm, cool it. Literally. Limit your physical activity. Loosen your clothes. Throw out the polyester and the other nonbreathing fabrics. Try topically applied 25 percent aluminum chloride tincture, obtainable in a drugstore and recommended by many dermatologists. And if the situation becomes really soaked, ask your doctor about tranquilizers.

Either They Hate It or They Love It

Cosmic battles have been fought over the cosmetic virtues of soap. Back in the days when most soaps were villainously harsh and irritating, I would have agreed that soap was not a wonder beauty treatment. But times have changed. Women wear makeup. Air has pollution which coats the face. It's important to *clean*, more important than it ever was. And soaps are so mild today that even the driest face will probably not react.

The experts are still split but I'm not. I think soap's great for anyone and especially for the big woman with the beautiful skin. Despite the rap against it, it works. It does what it's supposed to do, which is clean. There are soaps sold for all skin types, ranging from sulfur-medicated soaps which dry, to rich oil soaps which are supposed to leave a layer of moisturizer on dry skin. Between you and me and the rest of the gang, there's very little difference. Soap is supposed to loosen dirt and grime. If it does that, it's good. It's *how* you use soap that really counts. A quick soap pat and rinse or, worse, insufficient rinse, is useless and can even be quite drying. But if you use your fingertips to produce a rich lather and massage all over the facial area with your fingers or a soft cloth, now you're talking! Pay special attention to the crevices and oil-producing spots on the forehead and alongside the nose. Thoroughly and gently keep the cloth moving for a few minutes to strip the skin of dirt and caked oil. This also loosens blackheads. Rinse and rinse again to remove all soap traces with warm water followed by a refreshing splash of cold. That's it. A good soap and

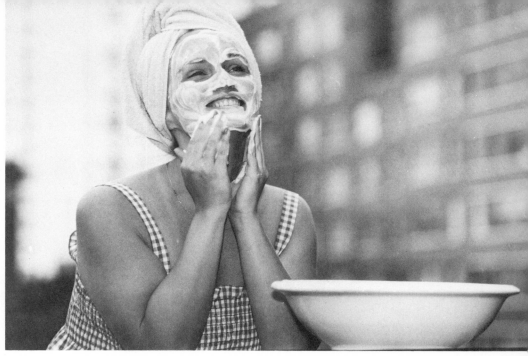

Clean skin is healthy skin! Work up a rich lather and massage facial area with fingertips or a soft cloth.

Rinse thoroughly with warm water to remove all soap traces. Follow with a refreshing splash of cold water.

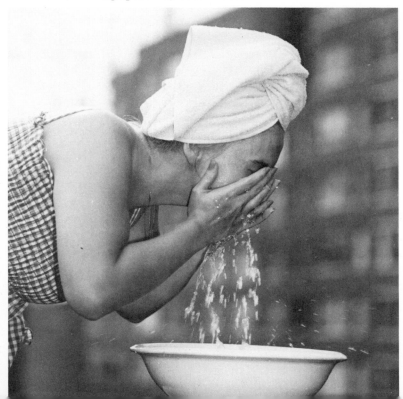

water treatment, regularly applied, is all most people need for fantastic skin.

And then, and then, there's the *other stuff.* The other stuff is fun. It smells good, massages your psyche and maybe, maybe helps a little to keep your skin supple and healthy. Most important, the other stuff makes you *feel* virtuous and shining.

Here's some of the other stuff:

Facial Masks

Nefertiti and her grandmother, you and your grandmother have all used facial masks at one time or another. (*You haven't?* It's time to try one.) They are said to cleanse and stimulate the skin and they give you the feeling that something good is happening to your face. How often do you mask up? Once or twice a week is refreshing unless you have dry skin, in which case you shouldn't do it more than once a month.

What do they do? As the mask dries on the skin, the ensuing warmth and tightening gives the sensation of rejuvenation. Most masks disguise but facial masks don't—no matter what you've been told. They will not erase the crow's-feet that smokers develop; they will not cause the blotchiness that comes from drinking too much to disappear; they will not rub out the tiny, spidery red lines so many big women seem to sprout. If you have an extraordinarily dry skin, facial masks can even be irritating. But if you *think* they refresh and rejuvenate (and who's to say thinking doesn't make it so?) here are some recipes for some super homemade mask preparations.

The Play With Clay Mask: Mix half a cup of kaolin (ask your druggist for colloidal kaolin, which is nothing more than a clay derivative), two teaspoons tincture of benzoin and enough distilled water to make a paste (a kind of loose one). Apply to face, leave on for ten minutes and rinse off with cloth dipped in warm water.

The Honey Mint Yogurt Mask: Makeup genius Adrien Arpel offers this mask. Combine one teaspoon honey, one half-cup plain yogurt, one tablespoon of Fuller's earth, two drops of mint extract and one pinch of bicarbonate of soda. Mix well. Apply mask to face

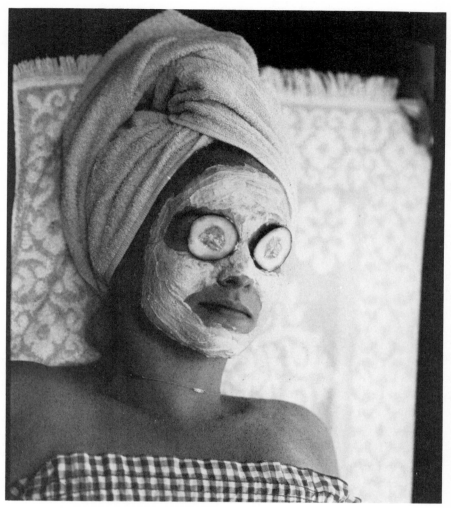

Facial masks cleanse and stimulate the skin.
Cucumber slices refresh tired eyes.

with fingers. As the yogurt softens your skin, the Fuller's earth and honey will pull impurities from it. Apply strips of dampened cotton over the mask until your face looks like Tutankhamun's before they unwrapped him. Leave only your eyes, nostrils and mouth free. Rest for ten moments, then remove cotton and rinse off mask.

The Lemon Egg Mask: The simplest of all masks calls for one half-teaspoon of lemon juice or vinegar and one fork-beaten egg white. Combine egg white with lemon (or vinegar) and smooth over face. Allow about twenty minutes for drying. Rinse.

After any mask it is always good to follow with a gentle acid rinse to restore the skin to its natural, bacteria-killing acid state. An easy acid rinse consists of one-eighth cup of vinegar and one and a half cups of water. After patting on the rinse, allow your face to dry in the air.

Steam Mists

Yum. I really love them. They definitely open closed pores to release dirt. An added plus is the nice boost that the warmth gives to blood circulation, which also helps the skin to expel impurities. And on top of it all, steam mists give your face a brand-new-baby kind of glow.

You can buy a steam mister for about twenty dollars. Insert some water in the water compartment, plug in, thrust your face into what is, in essence, a tiny steam room—and luxuriate! Or you can improvise a steam mister by filling a sink with very hot water and ducking under a terrycloth tent for a while. *Or* you can even use a teakettle with a long spout which aims the steam *away* from the kettle and the source of the heat and *toward* your face. Be very careful not to put your face near the burner part of the stove. After a steam mist, it's a good idea to pat an astringent like witch hazel on your skin. That closes the open pores and prevents makeup from seeping in.

Astringents

They're liquid pats for oily, *never dry*, skins. They close open pores and temporarily give a feeling of skin tightening and freshening. Good old witch hazel is a terrific and cheap astringent. Also unscented alcohol. Naturally, you can buy expensive astringents which come in prettier bottles. Astringents are particularly nice for large women who perspire a lot. They seem to inhibit facial perspiration a bit.

Moisturizing Madness

See chapter 3, Bathing and Beauty, and check out the comments from dermatologist Dr. Irving Abrahams earlier in this chapter. Moisturizers have many doctors saying *never* and many cosmeticians saying *always.* You have to read the pros and cons and decide for yourself. One thing is for sure: *very* oily skins don't love moisturizers. For every sixty beauty experts who would wither if you took away their moisturizers, another sixty will say that you just can't feed the skin from the outside—it simply doesn't work. The human skin, they claim, is nourished by nutrients carried through the bloodstream—just like every other organ—and the skin, thus nourished, gives off its own secretions to keep itself moist and pliant. Could you help an ailing liver or heart by applying something on the outside of the organs? Well, skin is an organ too, say the antimoisturizers, and cannot benefit from external lubrication.

Still, on a skin-chapping winter day, a moisturizer *does* feel good. I like it, I don't care what anyone else says. I feel that economically, a moisturizer saves me money because my makeup slides on easier and it takes less to cover the same area. I think of a moisturizer as a primer. I put it on before the paint. Then there are experts like Dr. Erno Laszlo, the late and very famed international skin specialist, who once said in an interview that dousing the skin with moist creams wasn't apt to help much. Instead, he recommended a high intake of Vitamin A which he felt nourished the skin—from the inside out.

You have to make up your own mind on the moisturizing madness conflict. Do it by trial and error.

Cleansing Creams

Cleansing cream is our oldest cosmetic, invented by a second-century Greek physician named Galen. Use it *before* your soap and water treatment to dissolve oily dirt and makeup. Cleansing creams almost always have fats and oils and maybe even some water in them. Heavy faces often produce more oil than thin ones, and cleansing cream should be removed *thoroughly* with soap and water on those skins. A good and inexpensive cleansing cream is any five-and-dime-store cold cream. Of course, you can double the price with any cosmetic company's name brand.

Facial Uglies

ROOTING ROSACEA

Rosacea, a disease of the oil glands expressed by severe inflammation and infection, seems to be a special beauty problem of the middle-aged, heavy woman because her supersweating clogs pores and causes excess oil-gland production. It looks like teenage acne but because of the blood vessel enlargement, the skin where the lesions appear looks unpleasantly red. Ever see a woman with a large red nose? She probably has rosacea. Diet helps! Give up spices, coffee, tea, milk and alcohol. Use a lot of soap and water. A dermatologist can help with antibiotics and even hormone treatment as a last resort, but try Sulforcin lotion before you see a doctor, says Bedford Shelmire, M.D., himself a dermatologist and author of many skin-care books. Makeup does not seem to affect the condition so try to mask the redness as best as you can. Emotional flurries and exposure to extreme climatic conditions often brings on an attack. If your emotions trigger rosacea, ask your doctor about a mild tranquilizer.

BLACKHEADS AND PIMPLES

Sure it's nice to say run to a dermatologist or to Georgette Klinger's every time you see a blackhead, but whom are we kidding? The fact is that you *can* squeeze out your own blackheads if you're scrupulously clean about it, ignoring your mother who invariably says, "I know someone who died from that." Wet cotton balls with very hot water and apply on the site of the blackhead for a couple of minutes to loosen the blackhead. Squeeze, slowly. When mission is accomplished, disinfect the whole area with alcohol. Make sure it's a blackhead and *not* a pimple you're squeezing. The latter should never be squeezed because *that* can lead to infection, permanent pockmarks and worse. You can *help* pimples to "come to a head," with hot-as-you-can-stand compresses on the site. The sun, which is terrible in almost every way for your skin, does dry up excess oils and helps to clear up pimples: so if it's summertime, and you have an important weekend date, risk the sun exposure for the sake of the pimples.

OTHER TINY UGLIES

If you are really despairing of covering the tiny red capillaries big women seem to get so often, and the moles and the other tiny uglies on your body or face—have them removed by a doctor. It's no big deal!

Moles are pigmented growths on the skin and can be removed painlessly and quickly by either a plastic surgeon or a dermatologist. They generally never grow back.

Warts are a different story. They are virus-caused and often appear and disappear no matter how many times you have them removed. Skin doctors use acid (painless, really), surgery, ultrasonics, freezing them off with liquid nitrogen and many other kinds of topical medicine to get rid of the pesky devils. No one falls down with shock if they reappear.

Dilated capillaries, again, are one of our biggest problems. The spidery red lines are only tiny blood vessels, though. Electric needles applied by doctors coagulate the blood and make the capillaries turn white. They also return, sometimes.

Stretch marks. Oh, those miserable yo-yo diets where we gain and lose and gain again! Our skin, being the body's most flexible organ, expands, retrenches and expands again. And stretch marks, which are really ruptures in the elastic fibers of the lower layer of skin, result. Besides rapid weight gain and loss, pregnancy, certain medications like steroids and certain hormones which increase in production during adolescence can also cause stretch-mark scarring. What can be done? Not too much. Try a corrective makeup product like Lydia O'Leary's Covermark. Sometimes the medical procedure known as dermabrasion can help make scar marks less visible. (It is performed by a dermatologist or plastic surgeon in his/her office.) There is an operation called abdominal lipectomy offered by plastic surgeons which can be performed to remove excess fat from the abdomen and also to remove severe stretch marks. This should be done only as a last resort and only if you are absolutely traumatized by the scars.

Can you prevent stretch marks? Opinions differ, but it can't hurt to rub lubricating oils like cocoa butter into the area. It helps not to gain weight too quickly, or lose too quickly. And last but not least, it does *not* help stretch marks to take huge amounts of Vitamin E and zinc, according to the Food and Drug Administration.

Facial Massage

Done vigorously, it's the biggest no-no!

Everyone says it feels good, but be careful. Instead of exercising facial muscles to prevent wrinkles, vigorous facial massage can actually break down connective tissue at the base of the skin and *cause* wrinkling and hanging skin. The weakened facial collagen fibers have broken and crumbled, and your pretty skin, the large woman's greatest asset, becomes disaster. The same principle applies to all those shining, stainless-steel machines you see at exercise spas. Great rollers and pummeling devices override your body, supposedly to stretch the muscles and work off the fat. All those machines really do is what a butcher does when he pounds a piece of meat with a mallet: he *flattens* it by breaking down the tissues. Mallets and machines and vigorous facial massages flatten and undermine the skin instead of tightening it. *Gentle* manipulation of the facial muscles and skin in an upward direction is blood-stimulating and feels good, but anything more frenzied should be avoided at all costs. Our weight has a lovely, skin-puffing effect which fills out wrinkles in the face and acts as a natural cosmetic. Try to enjoy it and *don't mess around!*

Nails

Manicured, reasonably long fingernails tend to make chubby fingers look slimmer, tapered and more graceful. Nails are almost a trademark of femininity, but *too* long nails look like Charles Addams nails. They become a liability, raking and scraping everything in sight. Of course, they are useful as lethal weapons in attack. Still, writing is handicapped, you can't pick up too many pins, and forget typing and telephone dialing. Anyone who makes love to you is brave.

For nice nails, wear protective gloves while doing housework and file and clean them regularly. What's more gruesome than a layer of dirt under nails? Nails are simply extensions of the skin and are able to pick up infections from dirt. Screaming colors like chartreuse or blood red are not sexy on nails, but soft colors and even colorless polish are protective as well as good-looking. Try to pick up your skin tones in your nail colors, using rusts and beiges as opposed to sky-blue pinks and fire-engine reds.

Diet

Many skin experts suggest that a diet without fats or oil of any sort cannot be terrific for the skin. If you have a dog with flaking, dandruffy-looking skin and you supplement its diet with a tablespoon of vegetable or peanut oil every night, voilà! no more flaky skin. The same principle works for people. Crash diets that exclude all vegetable and animal fats are not geared to produce glowing skin. Candy and chocolate mousse may not be terrific for your teeth or gums, but they will not adversely affect your skin—despite what you've heard.

Sunburn

Use a sun-*block* lotion, not just any suntan lotion. You will still get tanned, but more slowly. If this advice comes late and you're already fried to a crisp, wet compresses, cool, cool tub soaks and cold-cream body lotions will help. Don't try anything like cala-mine lotion which dries and induces peeling. One more thing: before you use *any* commercial sunburn anesthetic, test it in a small area to see that you're not allergic to it.

V Hairlines

She was a redhead, all right, there was no doubt about it. A flaming flirt of a redhead. God knows how many men had fallen for that gorgeous, silky mane of hair.

It was hard to tell what the rest of her looked like, though. There wasn't much else left of her.

She was the eighteenth-dynasty mummy of Hentawi, dug up recently by an enterprising anthropologist. Gone were her voluptuous curves, gone the eyes that had driven men wild, gone the intelligence, gone the flesh. Aside from a few paltry bones and some leathery stuff that passed for skin, all that remained in vir-

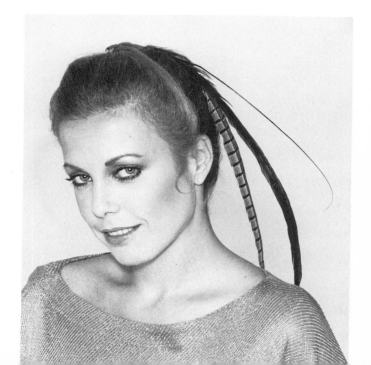

tual splendor was her magnificent head of red hair. But oh, what hair. It had withstood the weight of centuries. It had lasted for thousands of years, when every other human feature had faded.

Such is the nature of hair. It's pretty durable stuff. You can bleach, dye, straighten, curl, shave, shape, puff, pad, wave, frizz, cut, braid, thicken, thin and transplant it and it keeps coming back for more. It varies in type, texture, color and length not only in individuals but even on the body of one person.

And it's pretty romantic stuff. We have always had an obsession with hair. Poetry, folklore, myths and Broadway shows have lauded it. Whole industries have grown up because of it. Hair is a personal form of expression that seems to speak loudly no matter which era you've grown up in.

The ancient Greeks sacrificed their hair to the gods and today's kids sacrifice their hair to nobody. The latest inventions become outdated and kings and presidents come and go, but our fascination with hair remains.

Hairstyles have included African mud sets, Egyptian plaits, Greek curls, Elizabethan pompadours, British marcel waves, American bobs, adolescent ponytails, Afros and flips. We have encouraged topknots, toupees, postiches, spit curls, chignons, chous and pigeon wings.

Jackie made us crazy with bouffants, Audrey Hepburn made us cutesy with urchin cuts, Veronica Lake made us sexy with half our faces hidden in hair veils. Brigitte has had us long, blond and tousled, Mamie has had us banged. And the next hair fashion guru will lead us—where?

No one needs *good* hair advice more than the heavy woman. If our hair looks terrific, the rest of the body follows suit. And we've had more than our share of hair advice. Keep it gray; dye it. Cut it, let it grow, wash it, tease it; don't wash it too much, oil it, glue it, spray it. Take vitamins for it; use electricity and hot irons on it. Swallow monkey glands, female urine and God knows what else to keep it healthy. The Greek big women used goat's fat and swallowed swallow's dung to lighten their hair. Cleopatra, herself no lightweight, swore by bear grease.

And it stands to reason we've had our share of hairdressers. Some of them have been lunatics, some masochists and some geniuses. The first hairdresser of all time was a gentleman named

Champagne who curled and coiled away in the seventeenth century. He used to style one side of a lady's hair and demand a kiss before he'd undertake the second side, that rascal. Champagne would never take money for his services but he did okay in gifts from the adoring ladies, including ex-queen Christina of Spain, who gave him a coach.

There have been millions of hairdressers in millions of neighborhoods all over the universe. But there have only been a few legendary modern ones: true craftspeople whose fame has grown and endured because their skill and artistry have been unique. You will recognize their names: Alexandre of Paris, Alba of Rome, Masters of California, Sassoon of London, Moller of Hamburg.

And perhaps the greatest of them all,

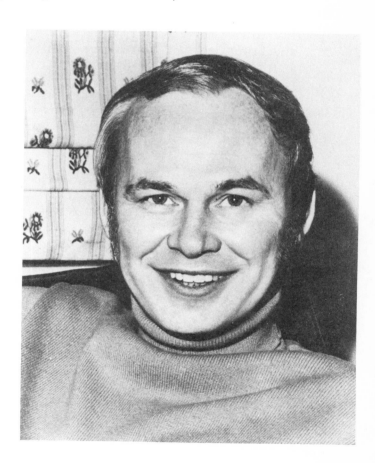

Kenneth, a legend in hairstyling.

Kenneth of New York

His office was huge, dimly lit except for the exquisite lamp on the massive desk which cast a marvelous glow on his own, beautifully styled, blond hair. His clients have included the most famous names in all the world. The hands which have held a thousand scissors played with a pencil as we talked about the particular problems of the big woman.

I had a million questions.

Me: Is there any style that is disastrous for the big woman?

Kenneth: The answer is excesses. *Anything* too much, too big, too long, too full, too clipped. My pet peeve for heavy women is the style that calls for the cropped look. I've seen it all over the country. Anyone, but the overweight woman in particular, looks terrible with her hair chopped off. They may call it a "boy cut," but no boy or man in the country wears his hair like that anymore. I'm not against short hair, obviously, but this butcher-cropped hair is bad hairdressing and a particularly poor choice for big women. The large woman should make the most of her hair—not sacrifice it in the name of easy care. It is appalling to see so many women devastating themselves like this, and worse, yet, never touching that cropped hair until they go back to their hairdressers for the next shearing.

You are famous for your haircuts. Why do you think women come from all over the world and pay large sums of money just to get their hair cut by a master technician?

Hair cut well, in feminine and natural styles, and kept immaculately clean is a pleasure to see and touch. It removes the need to set the hair in great ugly rollers all done up in toilet tissue every night which has to disgust everyone around you. A great haircut can make the difference between commonplace and really extraordinary good looks. It can make a plain fat woman metamorphose into a stunning big woman.

Shall I have my hair cut wet or dry?

It doesn't matter. Techniques differ. You must let your hairdresser work in his or her own way.

Which are more effective—razor or blunt hair cuts?

I have used razor cuts very, very rarely. I think generally they

are not effective. I *might* use a razor on a woman with an inordinately thick head of hair because only a razor could shape it in a
certain way. But razor cuts, unless done brilliantly, leave hair that
stands up and pops out as it grows in. True, they tease easier, and
dry faster and go around magnetic curlers very well. But a blunt
scissors cut looks ten times more natural and more appealing than
a razored cut which has been teased and set.

How often should one get her hair cut?

Hair grows a half an inch a month. *Everybody's* hair. It may
differ by a millimeter more or less, but count on six inches a year.
Now, if you have a hairstyle which depends on a very specific
shape or cut, three-quarters of an inch to an inch can throw it off
and make a difference. The general rule for this kind of mainte-
nance is a haircut somewhere between every four and eight weeks.

*The legendary hairdresser Alexandre of Paris has said, "The
base of the art of the coiffure is the cut, as the foundation of a
building is the base of architecture. A woman in our times is ugly
only if she chooses to be. Any unattractive feature can be dis-
guised by a good hairstyle." Do you agree?*

I suppose it's true. It's a question of illusion. If a woman comes
to me and has spent twenty years thinking "My ears are too big"
or "My chin is too short" or "I'm too fat to be pretty," and I change
her hair in some way that can really be terribly minor like putting
bangs where no bangs have been, or taking bangs away, then that
dissatisfied woman looks in the mirror—and she's someone else.
I have helped her to create an illusion that fast becomes a reality.
She no longer sees the ears or the chin or the fat. She thinks she
looks good. And you know what? She really does. Because she feels
prettier, she somehow *becomes* prettier. It works. It really does.
Not only she, but the world, sees a more secure, lovelier woman.
That's a certain kind of wonderful power an expert hairdresser has.

*Many hairdressers create new styles just for the sake of change.
Is that the kind of power you are talking about?*

Certainly not. My real power lies in being able to help women
discover themselves, not in *my* discovering them. Unfortunately,
the people themselves rarely create the changes today. Whole industries and publications have grown up based on falsely manipulated change for change's sake. I don't want that power that the
industries and even the women themselves try to thrust in my

hand and imagination. Take skirt lengths, for example—the whole business should have been dropped thirty years ago. Some women look good in short skirts and some in long, and they should stick with what's good for them, not what fashion and false change decrees. Never do anything to yourself that you don't like because someone else has decreed it's fashionable. This is particularly true with hairstyle.

Tell me about washing my hair. Can I do it too often?

No. Your hair soils more easily because you perspire more than a thinner person. You *must* wash it more often. It will not dry out even if you wash it daily.

What kind of shampoo should I use? Is an expensive shampoo the best?

A shampoo should clean, primarily. Many expensive and inexpensive brands work equally well. Often we identify a good shampoo by how much lather it produces and that's a mistake. The best shampoo I ever used was called Soapless. It wasn't really soapless but it was great and it really cleaned the hair wonderfully. The company went bust. Americans were used to Prell-type suds. More lather means more detergent which can actually dull and dry hair. Trial and error is the only way to find out what's the best for you —but don't be misled by the whipped-cream lather.

Should every woman use a cream rinse? The fashion magazines say yes.

I say no. Cream rinses were invented many years ago to facilitate combing through hair that, at that time, because of the newly invented double-processed hair coloring, was impossible to comb through. But if you have a fine head of hair, even a thick head of hair with fine texture, you so soften it with a cream rinse that it will not do *anything*. A cream rinse won't hurt but you must use your judgment as to how much, if at all, it helps. On the other hand, if you have very coarse, wiry, kinky, curly or thick hair, you do need a softening product and you can use an undiluted cream rinse to good advantage. Experiment. No one will kill you, either, if you don't follow the manufacturer's advice to use the rinse undiluted. Dilute the product about four times to the bottle. Comb your hair through, in the shower, with the diluted rinse and your hair will probably react well. It will not become greasy as quickly or stick together or lie flat against your head. And the bottle of cream rinse will last longer.

What about vinegar rinses?

Vinegar rinses take away soap-film residues. They help with long hair tangles although they do not soften the hair. But vinegar, like lemon, is acidic, and if you have color on your hair, you are liable to affect that color. If your hair tends to be dry, vinegar rinse might make it dryer.

What about eggs and lemon and balsam in hair rinses? Do they change the hair for the better?

Whatever you put on your hair from the scalp out does not permanently affect the hair. Your general health, a terrible emotional trauma, a physical change like a hysterectomy, or a pregnancy certainly *can* affect the living hair bulb and thus, the hair, permanently. But the lemon, eggs and balsam you speak of are temporary bandages for external conditions, based on your individual hair texture. Even if you permanented on top of another permanent, which is not recommended, it wouldn't look very attractive for a while, but when the damaged hair grew out, you'd be home free. You can not apply any living thing to the nonliving hair and have it damage or improve the hair root.

Is hair really responsive to emotional states?

When you are an excessively nervous person, your skin may erupt and any number of other physical changes can take place. Hair also reacts to strong emotional trauma with dandruff and hair loss. The reaction does not have to be permanent. Certainly hormonal changes such as those connected with menopause can affect hair. Enough studies have been done with balding men to show that adding certain hormones to their diet caused hair growth. Unfortunately, the same hormones often caused the men to grow breasts and other (for men) strange things. The problem of hair loss and damage has no simple solution.

What kind of brush is the best brush for my hundred daily strokes?

Natural bristles are probably better because they tend to be less stiff. They will not break the hair as they brush through any resistance. But anyone who still brushes her hair a hundred strokes a day is living in the dark ages. *No one* should be doing that anymore. When people had waist-length hair in the late 1800s and they washed it twice a year, women literally cleansed their hair by brushing it. They did not permanent-wave it, they rarely tinted or dyed it. They certainly never straightened it. Their hair had little battering. But why would you want to brush it one hundred strokes today? You're not going to make it grow faster and, I trust, you wash it more than twice a year so you don't need the cleansing benefits of brushing. Nothing inside your scalp will be changed by brushing the nonliving hair. To a certain extent, a brush *will* polish the hair and get rid of any excess hair spray and air pollutants that may have landed on you. But whenever you do brush, brush gently. Don't attack the scalp.

Will straightening or permanenting the hair too much damage it?

Sure. You're talking about chemical processes. The chemical formula is very close in formulation to a depilatory. Straightening and permanenting means softening each hair first, then putting on a neutralizer to chemically replace the molecular structure you've broken down. I don't mean to frighten anyone away from either process, but all things should be done in moderation.

What's moderation?

You shouldn't redo straightening or permanenting until the original process has grown out. Short or layered hair that's approximately three or four inches long should be straightened or waved no more than two, maybe three (that's stretching it) times a year. Long, one-length hair should be done about once a year. You must cut off the hair that's been straightened or waved. You should not redo it.

The big woman with a round face—what kind of hairstyle?

I don't usually go by shapes of faces or rules that have been made for a special few. What's important to me in style is proportion. If you're short, long hair tends to make you look shorter unless it's up in some way. If you're big-faced as opposed to small-faced, no matter *what* the face shape is, more volume of hair produces less of a face, so fullness *is* good for you. If you have a small face, more hair produces even a smaller face, so you have to have a style that carries your hair away from your face, to make it proportionately larger and more pleasing. Angles on exaggerated face sizes often help. Therefore, if you have a very big face, an asymmetrical line is better than a symmetrical line for you. It's a question of basic design to find hair shapes that complement the proportions of your face and body.

Okay. How do I go about finding a great hairdresser?

Start with other people. You can tell when a friend looks better than she ever did before. Does her hair move well, does it fit her head, is she somehow prettier? People are flattered to be asked about their hairdressers. Even if you see a stranger walking down the street with a marvelous hairstyle or haircut, *ask* her where she got it. Then call that hairdresser and tell him or her what it is

Hair by Victor Friedman of Kenneth's Hair Salon.

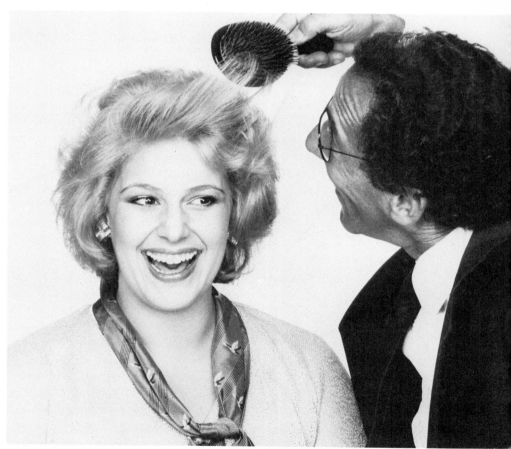

about Mrs. Cromwell's hair that you admire. Perhaps your hair won't fall in exactly the same way hers did, but it will give the hairdresser an idea of what *you* think looks great. Magazines are still another source. If you see a model with fantastic hair, check in the small print alongside the ad to see if the salon that did her hair is listed. It often is.

How do I choose a style?

Taking clippings from magazines of whatever hair you admire is a fine way. Be realistic. If you're blond, don't bring Elizabeth Taylor's picture to your hairdresser. It makes no sense—you won't be seeing yourself. A blond curled head and a dark curled head will not look the same because the light does different things to them. Clip pictures of hairstyles where the length and color of the hair are similar to yours.

What happens if a hairdresser says he wants to give me a certain style and I know I'll hate it, but he's very insistent?

Run, don't walk, from his chair. No one knows better than you what kind of hair you'll be comfortable with. Naturally, if you

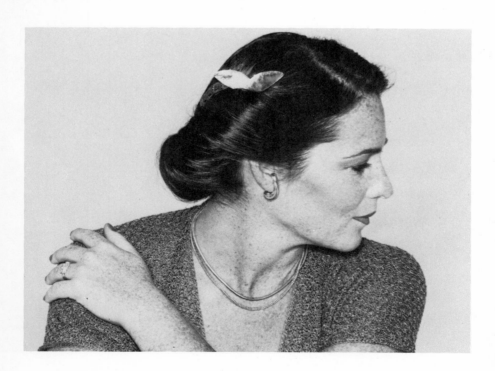

wish suggestions, be open to new ideas. But if you do not want to experiment, let no one browbeat you into bangs if you feel you look like a poodle in bangs. And if you do decide to take a hair-dresser's suggestion and it doesn't work, ask him about alternate ways you can work with the style until it grows in. If you haven't gone to a butcher or some insane person, you can always modify a style. Try to be open to new thought. I had an elderly woman today who came in with her granddaughter. She had been wearing a helmet of teased, sprayed hair all her life. It felt gritty—like sand. She left with her hair feathery, shining, soft and away from her face. Also twenty years younger, I think. If she had hated the style I chose, there were other ways she could have combed the finished hair. A good hairdresser always leaves you with *a choice.*

Can I blow-dry my hair every day, safely?

Yes, if the dryer is not too hot, if you do not bring it too close to the hair and if you do not use the brush too roughly. Think of your hair as fabric. A cotton skirt is made up of many threads. If you rub the fabric every day, rub, rub, rub, eventually you will get a hole in the skirt. Think of your hair also as so many threads, although each hair is stronger than any thread ever was. It does have to bear the attrition of your daily life. It gets rubbed on the pillow, gets battered by the wind and the soap and the brush you use. It can wear out, just like the cotton skirt. Blow-dryers, used improperly, are that much more attrition battering the hair. And your hair will wear out from the ends up, because that's the part that's been around the longest, that's the part that has taken the most battering. Those are called split ends.

How can I cure split ends?

Cut them off. There is no other way because nothing cures split ends. You can put creams on them to temporarily fill them in, but the creams are just a bandage. They are still split. It's very basic.

Can I take vitamins to give my hair health and body?

Vitamins for hair, as far as I am concerned, are vitafrauds. I'm not a doctor and this is a personal opinion, but nothing I have *ever* seen or read has proved to me that taking vitamins or any combination of vitamins has ever helped the hair. Certainly proper nutrition is essential for body health and thus in turn, hair health. But the consumption of isolated vitamins never did a blessed thing. One woman wrote me a letter asking me if she should put

Vitamin E *on* her hair—a very famous nutritionist told her it would be terrific. I told her she could put all the Vitamin E in the world on her hair and it would just lie there on top. It wouldn't do a thing in the world for the hair bulb which was the living part of the hair.

Any special tips for summer care when hair is a nuisance if it's not easy?

Decide on the summer length you like. If it's short, you can have a wash-and-wear cut. If it's straight, you can have a light body permanent to hold in the style. If it's long, you can wear it in a topknot, rolled at the temples or gently pulled back. All hair, and especially colored or straightened hair, needs to be protected from the sun. Hair conditioners are good, particularly in the summer, for this kind of protection. The all-time great conditioner is castor oil, the stuff your mother had to hold you down to take. A few capfuls combed through the hair gives a thick coating to protect. Wash it out well. Another tip: when you swim without a cap, the pool and the ocean do unpleasant things to your hair. If you have a can of soda water handy, don't drink it—pour it on your hair. It'll get rid of chemicals and salt until your next shampoo.

Why do you think women let their hair down at the beauty salon in more ways than one? I hear women confiding the most intimate details.

Not to me, they don't. I won't allow it. Women are at a vulnerable point at the hairdresser's and they may say things they very much regret saying later. It's true that many hairdressers do encourage this sort of thing. It is, in a funny way, a sort of weapon for them. It takes their clients' minds off what is being done to them. In order to do the job I am paid for, I need information from my client that has nothing to do with her sex or financial life. I need to know:

How does she want to live with her hair?
Does she want to do it herself?
Can she do it herself?
How often does she want to see a hairdresser—once a week, month, year?
Does she have any pet hates about her hair?
Has she ever had a hairdo that worked especially well? Why didn't she keep it?

Answers to those questions will produce the best results for the client (if the hairdresser is paying attention). It is more important for the heavy woman to play up her hair assets than it is for the fashion model. Look, hairdressing is a service industry. We don't sell fashion—we sell service. We *are* servants. That isn't a dirty word at a Kenneth salon even if it has come to be a dirty word in America. And in this business, you're only as good as your last movie—or in our case, your last haircut.

More on Hair

Kenneth is a master in his profession. But there are other experts and sometimes your best friend, your Aunt Sadye, your mother and *their* hairdressers come up with splendid ideas on how to make hair work. Be open-minded and experiment with likely sounding ideas even if they come from unlikely sources.

What follows are some hints and hair inspirations culled from a potpourri of professionals and amateurs who spend a lot of time playing with the hair of big, beautiful women. They know that even if you were born with a Twinkie in your mouth, your crowning glory *should* make such a difference in your appearance that, Twinkies notwithstanding, you look marvelous.

ON STYLE

It's funny. Ask any guy at all. It's the loose, natural look he prefers on women, every time. But the women—oh the women. Have they listened? No. Down through the ages they have always struggled with the beehives, the pompadours, the lacquered, sprayed, formal pomp of overdone hair, but no more. The times they are a-changing. Our lives are too full to fool with preposterous coiffures.

The big woman was never terrific in preposterous coiffures anyway.

Which means no sex-kitten tendrils curling down her back. And no ponytails. In fact, if you ask me, *no* woman over the age of fourteen should wear curling, waist-length hair unless she lives on Bali.

For some reason, extremes of any sort seem worse on us than on our thinner counterparts. Exotica is definitely silly. Although natural fullness which comes from a superb haircut is great to balance out the body fullness in top-heavy women especially, *bigness* of hair is disastrous. Bigness is *any* complicated, teased, wide nest that circles the scalp more than three inches out in any direction.

And take cleanliness: skinny Debby Boone can get away with oily tresses once in a while—even a flake or so of dandruff. You can't. I can't. So help me, our dandruff flakes seem larger. And whiter. Our little trick of perspiring heavily makes our hair look limper and get dirtier faster than a skinny kid's. So wash often.

Back to style: we don't look well in shaved heads. Or tight frizzes. Or Afros unless we're African, in which case, we look splendid! Or corn-row braids in many directions. Or milkmaid braids. As I said—extremes.

What's great is *sensible* style. When you are big, if your features warrant the severe look, you can wear your hair gently pulled back in an early Grace Kelly style. (Too tightly pulled back hair means certain hair loss: never use rubber bands: try the fabric-covered elastics.)

You can wear your hair softly curling around your cheekbones like a Raphaelite nude. You can wear it neatly shoulder length (no

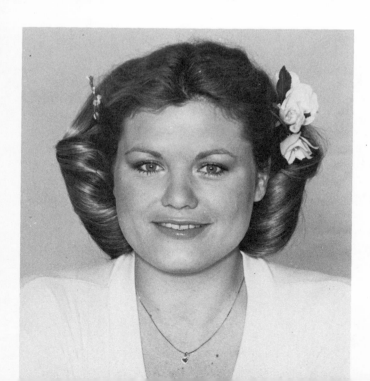

longer, please) in a soft, blown-dry fall. Your hair should flatter your bone structure: a good hairdresser will know how to find your bones even if they are hiding.

If your hair is thin or limp, you should *not* wear it long because the weight will flatten it out even more. If your hair is ringlet-curly you also should not wear it long unless you are Shirley Temple—or Patricia Herring, my grade school nemesis who got all the boys with her naturally curly locks while my locks wilted on the vine. Keep in mind that Shirley and Patricia were eleven at the time of their greatest triumphs, which lets out forty-five-year-old look-a-likes.

A heavy woman often has a short, bulky nape of neck: loose, sloppy ringlets curling over this nape do not camouflage it but merely call attention to an area that should be played down. Keep bulky neck napes hair-free! I know it sounds like a battle cry, but it should. Bulky neck napes can be as depressing as nukes or gas lines.

Remember always that for short hair, in particular, the superb cut is the secret to success. You can fool around with many styles, but as you get older, you will find softer edges, less sharp outlines, more flattering. Younger big women can experiment with gentle

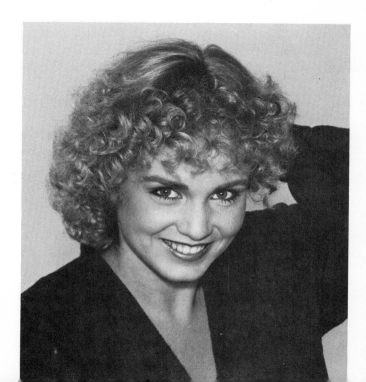

versions of the geometric haircut that Vidal Sassoon popularized, along with other more severe lines.

Bangs are not great if your face is very fat and round: they're just too cute for you. But by all means *try* them if you've always wanted bangs because choice is what we're talking about in this book. We are allowed to make our own choices no matter what anyone says is right for us.

Hint: Whatever hairstyle you do choose, it should meet one criterion: *you should not need gobs of hair spray to keep it in place.* In place is out of fashion, anyway. What's in is hair that moves and flies naturally and is delicious to see. Hair that is lacquered in place belongs on museum mannequins.

RINSES—GARBAGE OR GOOD STUFF? THE REAL SCOOP

If you've read that rinses can permanently affect the texture, control or health of your hair—you've read garbage.

If you've read that rinses can *temporarily* seem to add body to hair and make it easier to comb and manage—*right after a single shampoo*—that's good reading.

Rinses are for instant and not long-lasting effect. They have no permanent value, good or bad. There are:

Cream rinses. Neutralize static electricity and prevent flyaway hair. They seem to make the hair glossier and softer—for a few hours. They're especially good for bleached, curled or dyed hair. It's dumb to use them with limp or fine hair because *Vogue* tells you to do so.

Protein rinses. Some say they make the hair look thicker and even glossier for a short while. They do nothing permanent in terms of affecting hair growth or changing hair conditions.

Acid rinses. Lemon or other citric juices added to the final rinse water does seem to reduce soapy films left by some shampoos. But most shampoos today do not leave such films and so these rinses are almost always superfluous.

Beer rinses. Might give the appearance of thickening the hair, but do you love beery-smelling hair? I don't. Champagne is another matter, but I haven't tried it yet since I only go for the French kind and I can't bear to waste that on my hair.

Hair thickeners. They contain proteins, oil and other substances which coat the hair with an invisible film that seems to wrap around and stick to the hair shaft. They work by filling in the spaces—temporarily making your hair look fuller. They can't hurt, but sometimes they give a very unpleasant, sticky feeling to the hair. Try it—they only last until the next wash-out, anyway.

Homemade bonus. Stuff from your kitchen works as well as any $5.95 job and you get to play mad scientist. Try these:

- Raspberry Jell-O rinse (or lemon, lime and even apricot). A rinse in loosely prepared jello somehow makes your hair more manageable and adds temporary body. Apply it *before* it jells. Wash it out well unless you want your hair to mold.
- Swami's peanut conditioner. A conditioner touted by Donna Lawson in *Mother Nature's Beauty Cupboard.* The women in India, she says, use it to restore sun-dried-out oils. Use equal amounts of peanut oil (found at health stores and most supermarkets), lemon juice and yogurt. Massage the concoction into the hair and wash out thoroughly with a mild castile shampoo. (Health food addicts can use their own, self-ground peanuts instead of the peanut oil—yum.)
- Cider vinegar magic. Well, maybe it isn't really magic, and it really shouldn't work by all intelligent standards, but it does for me. I don't have color on my hair, maybe that's why. I mix about a half-cup of cider vinegar in a pot of warm water for a final rinse that seems to leave my hair shining royally!
- Castor-oil conditioner. Dry and brittle hair? This is your baby. Two tablespoons of castor oil, one tablespoon of olive oil. Warm together (do not make too hot—remember the old boiled-in-oil-torture). Massage mixture at a comfortable temperature into your scalp and then brush or comb it through your hair. *Then* wrap your head with steaming hot terrycloth turbans (keep changing them so they'll stay hot) for about twenty minutes. This allows all that moisturizing oil to penetrate deep into the hair follicles. Need I tell you to shampoo, *very thoroughly,* and rinse just as thoroughly to avoid sliding around on your pillow?
- *And an unorthodox tip*—unorthodox because I think I invented it. As far as I know, there's no medical evidence to back

it up. I got it from Benny, my co-author's airedale. For years, the vet has been telling Sherry to feed him small amounts of unsaturated fats to make his coat glossy. She does, and he has the shiniest coat on the block. Also, he seems to get rid of the dry, flaky white stuff that appears now and then on his coat (looks like dandruff) by ingesting somewhat larger amounts when necessary. Unsaturated fats are not the cholesterol-building-up kind. I cook with them and my hair shines up a storm.

STYLE

Simple is the big word.

If you're really fat, a too-small hairdo can make you look like a pinhead.

A too-big hairdo, with lots of curls or bouffant stuff, will make you look like 1955.

Keep the hair in proportion to the body. Balance is achieved by placing the width at the sides of the head to emphasize eyes.

A note of worth from Dr. Barbara Edelstein: Dieting can make your hair fall out. Really. Not always, but watch for it, and if you see any signs of hair loss, stop the diet immediately!

Hair: We should treasure its versatility, preserve its health and understand that it often serves as a badge for beauty, status, polit-

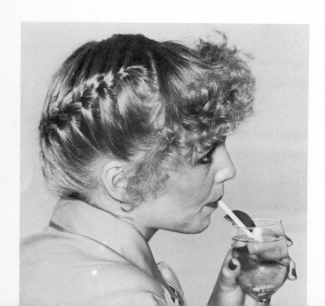

ical, and sexual appeal. Because it is composed of a marvelously strong and resilient fiber, hair can do many things well: you can vary its color and style endlessly. But be gentle and moderate. Experiment with a color rinse before you go ape with a permanent dye. Don't ever go too far from the color with which you were born. Try on a wig in the color you admire to make sure you don't look dopey in Titian red.

If you look in the mirror and your clothes are just right, your complexion is glowing, and your psyche is satisfied but your hair is a mess, you will not be happy with your clothes, your complexion or your psyche. Believe me.

Hair is your crowning glory—no matter what size you are.

VI Teeth and Mouth

When you were little, there was always the kid named Patricia or Melanie or Rhonda with the *teeth*. Sure she was chubbier than the rest of the fifth-graders and she didn't have your naturally curly hair, but when she opened her mouth to smile, twenty-two male fifth-grade cowboys dropped dead and lent her their best water pistols and baseball cards. God, what teeth that miserable Melanie had. Chiclets. Pearls of the South Seas. Her breath, when she whined, was like warm, sweet balm while yours was beginning to show the dragon-mouth tendencies which would fully surface later. When she giggled, all you saw was shining white, while your

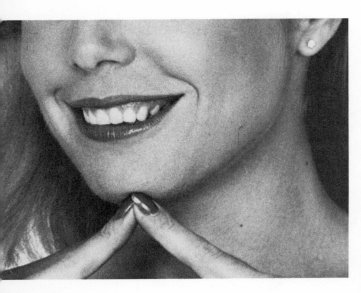

giggle revealed the little dental telltale spots of silver and gold. How come? Someone in Melanie's house knew about oral hygiene. All they knew about in your house was chocolate pudding, mashed potatoes and a quick sweep of a toothbrush.

Today, the art of gum and tooth care is so beautifully researched that, theoretically, no one should have too much trouble. Theoretically, you should be able to keep your teeth, or surely most of them, until your dying mouthful of chocolate pudding. Theoretically. In fact, though, no one pays too much attention. The relatively new science of periodontics and the relatively old science of dentistry have many answers. Really. But few women ask the questions until it's too late.

If you read this chapter thoroughly, and follow the advice herein, you really should go through life like Sparkle Plenty. I promise.

Here is a documented truth: the big woman is *particularly* susceptible to tooth and gum disease. Generally, big women eat big. And often, they eat badly.

It stands to reason that if you eat a lot you will collect more food particles in and around your teeth and gums. These bits of food furnish mouth bacteria with nutrients. Bacteria are particularly pleased when you feed them Lucullan diets of starches, fats or highly refined carbohydrates. And, let's face it, we often tend to be sneaky eaters. We don't want everybody to know that we're chomping away on a Baby Ruth so we tend to suck it or even gum it to death, instead of chewing it. Not only does this do bad things to the soul, but we're not even getting the good gum exercises of the chewing. When we suck candy, all that sugar gets drawn straight into the teeth. Chew forthrightly then, sisters, and brush afterward, if possible.

Foolishly, even tragically, the big woman who is so careful with her grooming, her fashion, her development of creative ability, neglects her teeth and gums, which logically get more wear and tear than a size 10's teeth and gums. And her smile is so important when she's trying to attract attention to her marvelous face. Try having a dazzling smile with puffy, reddened gums. Try eating with loose teeth. People who *really* enjoy eating enjoy it a lot more with their own teeth than with dentures. Studies have shown that dentures are only, at best, 25 percent as effective as natural teeth, which means that if you wear dentures you may not be chewing as well as you think: obviously, this can lead to digestive problems also.

The old adage "You are what you eat" is true. What you eat and how much you eat has a profound effect on mouth health. Primitive man did not have anything in his blood that was resistant to tooth decay even though the teeth in most fossil men have been found to be flawless. What fossil man did have were vegetables, whole grains, fish, fruit and very few Good 'n Plentys. He also had a stick, frayed at the end, as an antecedent to the toothbrush. Take a fossilized gentleman, feed him some French toast, Hershey Bars, orange soda and Danish and watch his teeth go, right before your eyes. A contemporary comparison of the teeth of civilized and uncivilized man by the anthropologist V. Suk showed that at the age of eighteen, only 10 to 15 percent of the whites living in metropolitan areas had perfect teeth, while among Zulus, it was 85 to 94 percent.

But here's the good news: most dental authorities maintain *positively* that even if you eat like a pachyderm and are a *very large person*, you can still have perfectly healthy gums and teeth. Keep in mind, though, that your body chemistry *may* be harmed by eating large amounts of carbohydrates and sugars and thus you may stifle the body's natural reparative qualities. And many nutritionists, like the famed Dr. E. Cheraskin, feel that proper foods and proper nutrients are even the key to *emotional* health. Still, when it comes to teeth and gums, you can almost always counterattack the terrible foods you eat by immediate and thorough cleansing. Pounds don't have to do with decay; care does. You'll have to work a lot harder and more meticulously at it than the woman who picks at her carrot soufflé, but you do have control, even if you're a large and indiscriminate eater. You can decide whether you'll have Melanie teeth or dragon breath.

Many very fine dentists and periodontists contributed to the information in this chapter, but we relied most heavily on the information provided by Dr. Leigh Levitt, dentist extraordinaire, and Dr. Burton Langer, associate clinical professor at Columbia University School of Dental and Oral Surgery. Both doctors have extensive and respected private practices and both have many women patients who are size 18 and over.

Okay. First bit of advice. Don't suffer because the dentist's chair is built for Twiggy. Almost every professional chair has an arm that goes down. Ask your dentist to put it down and leave it down. You won't fall out. You're not condemned to hugging your body with your arms as if you were in a theater seat. And if the dentist has a good bit of trouble reaching around your Rubens form, ask him to try working from behind. Believe it or not, he may not have thought of it. With dentistry, the view is as good from that angle as from the side. Your regular dentist will deal with problems of toothache, dental cosmetics, tooth decay and dental hygiene. If you have serious gum problems, you will need to see a specialist.

Who is the real villain in the tooth and gum decay drama? Why, as the dentist who came to talk with our local kindergarten put it, he's none other than Mister Plaque.

Mr. P. wasn't even identified as the bad guy until 1972. Before that, we thought sweets themselves somehow went directly into the tooth to cause "cavities," as we liked to say. Now we know that plaque is a colorless film that forms on teeth and gums. Bacteria love to adhere to plaque colonies on the teeth. And bacteria just eat up carbohydrates and sugar as they create tissue imbalances. So Mr. Plaque is bad news, but he's been around a long time. Shakespeare had plaque. So did that nice kid Joan of Arc. Warren Beatty has plaque. Jane Fonda can't do much about it either. Frank Sinatra, with all his money, has plaque colonies in his mouth. Even the Pope has plaque. Also Manachem Begin. Also Amy Carter. And her father. Everyone.

Some don't have much because, luckily, their parents didn't have much.

Some have a lot because of a propensity for Mars Bars and Fig Newtons. But listen: no one is telling you to stop eating. Just clean up your act a little. Like a smoker who puts sticky tar on her teeth, the eater with the lusty appetite has to brush more carefully than the eater with the stilted appetite. There is no way around the rule:

Big and/or sweets and carbohydrate eaters must be impeccable in their brushing and flossing routine because they are subject to greater plaque.

When plaque is ignored it turns into tartar, which is hard and very difficult to remove. But plaque itself is mashed potatoes to remove. It's soft and can be dislodged by brushing and flossing. It's *insane* not to learn, once and for all, the simple techniques required, and you'll find them near the end of this chapter. They take no longer than a sloppy and ineffectual toothbrushing. Don't, by the way, rely on a Water Pik to remove plaque. It won't. Water Piks are nice for removing chunks of food and for making your mouth feel refreshed, but they do nothing at all for Mr. Plaque.

Okay, how do you know when you are in trouble with your mouth?

1. Your gums may bleed. Bleeding is not normal. Bleeding gums are as pathological a symptom as a bleeding colon or a bleeding nose. Something is probably wrong. Do not accept the pink spittle in the morning as normal: someone should look at your gums to advise you. Sometimes, if bleeding goes unchecked for a long while, the body's healing or scarring capacity will remove the overt sign of blood and you think the problem's gone—*but the trouble remains.* The gum problem can then progress to a chronic state and you will have missed your chance to heal yourself without surgery. As the disease moves up the root of the tooth, it's very difficult to determine that a problem exists—and then you've lost precious time.

2. You may have bad breath. Ask your mother or your best friend to be honest and patient while you blow in their faces and ask them to *tell you the truth.* If you suspect that they're being "kind," check yourself. Did you wake up this morning with a bad taste in your mouth? The likelihood is that your breath is not terrific. Can you still taste the liverwurst from last night? Did you have a fifteen-minute catnap, shaking yourself awake with *another* dry and crummy taste? Gum problem warning. Fill a balloon with your breath and slowly let the air out under your nostrils. You're smelling a *better version* of what the world smells, so if the balloon breath is fetid—you've really got a problem.

3. Are your teeth or even one tooth slightly loose? Mobility of teeth is a sure sign that the gum problem which may have been marginal to begin with has become more advanced.

4. Do you have spaces between your teeth that you never noticed before?

5. Is there pus or any exudation coming from the gums or around the teeth?

6. Is there a swelling in any area of the gum?

7. Is there what looks like an abscess on the gums?

Remember that your gums may be reacting to normal or extenuating circumstances and, if so, they are not diseased in themselves. Sometimes, for instance, when women are menstruating, their gums become more sensitive and bleed more easily. Gums can react temporarily to drugs by becoming spongy and irritated. Dilantin, for example, taken by epileptics and people with head injuries, definitely affects the gums. Imbalancing hormones do the same. Birth control pills may create a gum reaction. Pregnancy may create sensitive gums and pregnant women must be especially careful about cutting down plaque.

However, if you have suspicious symptoms and you cannot attribute them to normal body conditions or necessary drug intakes, what should you do?

See Your Dentist!

He acts as quarterback of the dental system and will diagnose your condition. It is he who will decide whether or not he can treat the problem or whether it is more advanced and should be treated by a specialist, a periodontist. Clearly, the dentist will deal with any actual tooth decay. But a periodontist is someone who has been trained specifically in the diagnosis and treatment of gum disorders. If your dentist treats you for gum or loose tooth problems and they don't seem to be getting better, insist upon being seen by a periodontist.

How to Find a Specialist: Any large university or hospital can give you the names of qualified specialists. Your dentist will be able to do the same for you.

What Will the Periodontist Do?

If you've caught your problem early, you're in luck. Most gum disease consists of inflammation or chronic infection. Suppose you had a splinter in your finger. You'd have to get it out before an infection grew up around it. Well, gum infection is primarily a result of tartar (hardened plaque) on the teeth and in the gums, which has a terribly poisoning effect. Just as you'd remove the splinter, you have to get rid of the tartar and let the gum heal. The periodontist and his hygienists are meticulously trained to handle this difficult, time-consuming and precise procedure. You can't do it yourself. You need the skilled hands of the technician and her instrument. Consider the dirt under short fingernails. A normal nail-brushing will get it out. When your fingernails grow longer, you need an instrument to get out the dirt. Same with scaling and cleaning tartar from infected gums. The tartar is hiding under the gum, which is analagous to the dirt hiding under the fingernail. You need a tool to scrape it out. Does it hurt? Well, I don't love it, but then again, it isn't the worst thing in the world. The technicians and the periodontists are maniacally conscientious people who *love their work* and won't let you escape with a smidgen of tartar hiding on that tooth. Which is all to the good—I suppose.

Sometimes, this wonderful cleaning and a warning to return regularly for follow-up cleanings will be all you need. But if the problem has been allowed to fester, damage will have set in. Like what? Like plenty. The bones in your mouth may have become diseased. Almost surely you will have developed little pockets of skin, extra gum tissue at the juncture of the tooth and the gum. These little pockets trap plaque and food particles and normal brushing and flossing can't release them. What's next?

Surgery!

You've got to get rid of the pockets or spaces between the teeth and gums before bone damage occurs. You may already even need some bone surgery. All of this sounds worse than it really is. Don't be nervous. It probably won't hurt at all except for the uncomfortable period of a couple of days after surgery when the gums are healing. You can go about your daily chores during this time if you remember not to chomp down on steak bones for a while. And a bonus: most gum surgeons are so magically adept at giving anesthesia, you won't even feel the injection.

If you have already suffered bone damage, all is not lost. A gum bone transplant is a common practice. And a hopeful and little-known fact is this: modern periodontists now know that they often have the ability to stimulate the regeneration of bone. Only in the last ten years have such modern advances occurred in the field. If the gum bones in the mouth have decayed, sometimes clinicians can almost reverse the process of bone loss back to an earlier year. Unbelievably, the patient can often end up with more bone at the completion of treatment than she had when she first started.

There are almost no health or beauty books written today which stress the importance of periodontics. It is a relatively new and brilliant science. I tell you to get thyself to a specialist if you have gum disease!

If you are a very big woman, you must be particularly careful to see someone highly recommended by your dentist or a well regarded institution. No letting your fingers walk through the Yellow Pages for this job. If even minor surgery is required, you will need anesthesia and other drugs and your doctor must be thoroughly familiar with any possible side effects of those drugs, in your particular case. The big woman might need a larger amount of narcotics or barbiturates than her skinny sister. Systemic drugs, like painkillers, are regulated in terms of body weight. Certain large patients require more local anesthesia. Because many heavy women have breathing problems and a greater tax on their hearts, the wrong amount of narcotics, for instance, could depress the central nervous system and create ancillary problems. If very big women are to be sedated, *they must be sedated by clinicians who have the ability to monitor their cardiovascular systems.* Machines and trained anesthetists should be available to monitor heart rates and blood pressures. If such systems are not available, hospitalization for mouth surgery is certainly an option.

Many big women are plagued with diabetes. Diabetes has a clear effect on the breakdown of gum tissues. Diabetics have a reduced capacity to heal gum tissues and to regenerate bone. Heavy diabetic women, more than any other group, must be meticulous about oral hygiene.

The single most important thing you will learn at the periodontist's is how to care for your teeth and gums at home. Once you learn that, you are home free. It is different from the usual brushing instructions you've been getting all these years. It is simple and it is fast! Perhaps you're young and lucky and have not yet had to see a periodontist, because your gums and teeth are in pretty good shape. *Now, right now,* change your oral hygiene routine to the one which you will read below. It may save you thousands of dollars in mouth care.

Brushing

The most important part of brushing is getting into and sometimes under the gum collar that circles the tooth. The areas on the flat side of the tooth are generally cleaned by the actions of chewing and also rubbing the lips and tongue against the teeth. If you use a disclosing color tablet that your dentist will provide upon request, you will see that most of the plaque revealed by the darker color of the tablet will be up at the gum line and between the teeth. The last place you see serious plaque is on the tooth surface.

1. Use a soft (never hard) multitufted nylon brush. The individual bristles should be rounded and shaped in a straight-across fashion. Never fall for the propaganda that says "This toothbrush is round to fit your mouth." You will miss large areas if you use a rounded-surface brush.

2. Angle the toothbrush at a 45-degree angle into the gum crevice (the junction between the tooth and the gum). The bristles should be pointing at your nostrils.

3. Vibrate the brush (don't scrub because that will injure sensitive gum tissues) for about five seconds.

4. Pull brush down over tooth surface, sweeping away the plaque. First do the outside of every tooth in your mouth, paying strict attention to the back teeth. When you do the outside of the bottom teeth, the bristles should be pointing at your chin, and then you sweep the brush *up* the tooth.

5. Do the inside of your gums and teeth. (I have a friend who once unbelievably said to me, "You brush the inside? You're a fanatic!") Now, hold the brush *perpendicular* to your teeth, fitting the top tip of the bristles in the juncture between the gum and the

tooth. You really need use only the top half of the toothbrush for this. Vibrate and sweep down (or up on the bottom teeth).

Flossing

1. The rationale for flossing is that the brush cannot get between the teeth. Take a piece of unwaxed floss about twenty-four inches long.

2. Wrap it around the index fingers or thumbs, depending on what is most comfortable for you. Most people don't hold it short enough between the two fingers: the shorter the floss, the more control you have.

3. Put floss in space between teeth. The floss should touch the gum and not be jammed up enough to cut it. If it passively disappears under the gum, that's fine.

4. Pull it along one inside of the tooth, scraping the tooth, and then along the other inside, forming a C shape. The inside of the tooth should be shined by the floss almost as you would shine a shoe. If you get the area really clean, you should hear a squeaky sound—as when your hair is clean. Include the last tooth in the mouth, and behind the last tooth. Keep wrapping a clean area of floss around your finger so you don't use the same piece for the whole mouth.

If you have some fixed dentures you can ask your dentist for a nylon threader which looks like a large nylon needle. Thread it with floss, insert it between the teeth at the gum line and floss. Remove by drawing the floss through.

Disgusting tip: Think you don't need to do this? *Smell* the floss after it comes out of your mouth. Convincing? It should be! That's rotted material you're taking out.

Don't be concerned if you see some bleeding or if the gums are tender when you first start. Continue the routine. If your gums are healthy, the bleeding and soreness should disappear in about a week.

And how long should this all take? Would you believe five to ten minutes, once you've got the routine down pat. How often? Theoretically, if you brush and floss absolutely thoroughly, you only have to do it once a day. But who is so thorough? Therefore, to get the spots you missed the first time, two times a day is even better than one.

The Bad News: What should periodontics cost?

A marginal gum problem just affecting the soft tissue, with some bleeding as symptom, should run between $100 and $400 for prophylaxis and cleaning. A moderate gum problem involving cleaning and a few localized areas of surgery might run between $600 to $1,000.

Serious treatment with extensive surgery might range anywhere from $1,500 to $3,000, depending upon severity and involvement.

The "recall" which is the key to follow-up, consisting of an evaluation and cleaning, no less than two, and often four times a year, may run from $25 to $40 a treatment.

A Series of Theories, Orthodox and Un, About Toothpastes, Tooth Colors, Sweetness of Breath and Cankers.

CANKER SORES

The big woman's bane of existence. Some say they come from stress, some say they come from bacteria, some say they come from too many sweets. *They hurt.* Topical anesthetics like oragel, benzocaine, orabase and camophenique are good. Some people swear by a fixative agent like methyline blue, painted on by a dentist; it's as old as the hills, but it works.

Chloroseptic, currently popular, has anesthetic effects but tends to irritate canker sores with its astringent characteristics.

Tried and true kitchen techniques are milk of magnesia, which has a bland buffering effect, and plain old Karo syrup, which puts on a coating and takes away the sting.

CHEWING EXERCISE

Like everything else, teeth and gums need exercise to increase the blood circulation. So just don't eat. *Chew.* Stuff like carrots, celery, nuts and sunflower seeds. Some women even chew on Korean ginseng root which, they say, doubles as an aphrodisiac. Can it hurt?

BRUSH YOUR TONGUE!

Think about it. It's an important finishing touch!

OXYGEN ODDITIES

Bacteria that live without oxygen are called aerobic bacteria. They're the worst kind. Although there is no real medical evidence, many doctors secretly believe in the theory that stimulating the formation of oxygen in the gums discourages these bacteria. They advise the use of such substances as baking soda, salt, peroxide and glyoxide between the teeth to stimulate oxygen growth. Ask your own doctor before trying it.

TOOTHPASTE MEDIA HYPE?

No. Fluoride toothpastes really work to reduce decay by about 15 percent. Not a huge amount, but who's sneezing at it?

GRAY TEETH

It is normal for teeth to get darker with age. The color of your teeth is genetically created—like the size. If you smoke your teeth will get even darker; precancerous conditions in the gums may even develop from the heat and chemicals. Certain medications discolor teeth.

BAD BREATH, HALITOSIS OR THE CONDITION EVEN YOUR BEST FRIEND WON'T TELL YOU ABOUT!

Sherry once asked some 100 high school students, "If the guy next to you had bad breath, would you: (a) Tell him? (b) Write him an anonymous note? (c) Do nothing?" Ninety-seven students chose "Do nothing!" Here's this nice guy sitting next to them, terrific in every way except for the fact that his breath is fetid, and hardly anyone would help him out with the information! Why? Don't know.

Bad breath seems more embarrassing than gonorrhea. Last year, Americans spent about a quarter of a billion dollars on mouthwashes, flavored toothpastes and candy breath disguises. What is this condition that so many people hesitate to mention?

Halitosis comes from the Latin word *halitus*, meaning breath, and the Greek *osis*, meaning condition. It is nothing more than the normal mouth air that has been tainted by certain chemical compounds within the system. Halitosis, according to one study, often contains the same chemicals that give a skunk its smell—sulfur-containing substances. Think of it—skunk breath. Ugh! Several sources can be culprits.

- Something is decomposing in the mouth. (Have you brushed your teeth today?)
- A strain of bacteria called *strep* can feed on leftover mouth food and produce plaque.
- Decayed teeth can give out a miserable odor.
- Periodontal or gum disease will do it every time.
- Diseases of the respiratory tract like sinus problems, tonsils and infected adenoids can be at the heart of unpleasant breath.
- Dried out mucous membranes may leave areas infection prone and minus protective moisture.
- Bad breath can even come from the intestines. When garlic and onions are eaten, the oil from such foods gets into the bloodstream and comes back to the mouth through the lungs.
- Many other diseases can cause bad breath. Noted among them are gallbladder disease, ulcers, cirrhosis of the liver and kidney disease.
- Improper diet and certain blood conditions may do the trick also.

Had enough? There are more causes, but suffice it to say that bad breath is not a simple thing. Even nerves and anxiety can do it. How to cure it? Brush regularly, floss religiously and rinse faithfully. Brush everything (even your tongue). Watch your diet. Stop smoking; the smoke you're exhaling may seem delightful to you but smells foul to others. See your doctor if you suspect that your bad breath is caused by illness. If an infection is present, antibiotics eliminate odor. If the bad breath is caused by dryness in the air —very common!—provide water for the air to absorb. Put pans of water on radiators and other heat sources. If it disappears quickly, you just *know* that air is desert dry. Do mouthwashes and candy mints help? They don't cure but they camouflage. They can mask the problem for a while. Use fluoride toothpaste.

Mouth Sweeteners and Brighteners

Plain old table salt makes teeth gleaming white. Great for nicotine and berry stains. Great for breath. Salt rinses help sore or inflamed gums. (Half a teaspoon in a glass of warm water will do it.)

Baking soda and anything. Mix a quarter of a cup of baking soda with half a teaspoon oil of wintergreen, or oil of peppermint, or oil of cloves, or oil of cinnamon, for terrific tasting toothpastes. Marcia Donnan gives this in her book *Cosmetics from the Kitchen.*

Vodka mouthwash. It's great! Dissolve a pinch of thymol (a germicide you can buy at the drugstore) in one teaspoon of vodka. Dissolve a quarter-teaspoon borax, a quarter-teaspoon sodium bicarbonate and two and a half teaspoons of glycerin in water. (Warm over low flame if necessary, to blend thoroughly.) Add a teaspoon of oil of wintergreen or peppermint or a half a cup of spearmint tea for taste.

Peroxide mouthwash. Use 3 percent hydrogen peroxide and mix with an equal amount of warm water. Oxygen, in its bubbling liquid form, manages to get into hidden crevices and bringing oxygen to the gums kills off bacteria. Don't use more than a couple of times a day and don't swallow. It won't kill you, but then again you won't feel terrific drinking the stuff. Be careful with this one. Don't overuse! A condition known as black hairy tongue (sound like fun?) may come from overuse. Then again, if you want to discourage your boyfriend from coming around, black hairy tongue might be just the ticket.

Chlorophyll naturals. Fresh parsley and watercress, when

chewed, taste lovely and freshen the breath from their natural chlorophyll. They work better than almost any commercial breath freshener.

Preventive dentistry is the best word. Try to avoid foods that are rich in carbohydrates and particularly sticky stuff like peanut butter, caramels, etc., which stick to your teeth through thick and thin. Fluoridated water and toothpastes are great. Calcium foods are helpful.

A last word: If you have a particular problem like teeth grinding or true fear of dentists, any number of palliatives are available. Look into hypnosis and tranquilizers and, for the former, night guard appliances.

VII Big, Beautiful and Fit!

It's a lie: "Exercise will melt off pounds, honey. Join our group."

It's a lie: "You're too, um, uh, fat for an exercise program. Bad for the heart, you know."

It's a lie: "Lose weight—then talk about physical fitness."

It's a lie: "Come leap and bound and twist with Suzie Gymnastics. Acrobatics works for everybody!"

It's the biggest lie of all: "Fat women *can't* be fit. Fat women *can't* look good."

It's the truth: "Firmness and good body looks are *absolutely possible*, through exercise, no matter what you weigh. *Proper* exercise, that is."

First you have to cut through the muck. And is there ever muck. Almost every health faddist, club and book will try to sell you *thin*. There is no other way but their way. All I wanted was to find a plan that would allow me to be me and still provide for physical fitness. I'd renounced the yo-yo diets and the unrealistic aims of everybody who thought they knew what was best for me. I'd determined to maintain the weight that seemed natural to me, but the world was still trying to sell me machines, panaceas and thirty-day miracle weight-loss plans. It was looking pretty grim. Every exercise expert I met seemed to be operating under the "sell them anything if you can make a buck" theory. The consensus of opinion seemed to be that a fit and supple and strong body was not in the cards for me—*unless I lost weight*. The trouble was, I knew realistically speaking that losing weight was not in the cards for me. I wanted to make myself firm *now*. My size did not inhibit me

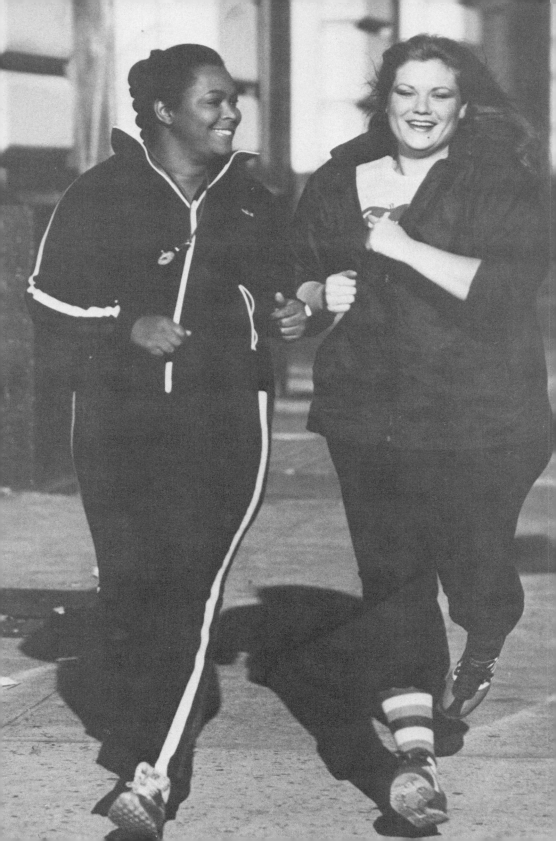

from doing anything else: why then was the world of physical fitness closed to me?

I knew I needed help. Honest help. Professional help. Intelligent help. I found him. He was a blond and beautifully soft-spoken young man who radiated honesty and intelligence from every muscular pore. Health, common sense and compassion flowed from him. Insistence upon integrity and tried and true and workable methods were ingrained into his philosophy.

Jamie Bourne used to be a professional dancer abroad and in this country. He began his commitment to teaching physical fitness to everyone, no matter what her weight, in the three world-famed Nicklaus studios he owned for many years. Now, with his own imprint upon the Bourne Exercise Studio in New York, he is fast becoming one of those cult figures whom everybody thinks she has discovered singlehandedly. People come from great distances to exercise with him. What he teaches makes good sense. His ultimate aim, moreover, is not to come up with the media gimmick that will make him a cool fortune, but to spread the word that fitness and litheness belong to everybody, regardless of size. Here is his philosophy on exercise and a program of exercises especially created for the heavy woman, as told in James Bourne's own words.

Fitness Is for Everyone

No matter how much fat covering you have, there is muscle underneath, and that muscle can be toned and conditioned. It makes absolutely no difference if you weigh 100 or 300 pounds: you can develop a firm, healthy and sound body. I swear it. I give you my oath. The exercises you will find in this chapter are not designed to make you lose weight. No exercise, without stringent diet, can do that. They are designed, rather, to change a loose, sedentary, clumsy body into a flexible, tight and proud one. If you lose some weight along the way, which is very possible, it is an ancillary benefit. The true direction is fitness, not thinness.

There are no gimmicks involved. No music, no shining silver machines. Just you and the floor—carpeted, preferably. If not, you can improvise a mat.

Everybody is beautiful. Every *body* is beautiful. Just the weight you are. We have been stereotyped into thinking that the television skin-and-bones image is the only correct one, but you can be vital, healthy and look marvelous no matter how much you weigh. You can learn, and you *should* learn, to cherish your own body as it is, this very moment, and for what it can be, all firmed and toned up. Developing muscle tone does not mean increasing muscle size. It means flexibility. Although there is no medical evidence that I have seen to back me up, I have observed through years of teaching that fat women are actually more naturally flexible than thin women. I don't know why—it's just there. An exercise program will firm and tone you. It will give you a greater sense of relaxation. It will increase your energy level amazingly. It will, by stimulating blood flow, change the condition of your complexion from doubtful to glowing. And it will, almost above all other things, release the constricting tensions that control your day.

Can exercise hurt you? No way. Not mine. Naturally, you should check with your doctor before you start any exercise regimen, but this plan that I propose for the heavy woman is just about danger proof—even if you have a tricky back. Most of the exercises are done on the floor purposely to protect weak back muscles. They are all also done in perfect spinal alignment, so there's no chance of twisting a muscle or part of the skeleton out of alignment. Heavy, fat, round, amply endowed women—whatever you wish to call yourselves—cannot do a lot of leaping and jumping around. It's dangerous for anyone but especially for one with a lot of weight to have that weight land forcefully on ankles, knees or feet. Exercises for heavy women must be designed especially for them because it may be dangerous for them to attempt to do what the uncaring, unthinking TV huckster is pushing. The extra mass of your body will inhibit certain movements and the size of your abdomen and thighs may not allow you to bend the way a size 12 bends. If you move quickly, your weight will cause you to develop a momentum of force which may cause injury.

With my plan, there will be no force momentum. Everything is done very slowly so you're only able to move as much as your muscles will carry. In fact, many of the exercises I teach are used in major hospitals for back therapy—they're that safe. If you remember to move slowly—to exercise *as if you were moving under water*, fluidly, controlled, smoothly—you cannot be hurt. And you *must inevitably* change in appearance and pride.

Where does pride come into this picture? Women must challenge themselves physically, no matter what they weigh. If you have a good sense about your body, if you like yourself, it shows all over. You're prettier. You're more appealing and more liberated sexually also, because a good feeling about your body comes with practiced movement. You must feel free to stand up and expose your supple self. If you're not afraid of your shoulders, your bosom, your genitals, your abdomen—if you're used to seeing and feeling them move gracefully, purposefully, your psyche and your attitudes are freed along with your physical self. Do you find yourself walking around with rounded shoulders, sunken chest and pelvis as you try to guard yourself from looking ungainly? If you checked in a mirror, you'd see that the opposite happens when you hide. You look more clumsy, ungainly—yes, even fatter. Change your attitude about your body—and you *can*, through exercise—and you see that pride, that inherent beauty, that psyche lift along with that stomach.

Exercise, in short, can pull you together, make you feel tight, healthy and mobile. Also noble. Use your body to express yourself. It speaks volumes. It is inseparable from your soul. It is the instrument of tasting, smelling, feeling, seeing better. A fit body is the height of sensuality.

It's a question of feeling alive—that's all.

It's a question of looking terrific—that's all.

Do you want to try? Stick with me.

Before You Begin

STICK WITH IT

There are several aspects of this program which you may find confusing at first. Do not despair if you are not able to coordinate all the movements and breathing patterns from the start. This will come with more practice and effort.

WHAT ARE YOU AFTER?

If it's to lose weight by exercise, don't waste your time. Only eating less makes you lose weight. If it's to look and feel better even if you never lose another pound, keep reading. These exercises are not in any way presented to induce you to diet. It may happen that you lose weight also, but the simple objective is looking good and feeling good—at your present weight.

THE BREATH OF LIFE

Practice it before you start doing the rest of the exercises. Oxygen is a necessary fuel for the body. The muscles need it. The brain needs it. With the prolonged, steady breathing pattern I will give you, tension seems to evaporate and your mind and body become prepared for your routine to come. As you breathe, try to relax and free your mind from distracting thoughts. This is your half-hour. Pamper yourself with total attention. Enjoy it. Love it. You might find the breathing difficult at first. You will probably exhale when the direction says inhale and vice versa. It will help you to remember that the exhalation is on the *exerting* movement and the inhalation is on the *relaxing* movement. The exhalation is always accompanied by an abdominal contraction, which pulls the abdominal muscle up and offers support to the lower back, preventing injury to that area. As you rhythmically expand and contract the abdominal muscle through breathing, the entire abdominal area is becoming flattened and strengthened. Sound complicated? Soon it will become as easy as breathing.

FLEXED FEET, MADAM!

Many exercise programs designed for women use a pointed foot: this is basically a carryover from dance classes. Although the point may be more pleasing esthetically, anatomically a flexed foot is more suitable and natural. Most of these exercises will call for

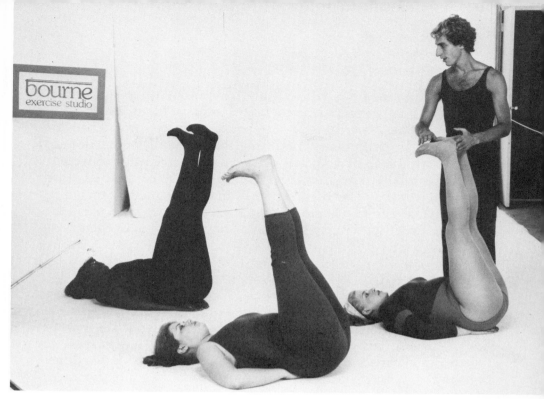

Flexed feet increase stretch in the back of the leg and help strengthen musculature of the feet.

flexed feet. Flexing your foot is accomplished by pulling the toe and the ball of the foot up and toward the knee. When you are standing, the foot is in this flexed position naturally. Most of the exercises are taught with a flexed foot because flexing increases the stretch in the back of the leg and enables you to create more tension. Heavy people carry more weight on their feet. Flexed feet also strengthen the musculature of the feet so that the familiar "aching feet" complaint of the big woman is banished.

BOUNCING, YANKING, JERKING, LEAPING

Very simply put, don't do it. The only thing accomplished by fast, jerky movements is possible injury. Move slowly and rhythmically. You will develop more strength, flexibility and control. Fitness cannot be forced or rushed. Tearing a muscle tendon or ligament is painful and very slow in healing. Even when healed, it will be quite stiff for a while. Another consideration is the fact that in the healing process, scar tissue forms. This is a hard, rubberlike substance with hardly any elasticity. Not wonderful for muscles. It is particularly essential that heavy women do not bounce, yank, leap or jerk. It's dangerous to have a lot of weight landing on ankles, knees and feet. And if it happens, as it so often does, that you have been particularly inactive or sedentary up to now, suicidal acrobatics are not your ticket. Floor exercises that are basically antigravity and resistive programs are your ticket.

CUSTOM DESIGN

These exercises are designed to give you more room to move, so that the extra weight of abdomen and thighs does not get in your way. You will find that putting your legs straight out in front of the abdomen causes the thighs to rub and impede action: so directions will call for making V's with your legs, or bending the knees slightly so the abdomen has a place to go. Don't worry. You are still giving plenty of stretch to the hamstrings and the lower back.

NO FLOUNCED SKIRTS

Don't cover yourself up. Get a good look at yourself and see exactly what kind of muscle tone you have and what you would like to have. If your flesh jiggles, so what? It won't jiggle for long after you practice this routine because it is *inevitable* that these exercises will work. So wear leotards and tights. In fact, you can even leave off the tights for better reality. If you do the routine daily or even three times weekly, *you will see a difference.*

I VANT TO BE ALONE

Don't be a groupie with your exercises. You will develop a better relationship with your body and be less likely to kibitz in your own room. It's a time for *you* to examine *you.* Remember: no matter what your weight, fatness can be fit.

USE YOUR JUDGMENT

Naturally, you should check with a knowledgeable physician before starting any new exercise program. But hear this: even if the doctor says a program sounds just great, you may find one or two of the exercises intolerable for your own particular regime. I doubt that this will happen with the exercises presented here. But if it should, *you* are the best judge and should scrap whatever doesn't work. Don't torture yourself—ever. One suggestion: if you are confused at any point about whether you are doing the right thing, write to me, personally, at the studio and I shall make sure you get straightened out. If you call, I will speak with you to clear up your questions. The studio telephone number and address can be found at the end of this chapter.

THE SEQUENCE IS THE ESSENCE

Do the exercises in the order given. They are purposely prepared to warm you up slowly, develop your maximum muscle and toning control, and gently bring you down to a sense of relaxation and a feeling of true exhilaration. If you were to graph the action, it would form a bell curve.

warmup   work   relax

When you've finished the routine, you've really worked the body *but you should not feel exhausted.* If you do, you're doing something wrong in your timing or performance.

MUSCLE TONING DOESN'T MEAN GETTING THE BIGGEST MUSCLES ON THE BEACH

Muscles are formed according to the tasks they're asked to perform. It is true that some exercises will develop muscle bulk, but they are not among the ones I suggest in this book. My exercises will strengthen, elongate, condition the muscles—period. Most women will not develop large muscle bulk anyway because the hormone that contributes to muscle building is present only in a very low level in the female metabolism.

JUNK THE JUNK

You don't need bicycles, jogging machines, belts or any shiny silver stuff. It breaks, anyway. All you need is *you*, which is always ready and which will have a greatly reduced chance of breaking if you exercise regularly. Junk is a media hype. It doesn't work. It's not possible that belts pounding at you can improve muscle tone. It's not possible that rollers rolling on you will roll off fat. The mentality that says the machine can do the work is a deluded mentality. Only you can do the work. Believe me. Everything else is salesmanship. Nothing less. Another thing: with just you to worry about, you don't have to be enslaved to certain hours, places, people, *things.* A floor is always available. You don't even have to exercise at the same time every day. Or even every day at all, for that matter. Be human. If you miss a day, the program isn't shot to hell. Honest.

WHOEVER SAID "CONSISTENCY IS THE HOBGOBLIN OF LITTLE MINDS" DIDN'T DO EXERCISES

The most important aspect of exercise *is* consistency. Which doesn't mean you can't miss a day or so. What it does mean is you must work slowly, over a long period of time, rather than fast or furiously for a moment. If this is your first attempt with an exercise program, don't even try to do it every day. You'll get bored and frustrated. Start with twice a week for a month, then increase to three times: by then you'll be devoted to your body and fitness and you'll probably never stop. Instant results are silly to expect. Your body is a living organism and responds naturally, not as a result of force or speed. Don't be fooled by advertising that promises immediate beauty, health and vigor. As long as you make the effort and are patient, you cannot miss dramatic results.

If you think you're unattractive because you are fat, reach for your toes! Stretch your frame! Stand up tall! Roll up—roll down —fairly shout—*I can do that!* My body is *ALIVE!*

A Fourteen-Point Exercise Program for the Large Woman

Here's my exercise program, especially developed for you. It takes *twenty-two minutes* to do.

1. BREATHING

Supplies necessary oxygen to the muscles, releases tension.
Lie on your back, knees bent and separated about eight inches apart, toes slightly turned in. Back of neck is resting on the mat, hands are resting on your lower abdomen. Inhale through your mouth for two slow counts: your abdomen rises as you inhale. Then exhale slowly, contracting the abdomen into the back. This bellowing action of the abdomen strengthens and firms the abdominal muscles. It also flattens the stomach. Repeat five times.

2. SINGLE HAMSTRING STRETCH

Stretches backs of legs, lower back muscles, inner thighs. Strengthens abdomen.
Sit up and separate legs about two feet apart. If you have a large abdomen, this will give you a greater forward-bending reach. Keep left knee bent and place sole of foot on right inner thigh. Right leg is straight with foot flexed, hips aligned. Inhale, reach up to the ceiling with both arms, chest lifted, then drop head forward, pressing the chin into the chest. Exhale slowly, reaching forward and out past the flexed foot, keeping arms parallel to ears. Begin to inhale, reaching all the way up again, and repeat five times. Although you are heavier, you are not any less flexible than a thin woman. With practice, this exercise will come naturally.

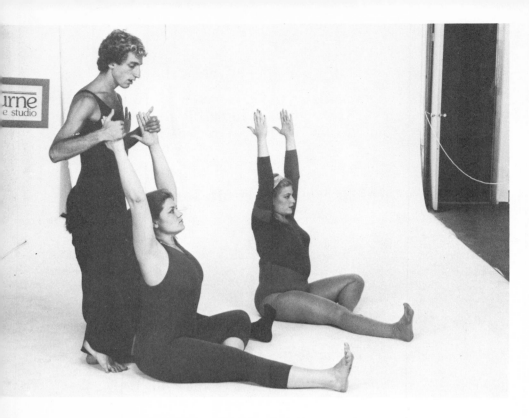

The Single Hamstring Stretch strengthens the abdomen and stretches backs of legs, lower back muscles and inner thighs.

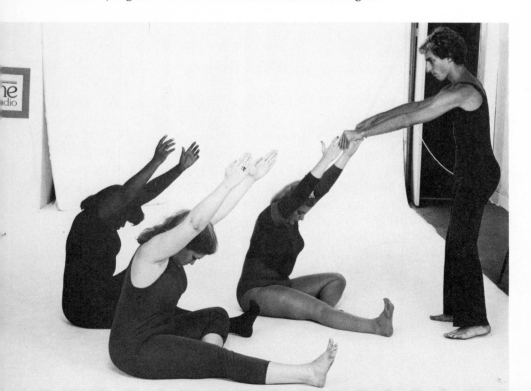

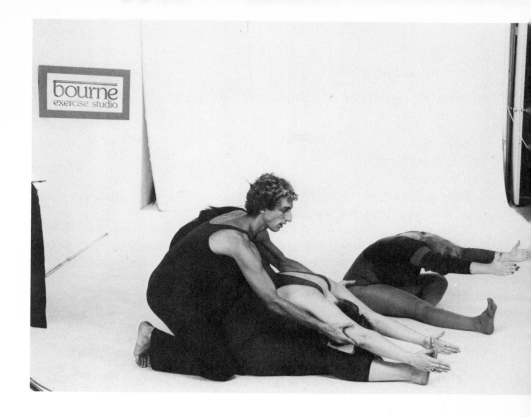

3. PELVIC TILT

Firms buttocks and thighs, tones inner thighs as well. Releases tension from lower back: great for lower back pain. Provides great sexual flexibility.

Lie down in "breathing" position, hands by your side. Slowly inhale two counts, allowing the abdomen to rise, then exhale, contracting the abdomen, and tilt the pelvis forward, buttocks tight. Keep the waist pressed down and the lower back on the mat, inner thighs pulling toward each other (not touching). Feel the stretch in the tops of your thighs. Inhale, roll down through the spine until the pelvis is resting again on the mat. Repeat eight times.

This is definitely a sexual movement whose roots stem from the natural childbirth motions that women have been practicing throughout the ages. The LaMaze method of natural childbirth deliberately teaches it to its women followers. For greater body flexibility, loss of inhibitions and increased sexual satisfaction, the pelvic tilt is terrific. Heavy women are particularly adept at this exercise.

4. V-STRETCH

Tones and firms inner thighs, flattens and strengthens abdomen and develops strength in thighs and buttocks.

Lie on your back, bend both knees up onto the chest, hands resting by your side and chin down. Back of the neck is on the mat. Inhale, straighten the legs, point them up with heels pointing toward ceiling. Slowly exhale, opening the legs apart into a V shape. Inhale, bring the legs back together. Slowly exhale, lift your head, contract your abdomen and lower your legs straight forward to about 45 degrees from the floor. Inhale, lift legs straight up again, lowering head. Exhale, bring the knees to the chest. Repeat four times.

This is one of the most difficult exercises in the group because the amount of muscular support a big woman needs is going to be greater because of the weight she must move. Still, it's an all-around great exercise to strengthen the body and set the stage for good posture. Start off with only one or two repetitions and build up to four gradually.

5. HALF ROLL-UP

Flattens stomach, strengthens upper and middle back. Relieves back and neck tension.

From basic "breathing" position, lace fingers together behind your head. Relax, inhale two counts, let abdomen rise, then exhale, contract abdomen and roll halfway up, pointing elbows toward your knees. Don't let the abdomen "pop out" as you roll up. Stretch the back of the neck slightly, then inhale, roll down to beginning position again. Repeat eight times.

6. HEAD ROLLS

Relieves tension in upper back, neck and shoulders. Firms up neck area to eliminate sag and droop.

Sit up, cross-legged, spine straight, shoulders down, head dropped forward, chin on chest. Inhale, bring right ear over right shoulder, then roll head all the way back, chin up. Exhale, left ear passes over left shoulder then chin, down to chest. Continue three times right, three times left.

There is no reason for heavy women to be loose heavy women, and the chin and neck areas seem to show fat first. That droop can really be firmed.

The Head Roll relieves tension in upper back, neck and shoulders.

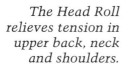

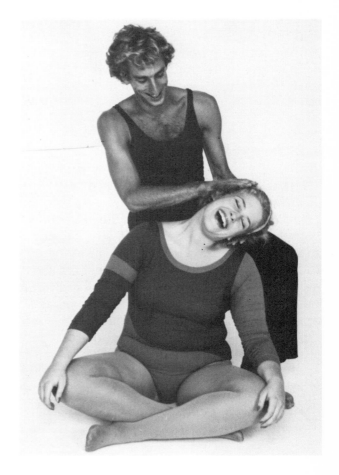

7. ROLL-UP (SLOW SIT-UP)

Strengthens and flattens abdominal muscles. Stretches back muscles.

Sit up, legs straight out in front of you, with slight space in between to eliminate thigh rub. Flex feet and grab under each thigh with hands. Lift chest, inhale, drop the chin to the chest. Exhale, slowly contracting the abdomen, and roll down along the spine to the floor in four slow counts. Don't let abdomen distend as you roll. To repeat, inhale, lift head, keep hands under thighs. Exhale, contract the abdomen as you roll up in the same manner. Do five sets (five roll-ups and five roll-downs).

Holding your thighs helps lift your weight. Eventually you will do this exercise without holding your thighs because the abdominal muscles *should* be able to support whatever weight you are, with practice. When you reach the "no-thigh-hold" stage, instead of grasping your thighs you will instead reach up to the ceiling with both arms, lowering them to your side when you roll down to the floor.

8. SIDE LEG LIFTS

Firms and tones outer thighs and buttocks. Fights against "saddle bags."

Lie on your left side, your head propped up in your left hand, both legs straight in front of you, 90 degrees to your body. Feet flexed, right hand flat on floor six inches from your chest. Inhale, two counts, as the abdomen expands. Exhale, contract the abdomen, lift top leg slightly above hip height. Slowly lower and inhale, relax the abdomen. Exhale, contract the abdomen and lift leg again. Keep knees straight, feet flexed. Don't move upper body or hips. Repeat fifteen times. Roll over to your right side and repeat exercise.

Remember, move very rhythmically, slowly. Control is the key word. Doing the exercises fast to get through them fast utterly defeats the purpose.

9. FRONT LEG LIFTS

Firms and strengthens tops of thighs. Great for runners.

Sit up, straighten the right leg, flex the foot. Bend the left knee, placing the left foot flat on the floor alongside the right knee, hands laced together on the left knee. Keep your back straight, your chest lifted. (As you bend your knee, if the stomach gets in the way, straighten the leg a little bit forward to give yourself room.) Inhale two counts; the abdomen expands. Exhale, slowly stretch and lift the right leg. Keep the back straight and the chest up. Inhale, lower leg. Exhale and repeat fifteen times. Change legs and repeat the exercise. Isolate the lifting of the leg so the upper body does not "rock" back and forth.

Heavy women tend to do more of this "rock and rolling" because in the beginning their weight is difficult to pull up. Remember to sit up tall and lift that chest. You may have to work harder but you can do it! I know, believe me.

10. STANDING KNEE BENDS

Strengthens entire thigh and buttocks area. Tightens looseness in the area, also. (If you have bad knees, just bend slightly while performing the exercise.)

Start with feet separated, about twelve to eighteen inches apart, slightly turned out. Arms up in front of your chest, palms down. Inhale, push the buttocks out and behind you as you bend the knees. Your weight should be on your heels. If your heels lift, then you must stick the buttocks out more and keep the weight on your heels. Go into a sitting position. Your pelvis should be jutting backward as if you were sitting on a chair (minus the chair). Hold, then exhale and straighten the knees, slowly coming up into a standing position, lowering the arms to the sides. Repeat ten times.

This exercise is actually more efficient for a heavier woman than a thin woman because there's more to lift. I can't say it enough: even if it's difficult at first, your musculature should be able to support your own weight, with practice, no matter what it is.

11. OPEN V-STRETCH

Total body stretch. Stretches and tones inner thighs. Increases overall flexibility.

Sit up with the legs open wide apart, knees straight, feet flexed. (If the extra weight in your abdomen and thighs causes you to lose your balance when your legs are opened wide in the V, experiment, and open them as wide as you comfortably can to retain your balance. You will be able to increase the V opening as you practice.) Arms reaching up, palms facing each other, inhale, turn to face the right leg, drop the chin to the chest. Exhale, contract the abdomen, bend forward, reaching past the right foot with both hands. Keep the knees straight and head down as you stretch. Come up, inhaling, turn to face the left leg, bend over the leg. Exhale and contract the abdomen, reaching past the left foot. Repeat three times to each side.

12. OPEN V-LATERAL STRETCH

Stretches and tones outer waist area. Removes lumps and bulges from the waist.

The Open V-Stretch stretches and tones inner thighs and increases overall flexibility.

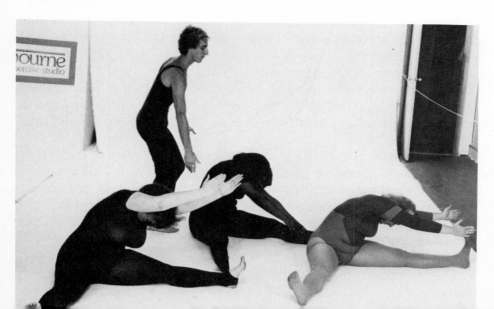

Same beginning position as the Open V-Stretch. Hands back to back, lace fingers together and turn palms to point to ceiling. Inhale, stretch up, pressing the palms up, then face left leg. Exhale, bend over to the right side, right shoulder inside the right knee. Keep the knees straight and feet flexed. Come up slowly, inhaling. Face the right leg and stretch over to the left, exhaling. Repeat two times on each side.

13. ANKLE PULL

Releases tension and stretches lower back and the backs of legs.
Sit up, both legs straight out and spread apart no wider than twenty-four inches. Flex both feet. Reach up with both arms, palms facing each other, lower back lifted. Inhale, reach up to the ceiling, drop the chin to the chest. Exhale, contract the abdomen, reach out forward and over the legs and grab your ankles. Relax, inhale, let the stomach expand. Exhale, contract and bend your elbows, pulling your head closer to your knees. Keep knees straight and feet flexed. Repeat five times.

14. STAND UP STRAIGHT

Improves postural alignment.
Standing up, feet separated twelve inches apart, palms pressed together six inches away from chest. Looking straight ahead, inhale, allow buttocks and abdomen to relax. Exhale, contract abdomen, squeeze the buttocks and bring your weight forward onto the balls of your feet, keeping knees straight. Repeat at least three times more.

Posture is a presentation. If you develop a confident, upright presentation, your body language says "I'm good, I'm pretty, I'm proud." Everyone, especially the big woman, must take special care to present herself in an assertive and poised manner. Slouching to conceal one's body is not only ineffective, it's sloppy. Good posture is more than a military standing at attention; it is looking great, conserving energy as you use your muscles more efficiently, breathing more freely as your lungs have more room to expand, and saying goodbye to miserable backaches! The miracle of the

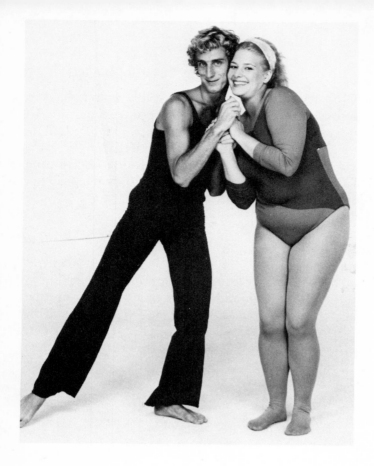

human body is that it's never too late to reshape its presentation —even after you've spent the better part of your life slinking and slouching and lazying around. Good body posture not only makes you prettier, it makes you more alert, intelligent, alive-looking!

If you have difficulty following written directions and would like the added inspiration and guide of a human voice, Bourne Exercise Studio has developed a half-hour tape to guide the big woman through her exercise routine. Listening to verbal directions makes it easier to learn the rhythm and the instructions. Fits any standard cassette recorder. Send a check or money order for $9.95 and request the *Making It Big* exercise tape from

Bourne Exercise Studio
  One Chase Road
  Scarsdale, NY 10583
  (914) 472-4144

VIII Invent Yourself: An Encounter Group

When a woman of high fashion asked Cornelia, the mother of the Gracchi, a Roman family of statesmen, to show her jewels, the worthy Roman matron put her arms around her children and said, "These are my jewels."

Here are mine.

They are six women I met on a winter afternoon and I can't stop thinking about them.

Six beautiful models—the American dream. They are wearing denims and lush wools, gauzy Indian blouses, velvet, wide-ribbed, citron-yellow corduroy. What cheekbones, what curves, what chic. Pretty? Are you kidding? *Gorgeous!* They're models, aren't they? Six stunning women who seem to have made it.

Not one weighs under 175 pounds. The largest weighs over 200 pounds. They range in age from twenty-two to forty-three.

They are clear evidence that there's a whole new world out there, waking up to the existence of the big, beautiful woman. They are big, beautiful women, all right, and they got together one Saturday afternoon to talk about the possibilities and the problems they face. Linda and Barbara and Debbi and Margie and Fiddle met at Marsha's brownstone garden apartment for a talk session. They were honest (painfully, sometimes) about their doubts, poignant about their failures and jubilant—positively exultant—about their possibilities.

Barbara: My mother was beautiful. She looked like Tippi Hedren. I was always this fat, awkward glop with bushy eyebrows and a mustache. My mother yelled at me for being fat. My father, being Italian, fed me more. "Oh, Barbara," the friends, the cousins would say, "you're so lucky. Your mom's so beautiful. Aren't you proud of her?"

Proud of her? I had double chins and tripped over everything. Also I was beginning to be suicidal. So I decided to invent myself. I decided to make myself beautiful. And I swear to you, girls, I completely transformed my face into what I wanted it to look like. I read *Vogue* and *Harper's Bazaar.* I experimented with hairstyles. I spent all my money on makeup. And shoes. I had more shoes than nine of my friends put together. Forget clothes. I never could find anything to fit. And it worked. You look at me and see pretty —but I know that I am an invention of my own. Anyone can do it. Honest to God.

I did lose some weight, but my doctor tells me that it's in my bones to be heavy. Cheryl Tiegs, never. But people turn around on the street to look at me now and I *know* it's because I'm attractive and not because I weigh a lot—even though I do weigh a lot.

Margie: Well, I can't say I invented myself. But I did somewhat change my thinking. I can hardly remember a time when I wasn't dieting. And when my emotions weren't raw from denying myself food. When I lived at home, I was constantly shrieking at my parents. When I got married, my husband and children were the targets for my frustrated anger. And I denied myself great pleasures —like cooking. I'm a great cook. But when I dieted, I couldn't taste, and how can you cook without tasting? So I didn't cook. The quality of my life, I guess you'd say, was really meager when I dieted. And I dieted all the time. And I gained back what I lost, all the time.

Now, I think I've broken through. Getting out into the business world helped a lot. Imagine me, a model! It gave me a great deal of confidence. Now I've got my weight down to what is realistic for me—about 185. I'd like to be thinner, but I'm determined to accept myself *now* for how I am *now.* If I happen to lose some weight, fine. If not, fine also. And I mean that. I'm not going to set impossible goals any more. If society doesn't like it, too bad. Sure I get depressed sometimes, but more often I am proud of my look. When I take the time to put myself together, I am a good-looking lady.

Marsha: I grew up heavy. Both my parents were heavy. In a family of eight—my luck—I'm the only one who's fat. I was always unattractive, with skin problems, hair problems, you name it. We were always very poor and ate mostly starch so no wonder I hated the way I looked. So what did I do? I joined clubs. I slept with every guy who asked me as a way of gaining approval.

Now, by hard work, I'm a model and an actress. In between I've scrubbed floors, waitressed, written. Everything but lose weight. Still, people tell me I'm attractive. I was featured in a full-color ad in a Macy's catalog the other day. I'm making it—life is easier. But you know what? I'd be lying if I told you different. I still feel ungainly, not pretty. But I'm working on it. I've come a long way.

Linda: I know how you feel, Marsha. Even though I don't feel ugly, I still am often self-conscious about myself. People automatically assume you're a slob if you're fat. They think you don't take care of yourself, you probably smell bad because everybody knows heavy people don't bathe so often. It's those stigmas we have to face. When you're thin and your life isn't working, everybody assumes it's tough luck—the world and outside influences are to blame. But if you're fat and your life isn't working, you did it all to yourself. It's all your fault that you can't control those childish oral impulses, isn't it? You're bad. It's so unfair, really. And so untrue.

Debbi: I'm thinking hard, and I really can't remember a time when being heavy has seriously gotten in my way. Except when I was a teenager. Getting dates was not easy. But now I have decided to be in control, take my life in my hands—do you know what I mean? If a guy tells me that I have such a pretty face but oh, such a fat can, I tell him, "Get lost, buddy, and goodbye!" Who is he to tell me to run and exercise? I like to eat. And I hate to run around. I'm not going to be a sprinter for him.

Fiddle: Resonance. That's the word. Resonance in life. And the people who have had impact in my life are those who see and make resonance. What the hell do pounds have to do with resonance? Extraordinary people are just not threatened by fat. I will not go

through my life wasting time and being less just to make some-
body else be more. I will be myself. Society says I'm a few pounds
on the other side of what they want me to be? The hell with
society. The other day, I read an article about this fashion show for
big women in California. They were showing their usual navy-
blue polyester tents when a woman got up and shouted—fairly
shouted to all the manufacturers who were sitting in the audience
—"*God damn it!* I'm a wealthy woman. I like being a woman. I
have good taste, I have money and I'm big. What are you trying to
pawn off on me? I can afford *good* clothes. I will not wear this
polyester garbage. I *deserve* to look fashionable—and I'll pay for it!
When are you manufacturers going to wake up?" How's that for
marvelous? I love that woman.

Marsha: Okay, you're right. And it's true that manufacturers *are*
beginning to wake up. But still there are the deeper problems. I
can't help being sensitive about my weight. When I walk down the
street and the Con Ed man calls out, "Hello, *Mama!*" I'd just as
soon kill him. I wouldn't feel one bit guilty for murdering him.

Fiddle: Oh, I *like* it when they affectionately call out to me. Sure,
I always *act* as if I were thinking, "You creep, you jerk," but inside,
I really like it. You know, it's just in this society that pounds are
not pretty. When a Latin man or an Italian man or an Israeli expresses admiration for voluptuous curves, for softness, he means
it.

Marsha: Well, it makes me feel cheap. If I were thin, maybe I'd see
it differently. I know it's reverse prejudice on my part, but I have
to admit, even if it hurts, that I think, "What's wrong with him if
he thinks I'm attractive?" You know what it really is about these
sidewalk Romeos—they aren't *choosy.* A dog could walk down the
street and they'd find it sexy. It's not flattering to me to be just
another piece of meat. And I think that comes from a strong feminist attitude as well as an insecurity about my weight.

Debbi: I feel that any man should be attracted to me, even though
it sounds like bragging. He'd be lucky if I'd choose him to go to bed
with. As one guy once put it, "I'm built for speed and you're built
for comfort." It's true. I'm soft and I'm imaginative and I'm fine as
a sexual partner. I think most big women are.

Linda: True. Once you break down the initial insecurity, sex and the heavy woman are very compatible. I do need to make sure I'm not being used. I *am* sometimes fearful that a guy will find a stomach roll or a fat thigh unattractive, but when I know a man who is beyond that stupid prejudice I, like many of my big sisters, am among the most sensual creatures alive. We are turned on to stimuli, to begin with. Our very natures are passionate. That's why we appreciate food so much, I truly believe. We are people who are turned on to life's pleasures, tastes, sensations, experiences.

Debbi: The only thing that bothers me about that is that many men are turned on to me sexually before they even find out what kind of person I am—what I think about. I hate that. I hate being seen as a sex symbol, even though I like sex.

Fiddle: It's the attitude of the men we choose that makes for a good or bad relationship, as with every other woman. Fat or thin, some men hold your hand and your hand is a rose!

Barbara: Where do I find that man?

Debbi: In Texas. You find him in Texas. Nothing like a Texas guy.

Marsha: Or a Latin. Latin men are great, intelligent . . .

Linda: Let's face it, any man who doesn't have his own handicaps which tell him to be ashamed of a big woman. Think of all the thin women who have problems—or *think* they do.

Marsha: You know what, I just thought of something. Modeling may seem like dumb work to some, but modeling for large-size fashion, as we do, is really making a political statement. It's striking a blow against the structure in America that says only skinny is pretty.

Fiddle: I'll tell you another political thing we can do. If it doesn't fit, don't buy it. Don't encourage the manufacturers to dump us with cheap junk. I'll tell you a funny story. I went in to a store the other day to buy another pair of these great-fitting Levis. Like a lot of my big friends, if I find something terrific, I buy it in twelve colors! The salesgirl whispered, "We don't have them anymore. There's an unspoken policy here that if a line starts to move really fast, the manager says, 'Get rid of it for a while.' He does that to make the other manufacturers happy. To help their old lines along." How do you like them apples? We are being manipulated by manufacturers who just don't want to spend money on research into what the heavy women really like. It's easier to turn out the same old junk. And the few designers who really do care, who try, are penalized if they are too successful. I'd rather wear stuff that's ten years old than buy any more black mourning clothes that sit on the racks. If we all refuse to buy junk, they'll get the message soon enough.

Linda: Do you mind if I change the subject? Here's something I'd like to talk about. It has always struck me as being rude and inconsiderate that people, even relative strangers, feel free to approach you and say, "You have such a beautiful face—it's too bad you're so heavy." I mean, they wouldn't come up and say, "You have a beautiful face—too bad about the acne." Or, "How come a nice girl like you limps?" Everybody feels free to announce that you're fat and that if you really wanted to, you could lose the weight, if you just used a little willpower.

Marsha: Oh, I understand. Somehow, when you're heavy, people feel free to approach you on many levels. We're more vulnerable. We accept their putdowns and it shows. We really must fight against that tendency to pitifully accept other people's judgments. Some people act as if they're doing you a favor to even talk to you. I hate this in myself, but when I meet that kind of a person, it makes me feel as if I *were* desperate. Oh, I'm working so hard to overcome that reaction.

Margie: No one has ever come right up to me and said anything about my weight, outright. Still, I always used to imagine they were talking about me. That's worse. One day—and I don't know where I found the courage to do it—I forced myself to go over to two women at a cocktail party who had been whispering and looking in my direction for about ten minutes and say, "Would you mind if I asked you something? Honestly speaking, were you just talking about how fat I am?" One of the women stared at me blankly, the way you know people do when they're being honest. "Your fatness?" she said quietly. "God, no. I was asking Lois here if she thought I ought to tip my hair blond, like yours." I felt like a jerk. I think of the incident often. We can drive ourselves batty with imagined slights. No one is really concerned with my pounds. All they care about is my value to them. Am I interesting? Amusing? A good friend? A lovely lover? A real person? My value is not in my size.

Fiddle: How many ugly, handicapped, pitifully bony people do you know who have made it because of *one* thing—attitude? Look at Barbra Streisand. She wouldn't have her nose fixed or conform to anyone else's idea of beauty. She insisted on feeling good about herself the way she is. We large-sized women must create our own markets if they're not already there. Take modeling—what we all do. If we didn't create a market for large-sized clothes, where would we be? You can find jobs and outlets in almost every area. [*Author's note:* See chapter 10, How to Get a Job.] My friend is Geoffrey Holder, the West Indian dancer-actor. He had some pretty tough barriers to break through. He was too tall, they said, too black, too inarticulate. But he fought them. And ended up famous. I will too. Do you think I'm going to let my pounds get in the way of living and looking good? No way. Look—this is the eighties we live in. Anything's possible. If we reach out to people in an honest way, they will forget we don't have candy-box faces and doll-figurine figures. As in the domino theory, when one barrier goes, they all will. We've knocked down a barrier against large-sized models —we can take them all on!

Barbara: You're right. Look around this room, all of you. Ten years ago, we would have been a bunch of dumpy, sloppy women. Now look at us. We're good-looking, functioning people. Sure we have insecurities and fears, but what six women in any room don't?

Debbi: We are able to make choices. We couldn't have done that thirty years ago. Times are really different. I'm really career oriented now. That's my choice. Social life, men, clothes, making friends—all come second to career, right now, for me. My weight is not in my way.

Margie: For me, it's still tough, but I know, as Debbi says, I can choose. I don't have to be the klutz. For instance, two years ago I went to visit some friends on Fire Island. They came to ferry us across the water in small boats. I got all flustered when I saw those rowboats—I just *knew* there was going to be trouble. Sure enough, the moment I hurriedly bounced in to get the thing over with, the damn boat overturned. I wanted to die of embarrassment. I arrived at the party dripping wet. Since then, I have worked on my psyche. I have decided I won't be a clumsy oaf even though I weigh 185. If I had to get into that boat today, I'd do it slowly. I'd lower my weight down in the middle of the boat and I'd make sure other people had entered before me so I could distribute my weight more easily before I plopped down. I wouldn't plop in the first place, I think, I'd take my time and not get nervous and embarrassed. That boat did not have to flip. I made it flip by my own insecurity. As Debbi just said—I could choose to be a different person from the one who was devastated by a rowboat.

Marsha: I'd probably still plop.

Fiddle: Oh, no you wouldn't. Fatness doesn't have to weigh you down. Fatness can represent a kind of freedom, a largesse, a generous liberality! It doesn't have to be a burden or even a protective cushion. Every society has its "Commies," its subversives. If we let them, the think-thin crazies will turn us into their subversives or bad guys.

Margie: Did you ever notice that fat people are never looked upon as desirable or interesting in this jogging culture? In fact, they're hardly ever looked upon at all. When was the last time you read a story about a fat person? Or saw a play about one? When I see another fat woman, I always feel I want to protect her. Fat people seem so vulnerable, so easily hurt—even in their anonymity.

Marsha: You're right. What we need is attention, I think. Everybody else wants us to hide. Once when I looked for a job waiting on tables at the World Trade Center, the manager told me, "You're much too heavy. We can't hire you. You'd attract too much attention and we can't have a waitress give that image. People won't order as much food because they don't want to look like you." If that happened today, I'd attract attention all right. I'd bring that guy up on charges of discrimination.

Imagine, the *sheer cruelty* of it! Another man once told me that I couldn't be a waitress in his restaurant because I couldn't fit between the tables—I'd knock things down. That's prejudice if I ever heard it. Blacks and women and gays have worked to change the system of such lousy prejudice. We have no choice. We have to work too.

Margie: Yes, we do have a choice. We just said that before. I am not a marcher or a fighter or a political animal. I choose not to get involved—that way. But I can still work to make my own life easier, even though I still find it hard to talk to my husband about my feelings. I am not comfortable yet with my fatness. I don't know if I ever will be. When I was little, I used to sit in our big love seat, munching Tootsie Rolls and pretending I was thin and romantic-looking. I was a 200-pound adolescent who fantasized being a butterfly. I never could talk about my fatness to many people, mainly because I think in my heart of hearts, my real body wasn't mine. It was a disguise. I was really this lithe creature, floating airily about. I didn't know who that fat kid was. I still don't. I don't know if I can ever acknowledge her.

Linda: Margie, you're too pessimistic.

Margie: Why pessimistic? I'm truthful.

Linda: Okay, in a way I do agree. Even if you do accept yourself and make yourself terrific-looking, it is hard to believe anyone who says they *Chose* to be fat. It isn't easy to be fat. I resent that kind of talk. You can make compensations but it's hard to believe anyone who says she chooses to be so far out of society's approval.

Fiddle: But the point is, do you play in society's ball park, or do you change the rules? You're more than a weight problem. You're a breathing, bleeding woman with joys and a face and an intelligence as well as extra pounds. And there are so many players on our team! I say you can make valuable contributions, meet great people, be a great person and still be sixty pounds overweight.

Linda: Put it this way. We play in their ball park because we *live* in their ball park. We don't try to change ourselves, but we try to make the best out of what we are. We do have to work harder at it, no getting around it. I work to search out the great clothes that will make me look attractive. I am *never* sloppy even though I love being sloppy. Sloppy is a 110-pound nymph in a torn sweatshirt and floppy dungarees. Sloppy and cute. At 190, I'm not cute when

I'm sloppy. It's not fair, it stinks—but it's true. Don't waste time thinking of how to lose weight, but time spent in thinking how to feel and look good is not wasted! Look, when I came here today, I felt like wearing my sloppy, stained T-shirt. But I stopped to think —is that the image I want to project? It isn't. So I dressed more carefully. And, I might say, it paid off. A very Ivy-League-looking lawyer who shared a cab with me on the way here asked if he could see me again—when it's not raining. I'm feeling good about that. I outweigh that guy by about twenty pounds. So what—I don't think he noticed.

Margie: I've been thinking about analysis to help me face bigness. Do you think it would help?

Linda: Sure it helps—*some* people. How can we generalize with big women any more than we can generalize with any other group? It happens that when I went through analysis, I was very thin, at the beginning. I lost a whole set of problems, but put on sixty pounds and another, different set of problems. Everyone reacts differently. You know, I believe that we have to find out not *why* we gained weight, but how to handle the weight. We gain for a number of reasons—heredity, glands, eating too much. All different kinds of studies have shown that big women are not *any* weaker or sicker or unhappier than skinny ones, to begin with. But what do we do after we gain the weight—that's the big problem. How do we deal with the world that wants to put us down? We have to find out not why we're fat but how to be fat and successful.

Fiddle: Good analysis! I know my problems come mostly from people telling me I should have problems. I bought that line and, worse, I owned it for a long time. It was hard to get out of the feeling I *should* be clumsy, I *should* be unpopular with men, I *should* be in hiding. But I did.

Margie: How? Tell me how to get away from feeling sad because of fatness.

Fiddle: Be the best you can be. Live. Get or create a job. Get in touch with your feelings. Try EST, TM, meditation. Try thinking. The problem is not getting thin. It's getting bored with life. Get *out of the house.* Survive!

Margie: Where do I start?

Fiddle: Be around people who are energy forces. Exaggerate your good points. Diminish your weaknesses. Be the best you can be. Now. Not next month when you may or may not lose a couple of pounds. Join a little theater club. Join a political organization. Go to museums. Listen to music. Call people up. *Push.*

Never apologize for what you are.

Never buy a three-way mirror. They're worse than a Roach Motel.

Barbara: What's a Roach Motel?

Fiddle: A product to kill roaches. The roaches walk into this little sticky box, see, and can't get out. And there they are—stuck in a box of dead roaches.

Three-way mirrors remind me of that. They stick you in a box labeled *fat.* It's hard to get out. Three-way mirrors are a killer. Who needs them?

Margie: Sometimes I think I'm more prejudiced against fat people than a skinny person would be. I hate buses filled with fat people crowding me.

Marsha: Me too! And I always stand on crowded subways. I never want anyone to feel that I'm taking up part of their seat, the way I'd feel if a very large person sat near me.

Debbi: Good, good—now we're getting to it. You really can't expect other people to accept you if you can't accept yourself.

Margie: Oh God, I know it. But how do I not feel guilty for always wanting to eat? My husband says he's full and is able to walk away from a hot fudge sundae. Walk away! Not me. And because I'm ashamed, I can hardly talk about the results. For instance, I'd love to put a larger tub in our house. Why shouldn't I feel lovely and sensual in a bathtub like everyone else? I can't even get enough water to cover my breasts, in our measly tub. But I'm too embarrassed to suggest it to my husband even though I can pay for it with my modeling money.

Fiddle: Would your husband be too embarrassed to suggest he wanted a new hairpiece for his balding head? Or new golf clubs because he ruined the first set with his lousy putting? Or caps on his teeth to hide tobacco stains?

Margie: No.

Fiddle: So?

Margie: So what? So you're right, I guess. I'm going to order that bathtub. I wish my body didn't sentence me to embarrassment.

Fiddle: Your body doesn't! Your head does. But your head can free you also. Tell yourself you're terrific. You are, you know. So am I. So are we all. I think there's a relationship between what we tell ourselves and how we really feel and act. You are a worthwhile person. Honest.

Barbara: Nobody has a right to tell anyone else how to live. I'm entitled to go to a good school and work at a good job and wear great clothes and make my face wonderful looking—if I like. I am coming to the point where I insist on those rights. Who is good enough to judge me? No one. It's a struggle, but I think I can do it. Sure I'm big, and sometimes I'm even fat, and sometimes I lose some weight and sometimes I don't. But I am always, always me. Which I happen to think is pretty nice.

Marsha: You were the one who said it at the beginning of this afternoon. Anyone can invent themselves, as you did. I like that line. It rings true. I am going to invent a stronger Marsha. Later. Right now, I feel like coffee and cake. Who else?

IX Life Situations

You feel like a klutz at parties? Your friends have come to pick you up in their Volkswagen and you're sure you'll get stuck in the back? Literally. You *know* everyone is watching you at the buffet table to see how much food you'll heap on your plate?

Relax. In order to glide in and out of the myriad life situations that were designed, it seems, just to plague us, you must first get your head together, as they say.

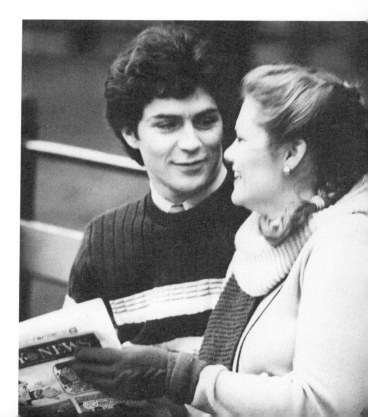

1. *Admit you are a large-sized woman.*

Now comes the hard part.

2. *Admit you are likely to stay that way.*

Once you can adjust to the fact of your heaviness, you can get on with your life. If you believed last year, and the year before, and still believe, even now, that you will one day be a size 12, you will drive yourself crazy. For years I had three different sizes of clothes hanging in my closet which were not even distinctly related to my real size. They were just hanging there, rather poignantly, just waiting for the day when I would fit into them. They would have waited till the millennium. Finally, I knew I'd found mental health the day I gave the 14s to my cousin Gloria, the 12s to my friend Barbara and the 7s to the Save the Children Foundation. How the 7s got there, heaven only knows. I don't even *know* any size 7s, having decided some time ago that they were all untrustworthy and no fun.

So you can't be a terrific big woman until you admit you are big. Big today and probably big all of your tomorrows. Once you understand that, you can get back to the business of living. Not eating no longer rules your every waking moment. Hostess Twinkies regain their proper value in life.

The full-time job of working on *thin* would take so many pleasures from my life that avoiding cane-seat chairs is very little sacrifice for happiness. Large-size women should say, "Hey, wait a moment! If anyone else backs me into a corner and hands me one more diet drink, I'll become violent!"

Look—of course I'd *rather* be thin. For one thing, it would make it easier for me to live in this gaunt-crazed society. But I'd also rather have a million dollars rather than the dollars I do have. It comes down to a matter of priorities, because I can't have either. Dieting for the rest of my life would make me obsessed with food for the rest of my life. I'm not going to make myself crazy over a lack of dollars *or* a surplus of pounds. There are more important things to do.

So—if you've gone on at least twelve diets in your life—and if you have gained forty, lost forty, gained forty, lost forty and gained it right back every couple of years—face it. One of the privileges in life you were born with is the privilege of *not* dieting. Claim that privilege and get on with the good life.

Now that you've faced the reality of your large and wonderful self, also face the comfortable reality that there are ways to deal with almost every uncomfortable life situation. *Everyone* has uncomfortable life situations. Some people stutter. Some are shy. Some are terribly nearsighted. They learn to compensate and to *handle* whatever problems arise. What follows are some potentially difficult places for the large woman—and how to manage them.

Automobiles

BUYING THE FAMILY CAR

Let the others kick the tires and check out the chrome. You try the seats. Can you get in and out comfortably? Are the seats too plush and soft? Can you reach the gas pedal? Can you slide in easily behind the steering wheel? If your pounds center in the abdominal area and if you are short, it is very hard to reach the pedals. Don't suffer. Pedal extensions for gas and brake are available. Don't hesitate to ask your automobile dealer. I have many *thin*, short-legged friends who have happily discovered pedal extensions.

Consider seat belts carefully. If they don't fit around you, you're going to buzz all the way to where you're going. Dealers can also provide seat-belt extensions, but if you have a tough time finding them, you can make your own. Cut off a set of belts that is least frequently used in your car. (The back set?) Then, overlapping the cut ends, stitch them securely together on a sewing machine, using heavy-duty thread, or have a shoe-repair place do it for you. The result is an adjustable lap-belt extender that can even be switched from one set of belts to another within the same car. I got this tip from members of the National Association to Aid Fat Americans, who insist upon their own safety, heavy or not.

Steering wheels can be a big problem also. The Saginaw Steering Gear Division of General Motors makes a wheel that tilts, telescopes and moves up and out of the way. Hooray for G.M.! You can also replace any standard steering wheel (15–16 inches) with a smaller (9–11 inch) racing-car wheel available at auto speed or part shops. If you're not mechanically inclined, get someone who is to install it for you so the wheel doesn't come off while you're zipping along at sixty on the highway. And that little racing-car wheel is pretty jazzy, also.

HITCHING A RIDE—WITHOUT TRAGEDY

Here come the Smiths to pick you up. They're terrific people but oh, their dumb two-door car. It's almost impossible for you or any other big woman to slide into the back of a two-door car and retain your composure, especially with a web of seat belts tackling you. So don't. *You have a right to the front seat!* Why not? Does it have someone else's name engraved on it? Handle the situation lightly, but insist firmly. Like this: "Uh, Smiths, someone else has to be prisoner in the back seat dungeon this trip. Sorry, but you don't mind, do you?"

It's as easy as that. If you don't say it, you'll wind up trying to maneuver 190 pounds through six inches. I've gotten into back seats thinking I'd made it only to find out that about forty-five pounds of me were being held up by a string. Everyone is happier when you assert yourself. And you can predict disaster better than the others because you've been there before: you *know* how panicked the Smiths will be when it's time to unfold yourself from the back seat and it looks as if you'll bring their whole car with you. So play it cool from the beginning. If your husband or lover ends up sitting with someone else, so what. You'll make it up to him when you get there.

GETTING IN ANY CAR, YOUR OWN INCLUDED, GRACEFULLY

Now that it's been established that you always opt for the front seat, how do you maneuver that effortlessly? Effortlessly, forget about. Even Grace Kelly can't get into and out of a car in one smooth motion. But there are ways to minimize the klutziness. In fact, this way is as close to graceful as there is.

If you're getting in the right side of the car, stand with your *back* to the door and sit down on the edge of the front seat. Both of your feet are still planted on the outside sidewalk. With your weight on the right front foot, which is still on the sidewalk, swing yourself and your left leg around and into the car. Then bring your right leg in. Simple?

To get out of the car: Swing both legs around and place firmly on the ground. You are now, once again, facing out of the car door. With your right hand or arm on the back of the seat for support, simply stand. You're *out!*

If you are driving the car and enter the car on the left side, sit down, facing out. Swing your right leg in first. Follow with the left leg.

At the Party

SITTING

The decor at the party may not match your decor. Don't panic. Just don't sit in anything if you think they'll need two people to lift you out. If you have artsy-craftsy friends who think pillow furniture is the last word, ask if you may use a kitchen chair—back trouble. You're pretty safe with a kitchen chair. Not too many people have breakfast on pillow furniture. If anything has a cane bottom, don't sit in it unless you want to make a basketball hoop. Use your head. Plead locked knees, plead slipped discs, plead *anything,* stand, but do *not* sit in anything you can't get into, stay in and get out of without embarrassment. Elegant women don't plop, fall through or get stuck. If you plan ahead, you can be stunning and always graceful. Look—there is no reason why you cannot be the general of your own war. And if the war does not include murderous dieting, it also should not include embarrassing situations. When you walk into a room, you *know* what chair you should sit in. Have a very accurate picture of you; clean the mental barriers out and stop thinking of yourself as a dainty little thing flitting through life. You are a big woman and your activities require some thought and control for the maximum in graceful living.

EATING—THE RIGHT TO SAY YES, I'LL HAVE THE FRIED ONION RINGS

Large-size women have to understand that people expect them to eat. There is no reason to starve yourself senseless into eclair deprivation because you are conscious that your plate is being watched. It is probably your imagination anyway. The skinny guy in back of you is just thinking of the moment when he can dig into the mashed potatoes au gratin. He doesn't care a fig what *you* eat. Don't take bird portions and mince and pick at your food just to prove you're not a glutton. It's silly, unliberated and besides you'll get very hungry. Taking minuscule portions merely calls attention to your size and does not convince anyone of your delicacy. You're a person. You've had a proper invitation to this party. *Eat* and enjoy. With one exception: if you know beforehand that the food is to be served buffet style and you will be required to eat from your lap, have a bite at home to take the edge off your hunger. It is difficult to eat a large meal from your lap mainly because you don't have much of a lap. Somehow, no matter how you slice it, a large-size lady looks ungainly doing a balancing act. You do not want to become an event. You do not want the shrimp jambalaya to slide from your thighs onto the oriental rug. Nobody should *be* a happening at a party.

GETTING UP FROM THE TABLE

It's a sit-down, formal dinner party. Everything has been going splendidly and you are making (you just feel it!) a lasting impression on the producer to your right who is casting for his next show. There's a part in it for you—he's hinting it all over the place.

Dinner is over and everybody rises from the table, including you. As you rise, you lean your weight on the edge (as you've done a million times on your own table edge), but true, unmitigated disaster strikes—the entire table tips. Plates, unfinished broccoli, wineglasses all go hurtling to the floor. You want to die. Nothing less than death on the spot will make you feel better. *How did it happen?* Your hostess has a flimsily made pedestal table which cannot take any weight on the edge. Or she has put too many leaves in an extension table and there are no longer four legs balancing a short table but four legs balancing a table which has been extended far too long in the center and easily tipped. *Never put your full weight on the edge of a table.* Use the support of a chair arm or seat or even gracefully extend a hand to your neighbor for support as you rise.

SMALL-TALKING AT THE PARTY

If the conversation is zipping around the room, don't expect any to zip your way unless you are aggressively friendly. In one way, being heavy makes you less foreboding looking. People trust and feel easier with warm-looking, large women. One marvelous advantage of pounds is the wildly wrong myth that surrounds them: other women don't think you're a threat. Hah. You can literally surround the most attractive men in the room and the other women don't worry. Let them dream on. *You* know how sensual a creature you are and you know how that appeal comes across best in a one-to-one, intimate conversation. You know that what attracts men is an aura that surrounds a woman who has a grasp on life—not an aura that surrounds a woman who is hungry or who is practicing self-denial. And furthermore, you know that many great loves have come from trusting friendships. You didn't know? I'm telling you. Believe it. Like yourself. Be an interesting woman, choose a life-style that's appealing and your own excitement will captivate strangers during a small talking session at a party. I personally think that a woman who is very young, very thin and very energetic would make even a man who's been dead for twenty-four hours feel nervous. Skinny women who jog in place because they don't want to waste time while the bartender is making them a drink make *everyone* nervous.

There are tricks to making great small talk and you can learn them. Don't kid yourself—it's a cultivated art. Mike Douglas once told my co-author, Sherry, that his best ad libs are the ones he prepares the night before. So *you* can prepare the night before by finding out what the other invited guests are interested in, what their professions and hobbies are. You can check out current newspapers and magazines for relevant items to drop that will captivate their attention. Ignore the weather and the hors d'oeuvres as topics of small talk. Ask someone what his first job was: that's a sure-fire opener that will cause him to reminisce and wax lyrically on his past. Wear a prop: someone *has* to ask you why you're wearing that Ronald MacDonald ring or the cuff links made of samurai sword handles. Ask someone who his heroes are or what he's done in the past year of which he's most proud. Circulate around groups: check out the conversation going on and break in after a while with a relevant question on the topic under discussion, directed to *one* person.

Not proven to make you the life of the party are endless jokes or details about your children, operations, and your cat who thinks it's a person. Kick-to-the-stomach-openers like, "How can you sit there enjoying that chopped liver when the boat children are starving?" are not calculated to make you popular. Nor is talk about the best sponges, mulches and ketchup brands.

Be a large woman at a party with something terrific to say. After the party, I guarantee you, no one will comment, "Hey, did you notice that size-42 woman?" Chances are he'll say, "Hey, did you talk with that woman who's made a study of transmigration of the soul? She said . . ."

On the Town

AT THE RESTAURANT

While you're waiting for the maître d', quickly scout out the joint to see which tables have movable chairs or benches—for easier access. And ask for them. Never try to squinch yourself behind a table where you'll have difficulty breathing out for the duration of the meal. Sometimes, the restaurants you choose will feature a banquette, which is a long bench that fits into or is part of the wall, and is usually upholstered. Aha, you say, that's the seat where I can spread myself out comfortably. Right? Sometimes. I've found out that spreading out is not always as important as sliding in. If the waiter has to pull out the opposite chair and table to somewhere in the foyer, the movable chair is easier for me to use. Then again, check *that* chair: if it looks as if it could be used as kindling for a very small Boy Scout fire, opt for the banquette. But you know your dimensions better than anyone else. Ask the waiter to pull the table away far enough, so your overflow in the back doesn't sweep all the silverware off the table. There is nothing more embarrassing than getting wedged in next to the quiche. Don't lean on the edges of pedestal tables or sit on flimsy, Tinker-Toy chairs. Find another restaurant if you think you're going to be subjected to a possible breakthrough or even discomfort. And once you get seated, anybody who lets herself be intimidated out of the hot fudge sundae by the scornful eye of a waiter better rethink her priorities. Be and order what you want.

AT THE THEATER

There's no getting around it: you simply have to know your theaters to find which ones have comfortable seating. After a show is over, one evening, zip upstairs and whip out your handy tape measure to canvass the seats in other sections. You may have to pay more for a box or a loge seat to get the extra seat width. Older theaters often have larger seats. Don't be ashamed to ask the box office salesperson to recommend the area with the widest seats. It's your money; no one has offered you guest passes. You're entitled to the best you can pay for in the theater.

SINGLES BARS

Although they're accepted these days as a rather legitimate way for young people to meet other young people, the *big* young person must be careful. *Bar stools are her enemy.* They are invariably the size of mushrooms and there is nothing more unattractive than rolls of fat oozing over a diminutive surface. Your bigness is attractive when you are sitting in a seat that fits. Or when you are standing with presence and poise. Bar stools do nothing for presence. In the movie *The Cheap Detective,* someone says to John Houseman, "How will I know you?" and Houseman answers, "I'll be sitting on the first two bar stools as you come in." Don't sit on two bar stools or overlap on one. Cocktail tables are available if you *must* sit at all.

ELEVATORS

Elevators are simple. All you have to do is *believe* that the reason the crowded elevator doesn't budge in an upward direction has *nothing* to do with your weight. And no one is looking at you or at the legend that says, "Only 3,000 pounds permitted in this elevator." Really. It's neurotic to believe otherwise. Understandable, but neurotic.

Home Sweet Home

You spend a lot of time at home. Don't allow yourself to be a victim. I know many families who play the game, Let's Catch Gloria Eating. If you make yourself a target for this game, even from well-meaning but misguided family, you do so from your own guilt and weakness. You are what you are. You'll eat what you choose, *when* you choose. You are *responsible* for your own life decisions if you're over sixteen. Don't forget it for a moment. If you refuse to assert yourself, you're doomed to be a Sneaky Eater. There is nothing worse than sneaky eating. First of all, it never works. Tootsie-Roll breath gives you away, every time. It makes you feel awful and it makes for a lot of crumpled papers and crumbs under the blankets. And if you're hiding Tootsie Rolls, what *do* you do with the wrappers after you've consumed the rolls? Can't throw them down the toilet—they stuff. Can't put them in a wastepaper basket—you'll be found out. You can't eat them— they're tough on the colon. So what do you do? You decide you will not be an oppressed target. You will not apologize for your size. You announce that fact to everybody. Do not take kindly to "suggestions" and other euphemisms for dictating your life-style.

In my house, it's heavy Mallomar country. There are only two kinds of Mallomar boxes—unopened or empty. There is never any such thing as a box of Mallomars with two left. And my family knows it: a long time ago, I whipped my hot fudge out of the closet and I've been happier ever since.

And shop sanely. A house without one Hershey Bar is an abnormal house. The days when I specifically leave all fattening stuff off my shopping list, I end up feeling like Ray Milland in *Lost Weekend*. I find myself looking for cookie crumbs in the chandelier.

I treat my family with respect and demand that same respect from them. It often happens that large-sized women have large-sized children. I have never made my children nervous, sneaky wrecks by visiting the same plagues on them that I remember from my childhood. Sure I teach good nutrition, but I do not supervise every morsel that enters their lips. Carrots and apples are available, but if they choose Chunkys, I will not make them hide their Chunkys in a dark bathroom. Chunkys don't give you pimples. Or destroy your psyche. Feeling guilty about eating them will. If you were a child food-sneaker, you'll understand.

SALT TALK

Throw out the myth that says you have to increase your salt consumption in hot weather. Sure, you do perspire more and lose *some* salt, but an extra pinch on your food will be much better for you than the salt pills you're used to. Salt pills can be very dangerous and can lead to possible dehydration and heat stroke.

CHUG-A-LUG

In the summer, this means much more water—not beer—than you usually drink. You perspire more than most other women *all the time*, and in the summer, you're losing pints of the stuff. Drink two and a half to three quarts of water daily, to compensate.

DOUBLES COVERAGE

More arguments come from "I'm too hot—*I'm* too cold" bickering under the blankets. Consider an electric blanket. It's a heaven-sent marriage saver for the big woman and her mate because it comes with dual controls. She invariably wants a lighter blanket because her pounds make her body temperature rise, and he is freezing. Big women are terrific to sleep with anyway. They are warm and soft and comforting with very few hard angles. If he's got a bag of bones for a companion, twin beds don't look like such a bad idea.

ALWAYS TIRED?

Have you been told it's because you're dragging all that weight around? Maybe. Maybe not. More likely it's because you are too sedentary. Modern researchers have found that heavier bodies, because of their genes, hormones or life-styles, tend to have a shorter supply of oxygen housed in ther lungs and in the blood that circulates the oxygen. Remedy? *Move.* If you feel very tired, don't take a nap. Get up and walk quickly around the block, scrub out the toilet, make the beds or do some exercises from chapter 7 of this book. Because of your particular metabolism, a feeling of tiredness *can* be caused by too little oxygen in the system and can be cured by a short period of strenuous physical effort. So forget the lie-down when you're bushed: it will probably only make you more tired.

Clothes

CLINGING POLYESTERS

On a hot day they really cling. On a cold day they can freeze your thighs blue, permanently. Still, even though the natural fibers like cotton and wool are much to be preferred, the polyester fan who *will not iron* swears by the synthetic fabric. Just for her was invented Static Guard. When it's sprayed directly onto the dress, it eliminates that cling-to-the-thighs-and-show-every-bulge syndrome. In the wintertime, fabrics that fairly crackle with the cold, lose their violence when Static-Guarded. As the expression goes, if you must wear polyester, let it all hang out.

TENNIS

Anyone can play tennis. There are no weight limitations as there are to say, being a jockey. But if you feel unhappy with bouncing flab, wear Supphose on the court. They're invisible and they control your thighs nicely.

THE GIRDLE REVOLUTION—THROW THEM OUT!

Support pantyhose, yes. Girdle attached, no. Heavy legs tend to trap, spongelike, any water you drink. Heavy bellies do the same thing. Girdles constrict the blood flow from the legs, allowing fluid to form a pool in the lower extremities. So don't wear them! If you tend to get a bladder infection easily, and your doctor suspects that nylon pantyhose aggravates it, wear a pair of cotton pants under the pantyhose.

If you *must* wear a girdle (hardly anyone jails themselves up anymore—and do you really think they make you look thinner?), powder the inside of the garment before you pull it on. It makes girdle removal a less than tortuous experience. Only buy a quality girdle. A cheap one will lose its shape and thinning ability after one or two rounds in the washing machine.

TO REACH THE IMPOSSIBLE PLACE

Bras are the nastiest. It's hard for anyone to contort herself into a figure 8 as she struggles with bra backs: for the heavier woman, the problem is magnified. So don't struggle. Buy bras that hook in the front. They do marvelous things for your shape as well as your comfort. And if your favorite bra has become too tight, bra extenders available at the nearest five-and-dime store are available and easy to sew on.

Shoes with buckles and laces are not shoes for me. I hate bending to buckle and lace every time I slip a shoe off for comfort. Pumps, the slip-in kind, are flattering and easier to manage. You can buy a *long* (about two feet) shoehorn to hang on a handy closet hook. Saves bending and bent shoe backs.

Rings that get stuck come off more easily with lots of lathered soap on the finger, or even some old-fashioned beeswax rubbed around the ring circle.

VAINNESS IS ONE THING, BUT YOU HAVE VEIN PROBLEMS

You're not alone. Many thin women also suffer from varicose veins, although we seem to be hit hardest. Like pregnancy, extra poundage aggravates the condition. Ditto standing a lot and no exercise. What exactly *are* varicose veins? As you know, veins carry blood to the heart. Blood in the leg veins has a particularly hard road to travel because it must go *up* against the force of gravity and against the weight of the blood above it. When you are fat, the constant weight puts added pressure on these veins which are nothing more substantial than long, elastic-walled tubes. They begin to sag, become weak and don't perform properly. Some of the blood traveling up begins to seep down where it meets the other blood traveling up. This back flow makes the vein dilate and causes a bulging, twisty blue vein—varicose veins, to be exact (varicose means permanently lengthened and dilated). They don't go away. They can be treated, however. Special fitted elastic stockings help. Surgery also helps. (It's simple, takes one day and is done under general anesthesia.) Exercise also helps (see chapter 7). Elevating legs helps also because the blood can move with gravity instead of against it. Therefore, whenever you can, use a footstool to raise the legs as you relax. And avoid tight stuff like girdles, tight boots, knee-high stockings (the kind that rubber-band your legs one inch deep). Keep moving as much as you can because the action of the leg muscles increases circulation through the veins.

If you have tiny, little spider veins—don't worry. They don't mean the varicose kind are on the way. Mostly they mean you're getting older. Sorry about that. The Pill and tight things don't help them, either. Leg makeup applied in upward strokes can cover them, sometimes. If they're really bothersome to you, see a doctor about injections to close up the vein. The injections are safe, but they don't always work.

Don't cross your legs—ever! No matter what you've been told

by your dancing teacher or your mother. Don't even cross your ankles. That impedes circulation badly.

HAZARDS OF WALKING—ONE IN PARTICULAR

Walking is marvelous in so many ways. And we usually do a lot of it, walking through our homes, supermarkets, offices, schools and the woods on summer evenings. But for the big woman, walking presents one serious problem—thigh burn. Sometimes it gets so bad that the skin on the inner thigh is rubbed raw. Which in turn makes you walk with your legs two feet apart. Handicapping, to say the least. Try a marvelous product called Chafeze put out by Warner Lingerie and available in any major department store. It's a soft, usually nylon tricot shield which kind of looks like an underarm perspiration shield. It comes with adjustable straps that fit around any size thigh and provides a protective covering for both inner thighs which tend to rub against each other as you walk. One drawback: the straps show under most snug fabric slacks and tight skirts, so wear them only with looser clothing. You shouldn't be wearing tight skirts to begin with. The Chafeze really eliminates thigh burn irritation, but if you're stuck without Chafeze handy, try some Vaseline. Warner's, sensitive to the problems of bigger women, also puts out a nice bra called No Exaggeration. It has a minimizing effect and takes away that projecting look which makes the large bosom even larger. It comes in sizes up to 44 D-D.

CROTCH SEAM TORTURE

You can end it. Exquisite Form puts out a stretch pantygirdle called Big Gal's Super Control which has no seams in the crotch or leg to irritate, irritate, irritate.

SHOPPING

If you have the bad fortune to enter a store where the salesperson is patronizing, overbearing and *will not leave you alone to make your own decisions,* politely but firmly explain that you prefer browsing to being force-helped. If she still won't take the hint and hangs around the dressing room fussing at you and pretending to love every ghastly thing you try on when you *know* she's just interested in making a sale, a little firm rudeness on your part may be called for:

- "Look—I know it's difficult for you, but I respond to a soft sell much better than a hard sell."
- "I know you're just trying to do a job, but I am not happy unless I am left alone to make a decision."
- "I'll call you when I need you. Please leave me alone."

Understand one thing. The salesperson's raison d'être is to make a sale. She really doesn't care whether you look terrific or like a sack of oranges. Very often, when women are large, they are assumed to be without fashion judgment and without confidence. Salespeople tend to take advantage of any indecision.

Another thing. You have probably been brainwashed to feel that since there is so little choice in your size you ought to be satisfied with the first thing that manages to slip over your thighs. This is no longer the situation. Make sure you find a store in your neighborhood or near-neighborhood which offers you a *selection.*

Some salespeople don't even want to see anyone over size 12. If you feel that you are being ignored because your size doesn't meet the salesperson's idea of chic, demand attention in a firm, quiet way:

- "I would like to see this dress in a red. Please, will you find it for me." No question, you notice. A statement.
- "I have only a few moments to spare and I am interested in a wool wrap-around dress in an 18. Please show me what you have in that style or others like it."

The moment you plead for service you take force from your request. Watch an insecure woman ask for the salt at a dinner party.

- "Please? Will you pass the salt, please?"

Watch an assertive woman or man do the same thing.

- "Pass the salt this way, please."

It makes a difference. A polite demand demands response. Big women for too long have been too *grateful* for anybody's attention. Reconstruct your verbal approaches.

If it happens that a saleswoman seems to be actively discriminating against you (you'd be surprised to see how often that happens) and you're certain it's because of your size, insist upon seeing her supervisor and explaining the problem. *Never, never* be a victim. Anywhere.

A personal tip: shop alone. Your own decisions turn out to be better, almost 100 percent of the time, than the advice of even well-meaning friends. You know you'll look good in the aquamarine shift when your hair is done and you have on high heels: she can't judge that. By the same token, you also know you're bizarre in pink bows circling the hem, even though she's fainting with pleasure at the idea of thirty pink bows. Don't let her or any clerk talk you into a size smaller when you know better but are too embarrassed to insist. Shop alone, carefully, and with great suspicion of salespeople who say you're gorgeous in froufrou and friends who really don't know what you're gorgeous or comfortable in.

Mail-order catalogs are good for ordering sheets. But be wary of ordering clothes for the big woman. It's difficult to judge from a picture. The slim-line size-42 skirt that makes the size-8 model look like a size 14 may make *you* look like a 48. Most mail-order fashion catalogs have gotten smarter and *are* showing their large-size clothes on large-sized models. If they don't go to the trouble of illustrating how a dress will look on you, don't go to the trouble of ordering it. A tiny dart in a size-8 dress will look like Highway 99 in your size dress. If you do buy from a mail-order firm, make sure it accepts returns.

One more word. Be prepared to spend more money on your clothes than your skinny sister. Buy less, if you have to, but buy good. You cannot get away with trendy, faddy, ill-constructed junk. Bargains are rare. Good clothes can be cleaned more often without falling apart, and because we tend to perspire more, our clothes hit the cleaners more often. Our clothes *do* get heavier wear at the seat, the inner thighs, the buttonholes. Shoddy stuff looks it, and lasts a tenth as long as quality stuff.

Medicine and Insurance

HE MEANS WELL, BUT . . .

Your tennis elbow is killing you. You can't hold the racquet and even the weight of a cup of tea hurts. So you go to your doctor for a shot or some elbow advice, and what do you get? You get a lecture on how you should lose weight.

You feel terrific, except for the elbow, you have no weight-related problems at all, and yet this old family or newly found doctor can't take his mind off your weight.

What to do?

Very gently focus on your reason for being there. Thank him for his concern and get back to the elbow. Understand that his entire training has taught him that fat is unhealthy, fat makes for a poor surgical risk, fat is not nice. Try to *hear* what he has to say, *if* you think he is genuinely concerned, and discuss your feelings and the new research that says fat is not as medically terrible as he's been taught to believe.

What if it doesn't work? What if you sense, like so many millions of fat women before you, that this doctor is really hostile?

Get dressed and walk out. It's not you who's crazy.

It's a fact that many doctors can't handle their own antipathy toward obesity. Even if they really don't see overweight as such a medical threat, their own sense of narrow esthetics makes them disgusted with extra pounds. And on yet another level, they may also feel threatened by their own inadequacy in getting you to lose weight. And their own ignorance on the subject of weight.

Dr. Jean Mayer, Harvard authority on nutrition, has written, "Not infrequently, usually dispassionate physicians and dieticians speak of their puffy patients in almost the terms used by proponents of lily-white supremacy for allegedly inferior ethnic minorities. Such a mood has, of course, the useful corollary (from the professional weight-reducer's point of view) that it makes possible projection on the patient of full responsibility for the failure of the program being advocated. Regrettably, it is true that 'weight control programs' meet with only very limited success." This means, of course, that the doctors can foist off the failure of their programs on you. If you don't lose weight, something must be wrong with you—not their diets or advice. A cop-out, to say the least. "Who would want to marry you?" asked the doctor of the prospective wife of Bill Fabrey, president and founder of NAAFA, when she came to him for the required premarriage blood test.

You are entitled to be treated by a doctor who is prejudice-free, knowledgeable about heaviness and willing to concede that there is more than one healthy way to live. If your doctor is down on *big* because of his own limited experience, do not tolerate for one moment his condescending attitude. Find a doctor with whom you can share an adult and working and sharing association. A doctor who can cure tennis elbow without being blinded by pounds.

Doctors Susan and Orland Wooley, psychologists in the Department of Psychiatry at the University of Cincinnati's Medical Center, suggest that physicians might do the following when dealing with their heavy patients:

- Advise the patient of the health risks of obesity but appraise the risk in terms of that individual, remembering that much needs to be learned in this area.
- Refrain from insisting on treatment the patient does not want.
- Try to relieve the patient of undue pressures to conform to social norms with regard to weight.

LIFE AND HEALTH INSURANCE

Having trouble getting it? Ninety-five percent of the big women I've interviewed complain bitterly about the discrimination of insurance companies against fat. But hear this: there are a few insurance companies which are aware that there is *medically no greater risk in insuring a heavy person, provided they are healthy,* and offer policies at normal rates. A pioneer in this kind of life insurance is Tom Nevai, who is vice-president of the Sullivan and Strauss Agency in Flushing, New York. They offer something called the Healthy Overweight Program. Perhaps your insurance company does also.

In terms of *health* insurance, which differs from state to state, if one belongs to a group of five or more in a company, often Blue Cross/Blue Shield and Major Medical policy companies will offer a "guaranteed insurability" plan which asks no medical questions of you. Again, this differs within companies, so check.

Check anyway, and *know your legal rights.* I've done extensive research into the insurance problem and I've come up with one big point: most people foul themselves up because they do *not* read their policies carefully *and* because they are not aware of their rights! Be aware of your legal rights as a consumer and you'll get better results.

For example: Did you know that the information you provide any insurance company as to doctors or past illnesses goes into a huge computer system known as the Medical Information Bureau, which keeps this data for all time? Any policy you wish to buy in the future is dependent on this information. Now, hardly anyone knows this, although it is *supposed* to be common knowledge and the insurance companies are *supposed* to give you this information (but rarely do). But who says you have to feed that computer the fact that you've had a diabetes condition and your doctor is Doctor Smith who can tell everybody all about it? You don't. New York State law (and it is the same in most other states) protects you, and the only way companies and the Medical information Bureau can find out about you is *if you tell them.*

Now, suppose you withhold the information that you've had a heart condition. You buy insurance and, within two years, die of a heart attack. The insurance agency has the right and will probably perform an investigation to determine if you did have the preexisting condition. They can refuse to pay on the policy. But suppose you die *after* you have had this policy for *two years.* In most states, your heirs are safe and the insurance company must pay up *even if you have misrepresented your state of health.* This is known as the "contestability" period.

Take the case of Mr. X who has cancer. The doctors have told him he will probably die within three years and he knows he is terribly underinsured. He feels great guilt at having to leave his family unprovided for. He applies for a life insurance policy and does not tell the company he has cancer or the name of his doctor. The company issues the policy. He dies in two and a half years and his beneficiary collects the full value of the insurance. If he had died before that two years, and the company learned he did have a preexisting condition, they could have refused payment of the insurance. They would, however, have to refund to his estate the total of all premiums he paid to them for the policy.

Is Mr. X guilty of fraud? Of immorality? Absolutely not! Your medical history may hurt your chances of obtaining insurance throughout your lifetime. Insurance companies know only what you tell them in applying for a policy. Once you reveal any information it will always be available to any other insurance company. You have every right to withhold such information.

Too many people, particularly fat women who are emotionally bludgeoned by unfair insurance agents and handicapped by their own legal ignorance, make the mistake of revealing things that their states, by law, do not require them to reveal.

The heavy woman is a victim of great misunderstanding and great uncalled-for prejudice in the area of life or health insurance. But the law protects her, if she will only take the time to investigate and understand the law.

There is a huge profit in insurance for the companies, and you have a duty to protect yourself and give yourself every insurance advantage. You have the right to get a copy of the insurance contract before you sign it. Read it carefully, at your leisure, and know where you stand. Be smart!

More Tips—For You

WHAT DO YOU DO IN YOUR SPARE TIME?

Play. What you play at or with determines your agility and grace. Face it. You are better at a sport, for instance, which requires skill and personal achievement more than it requires speed, strength and fabulous breath. If you're on the basketball or the tennis team, you are not going to be as much of an asset as a size nothing who runs as fast as the wind and can go on forever. But that is no reason for you to be sedentary. Choose a sport *in which you can compete at your own rules, speed and breath capacity.* You can sail, bicycle, hike, bowl, dance, golf, fish, walk and do any other number of things by yourself, or with others, but beautifully and without having pounds figure in your success—or lack of it. Get good, get even great at one thing. There's nothing like consummate skill to add pride and confidence.

BLACK MOOD AND DOWN DAY

It happens. Don't let anyone tell you that eating doesn't solve problems. For a true depression, nothing works like a binge. What follows is a day's menu guaranteed to wipe out the blues.

Breakfast

The Brazil-nut clam spread left over from last night
4 raspberry pancakes
Bran muffins
Chocolate milk

Lunch

Cold cucumber soup
Clams on toast
Tomatoes stuffed with cream cheese
O'Henry bar
Coffee (Sweet'n Low optional)
Handful of Jell-O

Dinner

Banana bread
Chicken livers Marsala
Spiced Persian lamb stew
White rice
Gingerbread man
Wintergreen and teaberry saltwater taffy
Tea

10 O'Clock Snack

Jujy Fruits and milk

X How to Get a Job

The law firm of Gardiner and Reeves needed a secretary. Fast. It looked as if Lauren Klausner was their woman. Her resume that came in the mail said she typed twice as fast as their former secretary, could draw a will and write a contract faster than most lawyers. On top of that, she had the loveliest and most intelligent-sounding telephone voice. Gardiner and Reeves could hardly wait to interview her in person. They all but offered the job over the phone.

The interview day came. So did Lauren Klausner and she was everything she promised—a dynamo, a whiz, an organizer, a creative thinker. She didn't get the job. Betty Lou Kelp did. Betty Lou had never worked before and opened her eyes wide just at the thought of operating the switchboard. But she wore a size-10 dress. Lauren's 175 pounds of talent began pounding the sidewalks. Again.

Unfair? Brutally so. True story? You bet it is. But facts are facts. It is harder for a heavy woman to find work than it is for a thin woman.

Sometimes, when she's lucky, the large-sized woman is a housewife, a feminist, a doctor, a lawyer, an OTB manager, a banker, a teacher, an entrepreneur, a real estate agent, a model, a singer, a writer, a telephone operator, an actress, a dog groomer, a decorator, a bartender. Almost anything. And she's usually very good at it. But sometimes, when she is not so lucky and too many people have said no to her, she does nothing. Or if she does get a job, she is sent to sit behind the ferns in the rearmost office, where no human being ever walks or talks. Limbo. And she's in trouble.

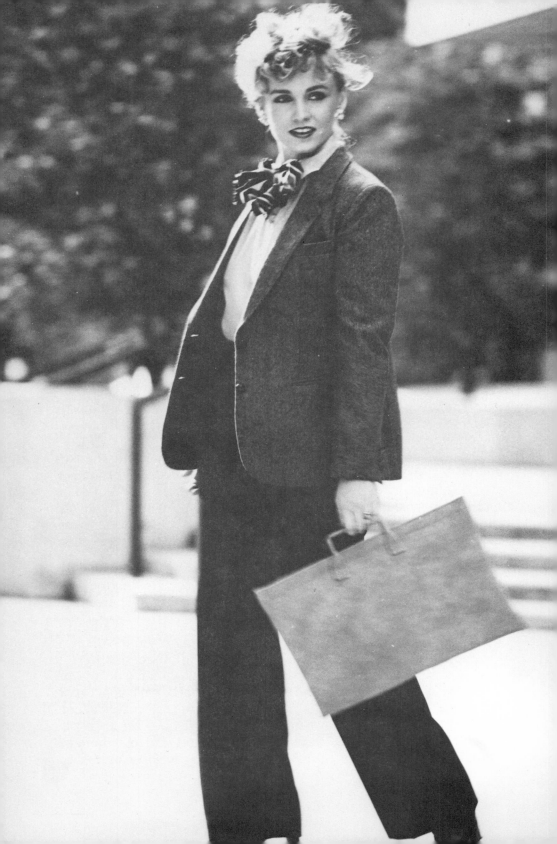

Everybody needs to work at something. Whether you're a home-maker or president of Baskin-Robbins, satisfying, fulfilling work makes for good sleep at night and alert, alive hours during the day. And then there's money. Make no mistake about it, this society judges you on whether you can wring dollars from your talents, and it feels good to know you are capable of bringing home those dollars.

Today, even many confirmed homemakers search for ways to combine their work with lucratively profitable sidelines that hold a promise for the days when children, and maybe even husband, have flown the coop in one way or another. Some of us have long ago given up homemaking as a sole profession and we have happily discovered the enticing world *out there* as a way to involvement and life-style.

Okay, first the bad news. It's tough to get a good job if you're very heavy. Where other walls of bigotry have fallen, the wall of fat rejection has not. Julius Caesar said, "Let me have men about me who are fat," but most employers think Caesar was batty. Everyone knows that fat is lazy and troubled and even stupid—right?

There's a built-in prejudice against fat people, according to Robert Half, owner of Robert Half, Inc., a worldwide chain of em-ployment agencies. "Anything not an advantage can be a disadvantage," says Half. "It's not an advantage for an executive to be portly. Corporations feel they don't have the proper image." He's right. Lumberyards, legal firms and marketing agencies say that their image is projected by who sits at the front desk. And the stigma that fat is bad gives the large woman many miles to go before she will easily be accepted for her worth—which may be considerable. Says Half, "A high-placed executive of one large company once told me, 'Don't send me anyone fat or from Brook-lyn. They both will steal.' Rampant prejudice of the worst kind," says Half. "Our sixty-four offices in the United States, Canada and England all make a point of hiring heavy women if they are quali-fied. It's sometimes a great advantage for the employer to do so precisely because the heavy woman seems to have so much trou-ble getting jobs. You just *know* she's going to be more loyal to you than anyone else."

An Office Temporaries spokesperson said, "It is much easier to get a position for a handicapped, black or unskilled person than it is for an overweight person. People just don't respect fatness. If you're fat, you're weak, and you probably won't do a good job."

And so the stereotypes fly and the biases against pounds remain even though many angry people have taken legal action against companies which they feel are discriminatory because of weight. Not an easy task: even the federal Equal Employment Opportunity Commission (EEOC) does not cover bulk in its charter although they've made many gains for blacks, women and the handicapped.

So much for the bad news. Are you ready for the good? Even though you do not have the inclination to fight political causes, you still should not be denied the right to work productively because there are many ways to go about scouring the existing job market and even creating new markets for your skills. Start out with the knowledge that Americans are definitely getting wider and growing all the time, despite what *Vogue* would have you think. In the early 1960s, the average American woman between eighteen and twenty-four weighed an average of 127 to 144 pounds. In the early 1970s, she weighed between 132 and 146. Prospective employers are getting somewhat used to the subtle increase and are starting to look beyond pounds if the applicant is neat, skilled and attractively aggressive. And things are definitely better for women in general. Many fields, from construction to politics, are opening up, and new attitudes are recreating society's view of women's role and value—which has to benefit the large woman's role and value in particular.

Where Do I Start?

With a list. What do you want in a job? How much money do you need? Will it be part time or full time? Indoor or outdoor? Manual, clerical or executive?

And another list. *What has your experience been? What are your qualifications?* What did you do in college? If you wrote for the newspaper, you probably have skills in copy editing, merchandising ads, layout, paste-ups. If you have never gone to college but have made some pretty terrific dinner parties for your friends, your qualifications may be excellent cooking ability, catering potential, food specialities (can you make the best quiche in town, the most chocolaty brownies, home-baked bread to beat any grandmother's recipes?). On this list should go your education (both school and life). What's life education? You may have learned to care for old people from a father who has aged under your loving and creative guidance; this life situation may well qualify you for a paying job in a nursing home or leisure center, and you surely did not need college anthropology to tell you how to do it. Writing your experience down on paper forces you to zero in, concentrate and come to some decisions as to what's a practical possibility and what's nothing more than dreams or wishes. But narrow down your field. If you've had experiences in a medical field, think about which kind of medicine you wish to pursue. Are you qualified to be a brain surgeon? Is it reasonable to judge that you might be able to obtain training in gerontology, physical therapy, veterinary medicine, research, nursing? Ask around. Talk to people already in a field that looks interesting. What are the rewards? The pitfalls? The hours? The responsibilities? The salaries? Will you mind being awakened at 3 A.M. to care for a wounded monkey? If you would, forget veterinary medicine.

Once You Have Yourself Down on Paper, You Can Start Your Resume

There's an old joke about the animal trainer who owned the best-trained mule in the world. Students of mule training from all over the world would come to observe him, and were shocked to see that before he even started with a novice mule, the master trainer would crack the poor animal over the head with a broad plank of wood. "First," the world's most famous mule trainer would say to his students, "you have to get his attention."

Same thing with a prospective employer. First, you have to get his attention. You want the person who is reading your resume to want to meet you; you want the employer to say, "Now that sounds like a live one." So you list your work experience with decisive and colorful language. Employers are busy, so the shorter and the snappier, the better. Your goal is:

- To make the prospective employer think you were *born* for his job.
- To make the employer think that by your experience, you were *bred* for his job.

Everything in your resume should point to that message. If you're applying for a job as television research assistant, don't list the course you took last summer in accounting.

Your opening should grab. Suck in the reader. If the employer isn't captivated by your resume by the time he's read three paragraphs, forget it. You've lost him. Your hard work lands in the wastebasket.

Your resume should be impeccably typed, with lots of white space showing (do not cram words together on the page). It should be short: the longer the resume, the less the applicant usually has to say. Because you are merchandising yourself, it doesn't hurt to make your resume physically attractive. An electric-color ink, a colorful envelope or folder to cradle it can't hurt. Be businesslike, though: kindergarten designs are not terrific.

There are a thousand books on the market that give examples of the authors' ideas of good resumes. Study a few of them and experiment with several suggestions until you come up with a resume that fits you and will grab an employer's attention. Don't expect to turn out a perfect product, first try. I used up a whole ream of paper until my resume was completed. You may also be told that you can use the same resume for a multitude of different job possibilities. *Wrong!* Sure, the basic information stays the same. Your phone number and name and address are constants. But if you are looking for a job with Avon, you will want to *stress* the fact that you sold encyclopedias door to door when you were nineteen, that you once wrote a beauty column for your local newspaper and that your theatrical experience in college plays gives you an edge on sounding as if you believed in every Avon product. Avon probably won't be too interested in the year you spent as an accountant for your father's firm or your job as a cage cleaner in the ASPCA.

Tailor your resume to the specific job you're looking for, even if you have to type a different version for each application. It pays off.

Every resume should, in one way or another, contain this information:

1. Name, address, telephone number.
2. Educational background. Include degrees and pertinent special courses you've taken.
3. Work experience, including names of organizations and dates you worked for them.
4. Positive results. Make sure you tell about the reorganization you inspired at the advertising agency, the contract the plumbing company was awarded because of your efforts, the new column the local paper began at your urging.
5. Your present job objective (the actual name of the position you want, if there is one) and how you are qualified to fill it.
6. A request to call for a personal interview. Don't wait for them. Say something like, "Unless you wish otherwise, I shall call you on the morning of December 3 to set up an interview . . ."

Don't mention your weight or your religion. They have no place on a professional resume.

A Covering Letter Sometimes Gets You the Job Before Any Resume Is Even Considered

Covering letters should generally introduce, be short and very, very appealing. A covering letter should always be addressed to one special person, usually the head of the department in which you are interested in working. A letter that mentions someone's name has a much better chance of gaining access to that person than one addressed "Dear Sir." The first few sentences, actually, should do the trick. Here are some first lines of three covering letters that paid off with personal interviews because they sucked the boss in with an irresistible appeal.

I work and play well with others, I follow directions, I even *give* great directions; I am dynamic, I am forceful, I am funny. I am Susan Crownmiller, and can you use me in your publicity department?

You will receive more resumes from your job offer than you can ever file. Still, I think you ought to pay particular attention to mine. It is different. I am different.

If people got points for modesty in this world, I would write a modest letter. However, it is hard for me to be modest about what I can offer your firm in terms of outstanding service and research.

Where Should You Look For a Job?

Try the want ads in the paper, but be careful. Any ad that seems to promise you the next-in-line-to-the-presidency job plus the fringe benefits of lunch with glamorous movie stars every day is very likely a come-on.

Trade magazines, newsletters and business newspapers also run want ads, or you can run your own. But again, be careful. Anytime you put your phone number in the newspaper, you are opening yourself up to many crazies who love to get their kicks by calling strange people who are job hunting. Anytime someone calls you from an ad you place in the paper and begins to ask you intimate details about your sexual proclivities, your family or your financial situation—back off fast! Even if prospective employers sound legitimate, check their firm names and numbers in the phone book to see if they are authentic as given, and confirm by calling them back. If you do place an ad in the paper, make it short, attractive and specific as to what you're looking for. Never put your name in the paper: either a telephone number or a box number will do.

Or you can go to a private personnel agency and hope for the best. You can sign up with as many as you wish—no one has an exclusive on your future. Keep calling them to remind them of your availability after the initial interview. And never tell them you'll settle for less money than you think you're worth. (Unless you have an inflated opinion of your worth; do you really think General Motors ought to start you at 100 grand?)

Or you can spread the word among friends and acquaintances that you're in the market for a new job. It's amazing what opportunities people have missed because no one knew they were interested.

Or you can check in with job-counseling agencies which may be sponsored by the job-placement office of your religious affiliation, your alma mater, the YWCA or any number of private counseling agencies.

A few suggestions regarding counseling agencies:

1. Your local chapter of NOW (National Organization for Women) can advise you of opportunities.

2. The *Directory of Approved Counseling Agencies* is published yearly by the American Personnel and Guidance Association, 1605 N. Hampshire Avenue, NW, Washington, DC 20009. These private agencies range in services, testing and fees. You can call the association at 202-483-4633.

3. A nonprofit organization for women specializing in career guidance is Catalyst at 14 East 60th Street, New York, NY 10022. Telephone 212-759-9700.

4. MORE for Women at 2 Lexington Avenue, New York, NY 10010 (telephone 212-674-4090), offers counseling for changing jobs and fields and for reentering the job market after absences of any length.

5. WOW (Washington Opportunities for Women) at 1111 20th Street, NW, Washington, DC 20036, is an agency for any woman of any race or any education (or noneducation). It is affiliated with the U.S. Employment Service.

Good written guides to job finding are:

Merchandising Your Job Talents, U.S. Department of Labor, U.S. Government Printing Office, Washington, DC 20402. Cost 25¢, stock number 2900-0136.

Job-Finding Techniques for Mature Women, Women's Bureau, U.S. Department of Labor, Pamphlet No. 11, 1970, available from the U.S. Government Printing Office, Washington, DC 20402, 30¢.

This Is the New York Women's Yellow Pages, published by St. Martin's Press, New York, is an invaluable source for finding counseling, placement, financial aid and other employment assistance.

Are There Job Markets Particularly Tailored to Heavy Women?

The answer is yes. Have you thought of being a model? No, I'm not kidding. Being heavy is a model job. The top designers are just beginning to design for the big woman and there is a frenzied call for attractive heavy women to model their clothes at fashion shows all over the country. Large-size manufacturers would rather have their clothes filled out by a pretty, heavy woman than have them drip, drop, drape-hang and bag off a size 10. Magazines and newspapers are beginning to show large-sized women in their ads. The pay is fine, you can do it part time, and you will feel gorgeous for perhaps the first time in your life. In fact, many size 14s and 16s have been told they're too thin—what wonderful words! One up-and-coming large-sized model agency in New York City is Other Dimensions at 393 Seventh Ave. N.Y., N.Y. 10001. Top agencies like Eileen Ford are beginning to hire large women to prove that stout can be stunning. You can be into fudge sundaes and high fashion at the same time!

You should know, of course, that being a model isn't the answer for everybody. Most of the women chosen to model do it part time because only the top models make enough to live on. The majority of women who model also type or hold down other jobs to fill in their incomes.

There are many other jobs just for big women. Dress shops catering to the amply figured woman are opening up all over the country. Large department stores like Saks Fifth Avenue and Lord & Taylor want attractive big women to serve as salespeople. As one heavy woman told me, "When I walk into Lane Bryant and a skinny size six tells me she knows what I need, I get furious! How can she know? I'd only trust *another* big woman to wait on me!" You can sell yourself and this reasoning to any intelligent person who hires for the woman's department of your local store.

If you are interested in the women's movement, there are organizations and women's centers all over the country that will bend over backward to hire or place someone who meets prejudice in the outside world. Call your local NOW (National Organization for Women) for details or buy a paperback book called *Woman's*

Work Book by Karin Abaranel and Connie McClung Siegel, put out by Praeger Publishers, 111 Fourth Avenue, New York, NY 10003. It's a directory of career-building women's organizations.

How about my job? You might say I make a great living off the fat of the land, and you can do the same thing in your area. I have eaten myself into a career of free-lance large-sized fashion show commentator. What I do is this: I check with the large-size departments of the local stores and arrange with them to put on fashion shows that do *not* feature undernourished models wearing fantasy fashions. Big women culled from the community walk down our runways wearing practical and affordable clothes, designer clothes and every other kind of clothes, from full size to 18-wheeler. I narrate the shows with humor, I think, and a snappy music background. At our shows we serve food and we do not slap the wrists of the women who reach for doubles in cupcakes. It used to be that a large-size woman who wanted designer clothes had to wrap herself in a Bill Blass sheet: No more. Gloria Vanderbilt, Pierre Cardin and Joseph Picone are among the big-name designers who have jumped on our bandwagon. It's a good job and one that you can create for yourself in Kalamazoo or wherever you live.

You can create your own business and open your own job market by being your own boss. Later in this chapter is advice on how to become an entrepreneur.

Have you thought of show business? Character parts for heavy women are always up for grabs. If you're a little nervous about the real thing, practice with a local theater group first. Television, particularly the smaller stations and cable TV (if your city sustains it), are particularly interesting possibilites. Commercials are a possibility. Acting classes are available in almost every area for beginners and also for people with some acting experience. (The New York Academy of Theatrical Arts, for example, requires no acting experience.) Check with the universities near your home to see what acting courses they offer, if you think the stage is waiting in the wings for you.

Here's a nifty idea: There are millions of heavy teenagers in this country who, along with their families, are aching for personal and career guidance. Who better to help such a teenager than *you*, who have traveled the same route. Find out from your local university what is involved in going back to school for a degree in psychotherapy or counseling. You are bound to be a success if you hang out a shingle as a specialist in counseling heavy teenagers—*not* how to lose weight, as everybody has been unsuccessfully counseling them, but how to make a good life *as they are* (the very point of this book!).

Start a Making It Big group. Jean Neiditch made a small fortune telling people how to lose weight. She had no special degrees, no medical expertise. Thirty million heavy women are just waiting for someone to come along to teach them how to make their lives successful even if they *can't* lose weight. Start a Making It Big group and watch it swell in membership *and* pounds. The trend is to "Size 16 is sexy," "Large is lovely." Be a leader.

There are endless opportunities geared for your size. Protect yourself from inside hooks that hurt, though. Any large-sized woman who goes looking for a job as a representative for a cosmetics industry deserves a doctorate in insanity. She must be realistic and understand that *that* whole industry depends on selling a skinny image. She won't get the job. If she applies for a job with an architect, however, any linear angles he's selling have to do with buildings and not people. She's much safer looking there. And take a tip: when you're out looking for a job, keep it a secret from family and friends until after you've gotten it. You'll feel better about not having to detail each failure (prepare yourself—you won't succeed the first time out!). And you'll feel wonderful about announcing your success when it finally happens!

Preparing for the Interview

Okay, you've located what looks like a very promising job opportunity. Now, how to get it. First, you must prepare for *a personal interview*. Here's how to go about it.

YOUR DRESS

Robert Half says that anyone who comes to look for a job in stretch pants won't get it—at least in any of the firms he deals with. "*No one* should wear stretch pants to an interview and that goes particularly for the big woman—it just looks terrible," says Half. "You must deny the stereotype that fat is sloppy by the way you yourself dress. Counteract your heaviness with your look and your attitude. If many people think that fat is unkempt, *and they do,* you must dress with perfect taste and neatness to put that myth to rest."

Lois Fenton, a professional fashion consultant, says, "Why is dressing so important? Isn't *what* you are more important than *how* you look? Certainly. But it takes months or even years to determine *what* someone is and only a moment to make a first (and often lasting) impression. It may not be fair but it is reality. If a woman wears a too tight or too short skirt to the office, it is obviously wrong and reflects poor judgment. Tight sweaters and pants, see-through fabrics, clinging textures, shocking colors, loud patterns, and seductive vamp sandals are all inappropriate and unprofessional."

The old sexist myth that women make their way to the top by taking advantage of their sexuality is no longer applicable. See-through and low-cut tops are fatal. You will not be taken seriously and you'll never make it past the interview.

As John T. Molloy, author of *The Woman's Dress for Success Book,* puts it, "Women have to decide between bedroom and boardroom." At least for the job interview, that is.

And don't lose your femininity in the effort to be businesslike. Even *Weight Watchers Magazine* agrees with me on this one. "That doesn't mean women should costume themselves in pin-stripe pantsuits, ties and derbies," says *Weight Watchers.* "You don't have to look like the president of IBM to want his job."

What you wear should depend on the job you're seeking. If you're going for an interview with a big law firm, the magazine recommends Molloy's favorite outfit, the skirted suit. If it's one with an advertising agency, "a more stylish outfit may be in order. Try to find out in advance how the people at the company dress."

The article quotes Carol Rivers, an advertising executive, on her secret for dressing for work: "Stand in front of a three-way mirror. Close your eyes, then open them. If anything immediately draws your attention, take it off or change it."

A carefully selected interview wardrobe pays off *more* than a twenty-pound weight loss. Conservative seems to be the best clue:

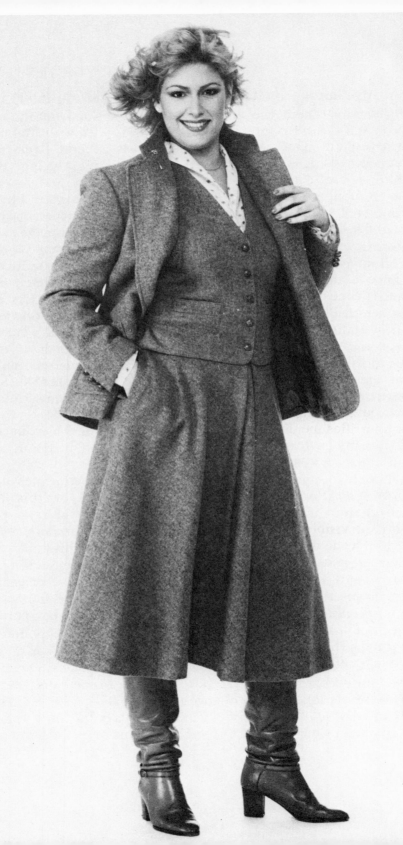

conservative but with panache! Navy-blue tents say blah, but put a stunning scarf on a navy-blue tent and you've just added *style*. No large woman should *ever* wear anything too tight—especially to an interview. Same goes for short dresses, far-out styles and low-cut blouses. If your taste runs to six rings and four bracelets clunking on each hand, leave the rings and bracelets home for the interview. (And probably forever. Big women look bigger in multiple layers of jewelry.) It seems silly to mention, but black-velvet flared pants, sandals that show off your purple toenail polish, and a feather boa are not terrific at the interview. Do not wear anything that makes you feel strange or uncomfortable. Try your outfit out at least once before the big day. You need all the assurance and self-confidence you can muster. Authoritative elegance gives a "thoroughbred" look. What is great for an interview? A tailored, well-made suit in a solid, darkish color or a subtle tweed; a blouse of silk or cotton with sharp lines and no froufrou laces or bows; a simple A-line dress with a good, "quiet" piece of jewelry (no costume stuff and no gaudy numbers). You are *not* interested in being the most fashionable and trendy interviewee of the day. Robert Horton, president of an advertising agency, has said, "Too much fashion terrifies me. I'm always afraid a fashion plate has her style more than my business on her mind."

NERVOUS STOMACH?

If you are visibly and horribly nervous with twitches and hands shaking and the whole works, ask your doctor for a mild tranquilizer to relax you. I'm not a believer in unnecessary drugs, but I see nothing wrong with a woman taking a calming precaution before an important interview. I'm not talking about three fingers of Scotch, which may not smell so reassuring to the prospective employer, or even three Valiums, which will promptly put you to sleep during the interview, but something milder and in between just to take off the terror.

And one more thing: if I ever get terribly nervous during an interview, I repeat this magic formula to myself: "One hundred million Chinese don't give a damn!"

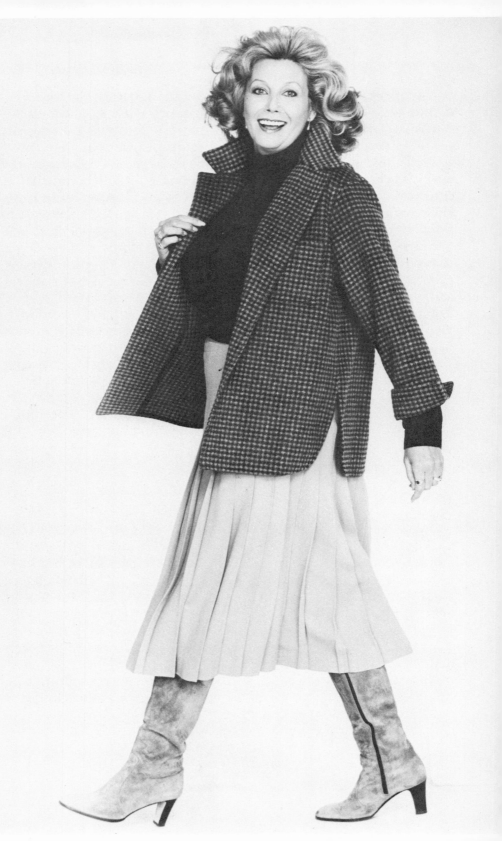

WHAT DO YOU SAY AT AN INTERVIEW?

Well, first of all you do *not* say, "Oh, hello! I'm pleased to meet you, and I'm so grateful you would give a clumsy, overweight thing like me a chance." Naturally, you would never say that, you are thinking. But don't be so sure. Sometimes your manner and what you don't say verbally are enough to radiate shame and defeat and get you a polite but definite refusal.

Walk in with head held high, with body held tall, with stomach held in (if possible) and with a warm smile on your face. Walk in with pride and dignity. Try walking around your house and ask whoever lives with you if yours is a walk of pride and dignity or one of shame and fear. Seriously! Your *presence* as a large person can be powerful or pitiful. Offer a firm handshake, making sure your hand is not (a) sweaty, (b) dirty-fingernailed, (c) limp. Women *are* allowed to offer a hand even if one has not been offered to them first.

Listen carefully to the interviewer's questions. Take your time answering them, thoughtfully. Use humor if you can, but never giggle nervously. Ask your own questions (which you have carefully prepared beforehand). Robert Half says to make sure you deal with any unspoken prejudice your interviewer may have against fat by subtly responding to the *unasked* questions. For example, a common fallacy shared by many employers is that big people are slow. Make sure you say at least two or three times during your interview that you are *not* slow or lazy—not in those exact words, of course, but in unmistakable messages, like, "I usually get more done in two hours than my co-workers do in six." "I've been a career woman all my life—I can't imagine not working hard."

Most companies like to hire healthy people, and they have been told by their insurance charts that fat is unhealthy, says Half. So be sure to insert in your replies something like, "I've only missed two days work in ten years." "Naturally, I do not advocate lying," says Half, "only putting your best, and healthiest, foot forward. Your prospective employer should come away from the interview thinking it will be to his distinct advantage to hire a big woman. It *will* be, also. Statistics have shown that heavier people are far more loyal to their employers than thin people. Perhaps because *getting* a job is not as easy."

Analyze the characteristics you think the interviewer is looking for. If you're looking for a job in a secretarial pool, aggressiveness and originality may actually work against you. The interviewer will probably think you're overqualified. But if you want to be a market research expert for General Foods, aggressiveness and originality might be just the ticket.

Dr. Arthur A. Witkin, chief psychologist of Personnel Sciences Center in New York, says, "If you want a job managing a group of taxi drivers, you need high aggressiveness, but that same amount of aggressiveness in a job managing a group of accountants will turn into oversupervision and will antagonize everybody." A conscientious, loyal person might be rejected as "unlikely to have imagination" in a creative arts organization. You can make your best impression if you're prepared and know what to expect.

One-word answers are calculated to drive interviewers crazy. Also verbose and rambling answers. Be specific and don't waste the interviewer's time by asking where the paperweight on his or her desk came from, although it is not a bad idea to get prospective bosses to talk about their favorite subjects or problems in the field. A lot is known about you from your resume: establishing a more equal footing by finding out something about the boss is often a good psychological ploy. Doing your homework before the interview consists in finding out about the article that appeared in *Time* magazine about the person or the field. Asking knowledgeable and leading questions shows perception and judgment.

It probably won't happen, but what if prospective employers come right out with an anti-fat statement? It is, after all, what they're thinking then, and should be dealt with accordingly. "Look," someone may say. "I see you're qualified but I'm afraid, honestly speaking, you may be just too heavy to move around our offices easily. You might tire easily and you just might project a wrong image for our company."

You *must* deal with it just as bluntly as they do. Humor helps and so does positive reinforcement of your own reliable track record: "I can make it easily around the office as long as no one is chasing me. I was the best waitress Schrafft's ever had, and you know how tiny and close together *their* tables are. And images are made by neatness, intelligence, friendliness and helpfulness, not by pounds. I guarantee you I can make your customers want to come back because they are welcomed so graciously. Fortunately, I don't add with my pounds so your bookkeeping is safe. And believe it or not, I take no longer than a size eight for lunch."

And there, it's out and dealt with! So if the employer does mention your weight, don't let it hang there like a major obstacle between you: clear the air; set the fears at rest! Say, "If you hire a skinny little person, she'll probably be nervous and edgy and cry a lot. I smile a lot. I have a marvelous health record and there's no fat in my head."

You almost force the employer to think, "She's not really *that* fat—and she's fun!" You've relaxed the interviewer; won the battle and the job.

Some other points:

- Don't overuse words like *great, wonderful, marvelous;* try practicing with words like *extraordinary, compelling, singular.* A varied vocabulary adds depth to your personality.
- Avoid cliches. ("I love people.") Who comes to an interview saying she hates people?
- Merchandise yourself. You don't win Brownie points for modesty. Sell yourself and your strong points. No one will do it for you.
- And watch for body language. If you see the interviewer moving restlessly about or looking at the clock, the interview should be ended. *You* can do it. Start getting your things together, sit up straighter or stand. You can be in control even if you're the interviewee. That shows firmness and direction.
- Watch your own body language. Will you perch nervously at the edge of your chair? Or will you *control* your environment by using the arms of the chair, by sitting back and looking relaxed and sure of yourself? Eye contact is good, but don't make interviewers crazy by never removing your eyes from their face. Staring at the ceiling or at your nails for long periods is disaster body language but it can't hurt to do these things for a minute, giving the interviewer a rest from your eye contact.
- Remember, above all, the logo of one Madison Avenue firm: *"Would you hire you?"*

SALARY, REFERENCES, PORTFOLIOS

Be sure to discuss salary before you leave. Any woman who seems as if she's not interested in her financial worth when applying for a job, gives a childish and nonprofessional impression. What should you ask for? Come prepared with a minimum that you'll actually take tucked away in the back of your head. Then *ask* for about 10 or 15 percent more. A word to the wise: Any *man* who goes for a job interview with hopes of making more than he presently does, knows he should inflate what he's presently making to the interviewer. It is not immoral, lying or cheating to do this: it's expected in the business world. Most *women,* new at the job market, are too scrupulously honest, which makes them naive and self-defeating. Very rarely does a prospective employer check with a past employer to see if your salary figures are accurate: it's hardly ever done. Even if they did check, they wouldn't be shocked out of their wits at your slightly inflated figure. They would be shocked if the figures matched exactly. If you ask for exactly what you wish to receive, plan on having that amount sliced substantially because the employer *figures* that you've upped your past salary and expectations. That's the art of negotiation. It's as old as the ages. Which is to say you should *never* lie about your experience or ability (well, maybe a slight exaggeration wouldn't hurt), but you should always be realistic when discussing salary. *And realism means the employer expects you will ask for more than you plan on getting.*

When you come to the interview, be prepared with a list of possible references, should you be asked for them. Naturally, be very sure your references will speak glowingly of you. People in the field as well as creditable character references are both acceptable. And, if possible, try to bring a portfolio. What's that? Simply tangible expressions of the kinds of things you've done. Perhaps you've never worked before but you've won two baking contest awards and have had your ethnic recipes printed in the local newspaper. Bring the awards and the newspaper. If you are applying for a job in the advertising or arts fields, bring samples of your work. If you have written, bring copies of published material. If you are looking for a job in a florist shop, bring a sample of a dried or a fresh flower arrangement that is smashing. If you are looking for a job dealing with teenagers or elderly people, bring samples of programs you have devised or used with them. In other words—show and tell! A visual presentation is dynamite!

Tip: Do *not* bring a trunkful of objects or a scrapbook of unrelated junk. Organize your portfolio as neatly as you organize your appearance.

AFTER THE INTERVIEW

Okay, the interview has gone rather smoothly. There is nothing to do but wait because the prospective employers have said they'd be in touch after they finished interviewing the rest of the applicants. Can you do anything in the meantime? You can.

While you're waiting for the decision, it can't hurt to write a follow-up letter. This is not the time to be obsequious or over grateful. They're the ones who are looking for a worker. Just be pleasant and say you were pleased to meet them or you enjoyed your hour together. Show enthusiasm for the organization. Express again your interest in joining that organization and briefly how you can add to it.

Then wait. If the wait is too long, say a week or so, it can't hurt to place another call to find out if the prospective employers have made a hiring decision. If they have not, the call may serve to refresh their memory about your qualifications being better than those of any other applicant.

What's to Do?

That depends on what you want. Let's go through it category by category. What if you're interested in making some fast money but you're not interested in investing your full time and imagination in a whole career? The children are away all day or you have odd days free from your present job and you wish to pick up a little extra cash. You're an actress with an uneven schedule and temporarily not working.

TEMPORARY OFFICE WORK

To be an office temp, you'll probably have to know how to type. According to one temporary office work manager, a junior typist should have accurate typing skills of fifty words per minute: a senior typist should be able to do sixty-five words. Without mistakes. Stenography should be at least eighty words per minute. If you can't type, you can still get a job that requires filing, telephone answering, receptionist work.

Benefits are: No personal commitment has to be made; different challenges of different jobs; very little responsibility.

Disadvantages include lack of benefits like vacation, sick pay and insurance coverage. Also you usually feel like a stranger in a new town. Temporary work is a good way for the woman who has been out of the work field for a long time, to ease herself back; it gives her an opportunity to improve her skills and her confidence. When you decide to take on temporary work, make sure you are clear about three things:

1. The salary offered and how you will be paid.
2. The distance you will be required to travel and the days you will be needed.
3. The nature of the work expected (before you agree to do it).

Sometimes you will meet interesting and appealing co-workers and bosses. Sometimes you will feel like an extra filing cabinet that nobody knows quite what to do with. It all depends on the job.

A PART-TIME JOB

The exciting part of the job revolution for us is that if we are primarily homemakers, we can still work part time and be home for the kids. Jobs that were once not available for us because someone didn't like our sizes are now opening up all over the place, and in the most familiar places. You can be a school crossing guard, a supermarket checkout clerk, a store salesperson during hours that are convenient for you. If you don't want a full-time job and are not a professional person, you can now have your pick of fulfilling "pink-collar" jobs. A great wedge to changing your life-style is to work part time, see how it goes and *then*, if you wish, enter the full-time job market. You can look for a part-time job at the bakery, at the dry cleaner, at the local Woolworth's. You don't need a resume: all you need is to sell yourself—in person.

VOLUNTEER WORK

Don't knock it as a great *start.* Even if you've heard that volunteering is out and making money is in, great emotional and personal benefits can be derived from donating your talents. And volunteer work is often a perfect bridge to a paying job. Take my daughter, Dina. She moved to a strange town and found herself deep in West Virginia without a profession. She had been a social worker in another state, so even though she was not licensed to practice her profession in West Virginia, she became the greatest volunteer in town. She was active on every committee there was. Even though she couldn't make a living at it, she would not be kept out of the field that interested her. At one point she was instrumental in getting a grant for a woman's crisis center. She was so good at doing it, she was offered a paying job, and today she is the executive director of that center. Score one for volunteerism. You have to start somewhere. If you believe in what you do, things have a way of working out. (Incidentally, my daughter is not built like Twiggy.)

SELF-EMPLOYMENT

What follows are ten ideas for your own business and ways to promote them. Check them out. One of them may change your life.

1. *Pet boarding.* First you have to love animals. There is a great need for clean and understanding homes in which to leave Fido or Paul the parakeet while their mothers and fathers are away. You have to be prepared to walk, feed, comfort, sometimes even groom

the little beasts. You have to have a home which is not noted for its meticulous nature. You also have to have a vet on standby call in case of emergency. Mrs. Fisher will be mad as hell if Spot Fisher develops cat virus and is ignored until he expires. You can set competitive rates by checking to see what the local (and often unsatisfactory) kennels charge. You can advertise for customers. There are 64 million households across the country, with two out of three harboring pets. Figure it out. (Once when I left Tao the Siamese with a Ms. Solomon, she insisted I drop her a postcard. To my persistent shame, I did.) *Dog walking* or *pet taxi* services are also viable money-making ideas.

2. If you are incredible in your kitchen and everybody says, "Hey, you ought to *do* something with this," do! *You can give Chinese-cooking or bread-baking or pasta-making lessons* in your own kitchen. Or make an arrangement with a local kitchen or gourmet shop. Figure out your costs and make them back plus a profit according to the number of students you get. You can cater for other people and either prepare homemade buffet dishes or arrange for whole dinners, hiring helpers to serve and help with the cleaning up. *You can write a cookbook* if you come up with an original idea. (A friend of mine wrote the *Day Before Cookbook.*) Write a brief proposal and submit it to cookbook publishers. (You can find them in *The Writer's Market*, a sourcebook of paying markets published by Writer's Digest, 9933 Alliance Road, Cincinnati, OH 45242 and available in your local bookstore.)

If you make the best chocolate chip cookies in the world (how do you think Famous Amos got started?) or the best cheesecake or the best jam, perhaps you can arrange to sell it to a local gourmet shop or department store. You can also go into the Health Salad Office Lunch or the Fried Chicken Picnic Basket or the Mushroom Quiche Gourmet Dinner specialty business. It's funny: when you are known for one smashing food dish, hungry businesspeople and starstruck picnicking lovers tend to find out about it and pass the word. You will probably need a delivery service for much of this. (It can consist of one enterprising neighborhood kid.) You can advertise by putting up notices in lunchrooms, cafeterias and universities as well as the local food stores. *Or* you can think about opening your own little cafe, coffee house or natural foods place with a limited but superb menu, for starters.

3. *Telephone stuff.* If you have to be home because of children, infirmities or other responsibilities, there's a lot of money to be made on your little old Princess phone. Many firms want to hire telephone solicitors: for example, they range from diaper companies, home-improvement firms, market-research firms, fire-alarm-system firms, magazine-subscription firms. For this job you need patience, a strong dialing finger (it may pay to install a push-button phone), a good voice and a selling personality. Look in the Yellow Pages for companies that might be looking for you.

Or, if you get up early anyway and have nothing to do between 6 and 9 A.M., *you can offer a wake-up service.* Some people are funny: despite all the alarm clocks, music-timing devices and clock radios, they need that friendly voice in the morning to make sure they get out of bed on time. *An all-day answering service* is a good business to start if you're home anyway because of illness or someone you have to care for. Clients such as the local roofer, plumber or carpenter list your number after theirs on advertisements, store doors or business cards saying, "If no answer, call this number." Or the phone company can install an extension of clients' phones to yours. This means that after someone rings, say, three times and the phone is not picked up, the call is then transferred automatically to your number.

4. *Do you have a special talent to promote?* Can you *create wardrobes for the big woman?* She's just coming out of the closet, as you know, and she needs help to build up her experience and security in the shopping and fashion field. If you advertise that you will "Dress *anybody* and especially over size 16s," you may find many customers willing to pay for your taste and fashion know-how. You will need to do some research on where the best shops, designer clothes, dressmakers and accessories for the large woman can be found in your community. And while we're in the shopping talent area, can you *provide a shopping service* for harried or unimaginative fathers who, because of divorce or travel, are separated from their children and wish to be reminded and helped with birthday, holiday and other special-occasion gifts?

Or can you *tutor?* Or can you write in italics and make a small business out of *addressing* invitations, announcements, etc.? Or can you offer your *reading services* to old-age homes and blind students? Make sure that it is clear you wish to do this as a business and not as a donation. If you're a *typist* you can type manuscripts, letters, or theses for a nice fee (from 35¢ to $1.10 a page). Or do you have a green thumb? You can rent yourself out as a *plant doctor* (no license needed) or a *plant supplier*. Two local women I know made a thriving business haunting the wholesale plant and flower market and selling at healthy prices.

Do you have a talent for *teaching knitting, macramé or needlepoint?* Check with your local yarn shop to see if they can use you, or operate from your own living room.

Are you a marvelous *photographer?* Go professional with a specialty in houses, kids or animals.

5. *Rent-an-Event.* Bonnie Schachter of New York has made a thriving business out of supplying *things.* She'll supply guests to perk up a dinner party (anything from a hippie to a stockbroker), a man in a gorilla suit for parties or conventions, breakfast in bed for friends or lovers (consisting of champagne, bagels and the Sunday paper), a belly dancer, a puppet show—the list is endless. It's a fun and easy business but you need an indomitable spirit to find events and people willing to be rented—for a fee, of course—and customers who wish to rent your wares. Advertising is the key to success here. Because of the original nature of the business, Bonnie has been able to place blurbs on radio and TV stations and in local newspapers. She puts out a sheet listing about 200 things she will rent to you.

6. Earlier in this chapter we mentioned Making It Big groups, a natural business for the large woman. Weight Watchers started out as a series of homey little encounter-group sessions with people meeting to talk about how they hated to be fat and how they hid the leftover noodle pudding by wrapping it carefully in tinfoil, ostentatiously throwing it in the trash and devouring it later on when no one was looking. The time is ripe for someone to start Making It Big or *Weight Wonder* or *Weight Worthy* groups. You might charge a minimum amount of money to begin with, hold the sessions in your own home and invite guest lecturers. The National Association to Aid Fat Americans (NAAFA) would be glad to send speakers. Writers (try me), fashion experts, etc., would be glad to come to teach how to be proud and beautiful and happy although heavy. The format of women sitting around sharing experiences and successes and failures is a "can't miss." Remember

how the consciousness-raising groups took America by storm in the 1970s? Before you know it, you'll have twenty chapters. Advertise for participants.

7. Are you a *"crafty"* lady? A friend of mine sells hand-painted garbage pails to gift boutiques to sell as "toy bins" for children. Another friend is a potter and is swamped with orders for bowls, flowerpots and giant-sized mugs. I know someone who hand-paints names and scenes and even messages on T-shirts and jeans: she can't keep up with orders. If you can make jewelry, carve wood for bookends, cheese boards, key chains—you're in business with local stores and individual orders as soon as the word gets out.

8. Be a *party planner.* There are some people who just throw up their hands at the thought of their child's sweet sixteen coming up, or the wedding showers they feel obligated to give. Others don't get nervous at the idea but are in the market for original ways to carry it off. If you have always prided yourself on a flair for entertainment, a creative bent of mind, you can start a business that capitalizes on your good taste and organizing ability. This is a business that can easily affiliate itself with other large concerns like a tent-rental company or a food caterer. I've heard of party planners calling themselves The Party Giver and Fete Accompli. You need to educate yourself in the areas of decorations, floral arrangements, music, photography, ethnic customs for weddings, bar mitzvahs, confirmation parties. A good business for an extrovert.

9. *Greeting card jingles.* At least a hundred times a year you say to yourself, "God, what a dumb card. I could do better than that." Well, don't just sit there—do it. There are many companies that buy free-lance suggestions. I list four of them here, but look at the back of cards you think you can compete with to see who publishes them, and give that company a call. Send about five or six or even more samples to each editor and enclose a stamped, self-addressed envelope for the rejection and the ideas returned—or the check. Address your ideas "Attention, Greeting Card Editor."

Hallmark Cards, Inc.
   25th and McGee Sts.
   Kansas City, MO 64141
   (Pays $50 an idea)

Rustcraft Greeting Cards, Inc.
  Rust Craft Road
  Dedham, MA 02026
  (Pays from $10 to $25)
Gibson Greeting Cards, Inc.
  2100 Section Road
  Cincinnati, OH 45237
  ($3 per line for poetry, up to $50
    for other)
Norcross, Inc.
  950 Airport Rd.
  West Chester, PA 19380
  (From $10 to $50)

It's a good idea to number each idea you send so the editor can respond, "I'd like to purchase idea 4, but I'm not interested in 1, 2, 3, 5, 6." Always *type* your suggestions. And get familiar with the market by reading greeting cards whenever you visit the local stationery store.

10. How about a *travel service for the heavy?* It's never been done before, and you can crash the field with suggestions as to which airlines, cruise ships and buses have the most comfortable seating; which hotels are particularly good for this group of people; which resorts, travelers aids and car rentals are recommended for maximum comfort, understanding and reliability. It's a whole new field, really, and you don't need a license. Perhaps you can even con a travel agent or an airline into giving you a job as their expert.

XI Travel

It used to be that we stayed home. Mostly in the kitchen or hiding out with the Mounds Bars in the bathroom. We were uncomfortable with any kind of travel because we always felt too fat, unpretty, unpopular. Airline seats never fit, we sweltered in our polyester pantsuits while everybody else wore gauze, and if we did go to an obscure hotel you might find us behind the potted palm at the pool, hanging out in our "mama" bathing suits—you remember, the ones with the skirts down to the knees.

Now it's different. We're different. Along with all the other options in clothes and jobs that are opening up, we're ready to see the world.

Listen—there *are* some restrictions. You can't go on the donkey ride if you weigh more than 190. And although women, unlike turtles, do not carry their hotels on their backs, sometimes, because of our extra pounds, it sure feels like it. Still, the far places beckon and anyone who can afford to travel is crazy not to. As a matter of fact, if anything is an ego boost for us, it's foreign travel. The good old U.S.A. is probably the only country in the world that worships *thin* so fanatically. Almost everywhere else you go, you will be appreciated and probably even lusted after, for your size. If you have never before felt stunning, delicious or gorgeous, go to Spain, to Israel, to Vienna—go almost anywhere else and you will find people not consumed with diets and weighing and measuring. The farther you get from American tourists, the more you will be admired for your hips, your shapely calves, *yourself*—with flesh instead of bones to touch. And somehow, when you're seeing new things, meeting new people in unusual places, even in our own

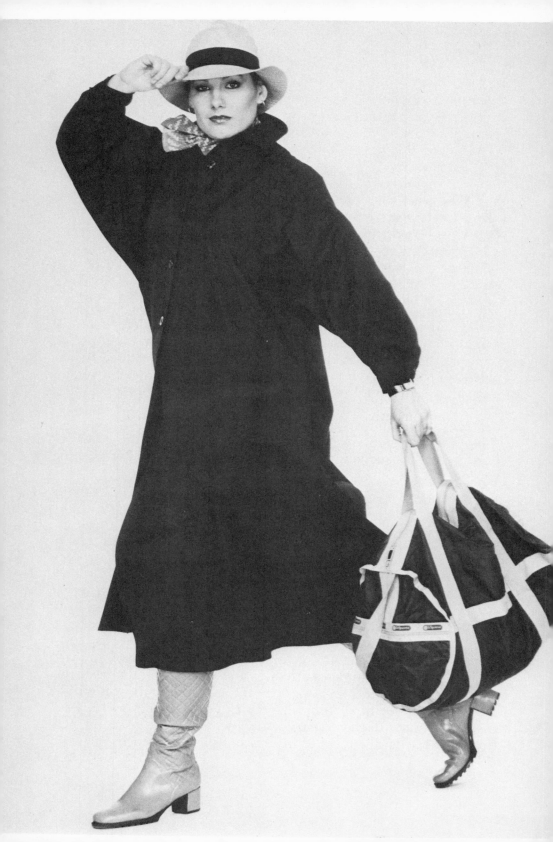

country, the whole issue of *fat* seems to be deemphasized. You're too busy, too exhilarated to pay attention to pounds. And a funny thing happens: if you're relaxed about your weight, everyone else is also. You'll never feel or look better in your life as when you're on the move!

Some general tips to begin with:

1. The only disaster that can crop up on an airplane is if the ticket agent puts two 200-pounders in the same two-seater. But speak up if that happens. You simply have to learn to demand your paid-for rights, and one of those rights is *travel comfort.* Cigar smoking was banned because enough people spoke up. If both of you large-sized people are too embarrassed to speak up and say the seat match is for the birds, you will have to suffer all the way to Pakistan. If you do assert yourself, this is what the airline can do:

- Change your seat to one with a more physically compatible companion.
- Show you how to raise an armrest to provide more room.
- Give you an extra seat. If you need two seats, CAB regulations state you only have to pay for one and a half. But if there happen to be two empty seats on your flight, you may request to be changed to those seats and ask for the refund of the extra half fare you've paid.

(Be sure to request two seats *next* to each other when making advance reservations.) Don't be shy to ask! You don't get a medal for being nonassertive and pain-swallowing. Not one person cares if you're a martyr. Only you suffer.

2. There is no reason why you have to be tortured with a too-tight *seat belt* or risk your life because you're too embarrassed to say the belt's too small. Airlines are *required* to carry seat-belt extenders. Ask for one.

3. If you *feel cramped* on a plane or bus, make sure you've determined exactly where the problem lies. We are apt to be very hard on ourselves. "Oh, boy, I'm so fat, I sure am fat, I'm too darn fat," you berate yourself when your bottom feels cramped. But if you're like me and many other big women, your sense of direction goes nuts sometimes. Even when trying on a dress: if a sleeve is too short, I'll think the neck is pulling. And when my feet are cramped, I could swear it's my fanny. Try stretching your legs out

or taking a little walk when you feel the seat encroaching on your bottom. Sometimes stifled legs are worse than stifled backsides.

4. You have a *right to preview* any bus or train on which you plan a trip. Walk up and down the aisles. Check out the leg room. If you're planning a longer trip, be sure to see if you can turn around, sit down and get out of the postage-stamp restroom. Chintzy bus companies have been known to stint on seat room just to get four extra passengers aboard. Rest assured, the *bus driver* has enough space to breathe. You *pay* for your seat. You're entitled.

5. *Capes* are quite a travel invention. They can serve as blankets, as pillows when folded, and as raincoats. They can disguise you when you want to be anonymous and they discourage pickpockets when you carry your purse underneath. They're loose and they're lovely.

6. We large-size women *perspire* a lot. You may have noticed. *All* our places perspire more than the regular perspiring places in skinny minis. I always carry a package of Wash 'n Dris for my neck, face and hands and a package of Bidettes for the other place. A wipe for every place, you might say. Nothing is cooler or more refreshing.

7. If you wish a special seat or train compartment which will make your large and beautiful self more comfortable, *a letter from your doctor* might add clout to your request.

8. If you have a special medical problem like diabetes or heart disease or a medical allergy and it is conceivable that a crisis might occur in which you could not talk, register with the Medic Alert Foundation International at P.O. Box 1009, Turlock, CA 95380 (telephone 209-632-2371). For a $10 lifetime membership you get a bracelet identifying your condition with Medic Alert's telephone number, where instant information on how to treat the emergency is stored.

9. Use a *travel agent.* They're free because they earn commissions from the airlines, hotels, cruise ships, car-rental agencies and wherever else they book you. Travel agents are among all the other best things in life that are free. Among other services they offer, they can:

- Plan a whole trip for you in a single visit, doing all the leg work, making local and long-distance phone calls.

- Use their clout to get difficult reservations and peak bookings.
- Supply tips and ideas on out-of-the-way places, that perfect little hotel you'll never forget, that cheap and gloriously gourmet restaurant, that secluded beach . . .

If you want to do the trip totally ad lib, a travel agent can still book your transportation so you'll get the most spacious accommodations.

If you don't have a favorite agent, the American Society of Travel Agents (ASTA) at 711 Fifth Avenue, New York, NY 10022, can supply one.

The first thing you have to know before you plan a trip is . . .

How to Read a Brochure

There was this lawyer who rushed to his office every morning, stopping only to put some change into the tin cup of the blind man who, with his faithful dog, sat in front of the lawyer's office building. One morning, the lawyer rushed up to his office and found the blind man drinking coffee from the tin cup and reading a magazine.

"Hey!" shouted the furious lawyer, "I've given you hundreds of dollars, thinking you were blind. And now I've caught you reading a magazine."

"Calm down," said the blind man. "I'm not reading. I'm only looking at the pictures."

Which illustrates something about travel. When you buy travel you buy blindly and, like the lawyer, you may be taken in by lies, promises or even omissions. Looking at the pictures may be a rip-off also. You can decide to go to a magnificent, sun-drenched beach you see in a travel photograph, but only the photographer knows that the picture was taken on the one sunny day in that usually tornado-prone area, with the cactus plants cleverly out of camera range.

Be careful to read between the lines when you check out travel brochures or touring promises. You would never pay for a restaurant meal before it was served or a chair before you sat in it, but you are asked to buy promises every time you travel to a new place. Brochures are promotional material, like commercials, with one aim only—to *sell*. You can easily buy tickets on an airline whose seats will not accommodate you easily and send a deposit to a hotel before you know if it is near or *on* the beach.

Here are some examples of media hype and myth—what they say and, in the second column, what they really mean:

"$45 and up for a single."

It's always "and up." Figure at least $55 for the only single they have left.

"Famous Blackbeard's tower said to be that legendary pirate's private dungeon."

It isn't. It's more hype. Probably the hotel built it last year. Key words are "said to be."

"Day on your own, at leisure."

Whatever you do today will cost extra.

"Explore and enjoy Paris for only $128."

That's how much it costs to go on land exploring Paris. How much does it cost to fly there? It's hard to walk to Paris.

"Luxurious, spacious seating."

For a very thin child.

"See twenty-two cities in all!"

Hurry, look quickly; there went Salzburg. Whoops—there goes London.

"Your hotel will face the aquamarine Caribbean Sea; your gorgeously spacious bathroom (with air conditioning) will have every modern appointment; orientation sightseeing is included free of charge."

Your hotel will face the aquamarine Caribbean, all right—from four blocks away; if you want air conditioning in the mouse-size bathroom, it will be double price, and the door leading to the bathroom will open *in*, effectively blocking the modern appointment, which is a noisy toilet. We will point out the sights on the way from the airport to the hotel for free.

"After dinner you'll be escorted by bus to the theater and then to a native restaurant for a gala meal."

You might have to spend an hour and a half on the bus while it picks up everyone (at twelve different hotels) it will escort to the theater; the native restaurant will be a clip joint for tourists and the gala meal will be chicken and one tostada.

"Only $459 for a week in a lovely stateroom on the S.S. *Huckster.*"

The stateroom is three-by-three with no porthole. You will be nauseated for the entire week.

"Cost of rental car is $110 for the whole week."

Plus gas and mileage charge. Plus supplemental charge for each additional passenger. Plus insurance. Also, the rental car is designed for Tom Thumb.

"Small escorted group."

Small by whose standards? Fifty people doesn't look small to me.

You can see there are many pitfalls. Ask your travel agent or the tour group arranger or the public relations person on the airplane, bus or train you choose *many* questions. In fact, make a list of terrific questions and don't leave until you are quite clear as to what's provided, what's omitted and what you're actually entitled to. Some of those questions might be:

1. Is tipping always included in the overall price?
2. Is the hotel actually *on* or just *near* the beach?
3. Can you obtain a bulkhead or exit-door seat on the airplane for me?
4. What meals are included in the price?
5. If I find the beds in my room are too narrow, can I request a larger bed?
6. Are the seats in the dining room movable or placed close together?
7. How far is town? Will I have to take taxis or does the hotel provide them?
8. Is the price you have quoted me the off-season rate or the rate I will actually pay?
9. Will there be any extras other than those you've mentioned?
10. What kind of automobile comes with the fly/drive trip? Can I get seat-belt extenders? Is it two- or four-door? How large is the trunk area for luggage?
11. Does the hotel have elevators? I notice my room is on the sixth floor.
12. Can I get the special diet I require (salt, sugar-free, kosher, etc.)?

13. What credit cards will be accepted where I go?
14. What kind of clothes shall I bring?
15. Is there any limitation on baggage?
16. Is there a rainy season where I'm going? Is this it?
17. Will there be a doctor available if I become ill?
18. Do all rooms contain a bath and shower? Or a bath *or* shower?
19. Who made the quality ratings in the hotels you're suggesting, an independent source or the hotel manager?
20. Are the rooms air cooled (fan) or air conditioned? I know there's a difference.

Suppose you decide to go . . .

On a Cruise

Sure, a large-sized woman might feel funny about being on a cruise ship where she will be held captive for a week or more with the same people, who may or may not be congenial. But stop blaming your unwillingness to take a chance on your size. The woman who has just had a mastectomy feels funny at first about public appearances. So does the girl who is flat-chested and all skin and bones. So does a stutterer. Or a person in a wheelchair. Or a painfully shy young woman. Everyone's got differences she doesn't love and hasn't yet learned how to cope with. But we are all still members of the human race and everyone who goes on a vacation takes her fears along with her expectations. Maybe you do take up a little more room, but no one but you is looking. You take the same chances on a cruise as anyone else. Listen, you may just luck out with the most interesting people on board while the size 8 who chews gum and talks dumb may be miserable.

Join in everything with zest and anticipation. Who doesn't want to be near a positive and happy person? It's contagious! It is possible that you are not thrilled with your image in a bathing suit lounging around the pool no matter what you read in this book. If so, bring a smashing coverall. Or get your suntan on a quieter, upper deck. But when it comes time for the shuffleboard or the dancing or the "horse racing" or any of the other things you love to do and do well—appear and partake! With joyfulness!

Apologies for size are definitely gauche. If someone compliments you on your great violet eyes, he doesn't need you to say, "Yes, but look at my hips." Mealtimes are also no time to discuss your or anyone else's weight or your noticeable lack of success with diets. Counting calories out loud puts a definite freeze on the party and doesn't do a thing for your image. Taste, try, *exult* in everything offered!

And although you've heard that cruises are splendid for meeting the man of your dreams, don't ever go on a cruise for one specific reason. To meet a man. To get a suntan. To get rid of your headaches. To find the answer to life. If you push for one result, it won't happen. But if you go simply with the idea of having a good time and you talk to everyone you can, take advantage of whatever the ship (never say boat) has to offer, flirt shamelessly with the first mate—you'll have a splendid vacation. Romance does lurk a lot on cruise ships, but if you've come just to meet a man, it's written all over you. You laugh too loud, look too tense and concentrated, appear too anxious to please. Relax. Have a ball. *Feel* that ocean, commune with that night sky. Whatever you're *not* looking for, too hard, you'll probably find.

Absolutely check out the cabin situation while the ship is in port on another trip. You will be surprised to find that sometimes the more desirable cabins (the outside ones with portholes) are smaller than the inside ones. Still, if you have a tendency to *mal de mer*, you'll want to opt for the cabin with the window so you can concentrate on the horizon in times of stress. The ideal, of course, is a large outside cabin. With a large bathroom. There is *nothing* more conducive to claustrophobia than for a big woman to be stuck in a two-by-two bathroom, 100 miles out to sea.

There's no better ship on which to cruise than Cunard's *Queen Elizabeth II*. Besides being the largest passenger ship in the world, (1,700 passengers, 1,000 crew), the *QEII* has space and flexibility in its staterooms and also in its public areas. You do not feel cramped, ever! Food is incredibly lavish, with the finest chefs in the world preparing the most succulent dinners and the most imaginative of desserts.

WHAT WILL IT COST?

What does the cruise price you've been quoted include? It includes the trip, food, room, entertainment, movies, lectures, sometimes wine. If the price includes tips, some people add more anyway for especially good service.

It does *not* include drinks, sauna, massage, steam baths, anything you do in port, beauty parlors, gambling on board. Tipping is expected. Ask your travel agent to give you an idea of the going rates for your particular ship.

Some of the biggest cruise lines are listed below. Also know that some cruises are sponsored by schools like the New School in New York City. You can actually get credit for a sail-and-learn session. On Prudential Line's South American cruises, passengers are briefed to spot whales, dolphins and sea otters as the ship cruises through the Straits of Magellan. The data gathered by the passengers is part of a zoological project conducted by Chile's Institute of Patagonia.

Cunard Line
  555 Fifth Avenue
  New York, NY 10017
  212-983-2500
Flagship Cruises
  522 Fifth Avenue
  New York, NY 10036
  212-869-3410
Holland America Cruises
  2 Penn Plaza
  New York, NY 10001
  212-760-3800
Home Lines, Inc.
  1 World Trade Center
  New York, NY 10048
  212-432-1414
Prudential Lines
  1 World Trade Center
  New York, NY 10048
  212-775-0678

Norwegian American Line
  29 Broadway
  New York, NY 10006
  212-422-3900
Oceanic Society
  240 Fort Mason
  San Francisco, CA 94123
  415-441-1104
Royal Caribbean Cruise Line
  903 South America Way
  Miami, FL 33132
  305-379-4731
Sitmar Cruises
  10100 Santa Monica Blvd.
  Los Angeles, CA 90067
  213-553-1666
Carnival Cruise Lines
  820 Biscayne Boulevard
  Miami, FL 33132
  305-358-2501

If you are interested in taking a cruise, write to one or all of these lines, asking for information on cruises being offered around the time you shall be ready to vacation.

If you decide to travel . . .

By Air

When you reserve your economy ticket, request either the bulkhead seat or the seats by the exit or galley doors. These are invariably much roomier on any airplane. On smaller planes, if these seats are not available, request any aisle seat even if you like to look out the window. The extra comfort you will reap by not having to climb over three others to go to the restroom is worth the window sacrifice. If you are flying on 747s, DC-10s or L-1011s, the wide-bodied planes, the middle seats are usually wider by an inch and a half, but you may still feel too closed in, in the center. For a complete list of seat sizes, see the airlines seat chart in this chapter. Airline aisles, for your information, are usually no wider than twenty-two inches.

Naturally, it goes without saying that first-class seats are more roomy in leg and width room than economy-class seats. Also very much more expensive. Keep in mind, though, that the cost of a first-class seat is usually less than a seat and a half in coach.

Get to the airport as early as possible to get the best choice of seats. If the flight is not crowded, ask the check-in clerk to leave the seat next to you empty—to "block it out." This will assure that the seat next to you will be the last seat assigned and if no one claims it, you've got your extra space free.

How do you determine which size seat will be most comfortable? Sit down in an armchair that is not at all spacious—indeed, just snugly okay. Measure the width of that chair at the narrowest point between the arms. Do *not* choose an airline (after checking out our chart) that only has seats *smaller* than the one you've just found barely comfortable. Otherwise, your trip will be most unpleasant.

Be sure to check all your luggage through so you can climb on board the airplane and down and up "thin" escalators at your destination, gracefully. Awkward luggage makes you feel fifty awkward pounds heavier.

Notice that miserable little food tray and how it won't ever rest flat? Tilt your seat back just a little: the wide-bodied planes, in particular, give plenty of space between you and the person in back so you don't end up in his or her lap.

If you are very large, you hate the airplane restrooms as much as I do. Even very thin people have trouble turning around in them. Try to use the bathroom at the airport before you leave. You can also temporarily dry yourself out so you can avoid the bathroom altogether during the flight by drinking nothing for at least six hours before boarding the plane. Upon your doctor's advice, you can take an antidiuretic pill or a medication like Probanthine which reduces bladder contractions and thus discourages urination for a time. For bowel control, don't eat any salads or bran foods for two days before your flight. Lomotil is a medication used to control diarrhea (more colorfully known as Montezuma's Revenge or Delhi Belly) which many travelers get from impure waters and foods. It can also be used to prevent bowel movements during a flight, if your doctor agrees. It is always best to avoid medication, but if the airline's bathroom is a traumatic experience for you because of its claustrophobic size, use the medication cautiously.

The steward or stewardess will bring you everything from magazines and writing paper to chewing gum, beverages, pillows and blankets.

Be sure you do not fly anywhere for at least twelve hours after you've had any dental work like drilling, root canal or periodonture performed. These procedures can leave an air bubble trapped inside your tooth or root canal which, at increased altitudes, will expand and put great pressure on nerve endings. It is also not a terrific idea to fly with a cold because the altitude tends to cause great sinus and head discomfort.

When you make your airplane reservations, do you know that you can request special meals? Vegetarian, kosher, salt-free, diabetic, Muslim, Hindu and cold-plate meals are all available at twenty-four-hour notice and are often better tasting than the regular fare. Eat less when flying because pressure changes can cause indigestion in flight.

Try to book nonstop flights so you don't have to get off and walk interminable extra airport miles to lounges.

If you do have to change planes because you can't get a direct flight, try to stay with the same airline. You probably won't have so far to walk and your luggage has a better chance of staying with you.

It's not the worst thing in the world to be "bumped" if the flight is overbooked, a problem becoming increasingly worse. You may even be placed on a less crowded flight and get paid for it, to boot.

An old cabin-staff trick for doing away with "popping ears" during takeoff consists of yawning and swallowing, followed by pinching both nostrils, closing the mouth and blowing. Chewing gum or sucking candy, which the stewardess will give you upon request, might also help.

We are subject to swollen ankles and nothing does it more than sitting in the same seat on a long flight, which puts continuous pressure on thigh veins. If you have varicose veins, you might be subject to this problem even more than others. Solution? Wear loose, roomy shoes (preferably lace-ups which you can undo if you have to) and walk up and down the cabin periodically.

If you leave home feeling tired, you will probably arrive feeling more tired. Don't work on departure day. Before dressing to leave, take a relaxing (not too hot) bath. Wear loose-fitting clothes because water retention makes the body swell during flying. Sandals are nice to allow your damp, sticky feet to breathe. There is no humidity during flight and the air is terribly dry. Drink at least one glass of water or club soda every hour during the flight *if you can manage the airplane bathrooms.* Exercises to keep circulation near normal and minimize edema (swelling) during flight of feet, hands and legs are these: hold out legs at full length and make small circles in the air; extend both arms and clench and unclench fists regularly: walk around the plane as much as possible.

If you're in for a long flight it's a good idea, says travel author Myra Waldo, to take an antihistamine like Dimetane, that induces drowsiness, so you will be able to conk out for a while. Never, says author Waldo, use the night shades the airlines distribute because they prevent the eyes from blinking (something that goes on even during sleep) and this causes circles under the eyes the following morning.

AIRLINE SEAT WIDTHS
(In inches with arm down)

First-Class Airline	707	727	737	747	DC-8	DC-9	DC-10	L-1101
Air Canada (ARR)		20		20.25	20.9	20		20.25
American	20.5	20.5		21			21	
Continental		21					21	
Delta		17			18.5	29		17
Eastern		20.87				20		20.87
El Al	16–17			21				
KLM Royal Dutch (ARR)				20.5			20	
Lufthansa	28.3	28.7	28.7	28.3			28.3	
National (ARR)		21		21			20	
Pan American	22			21			21	
SAS				21			18	
Swissair (ARR)				21			21	
TWA	20.9	21		21			21–22	20.9
United (ARR OR FAAR)		21	21	21–22	20–22.5		21.75–23.25	
Western	19.25	19.25						

Economy Airline	707	727	737	747	DC-8	DC-9	DC-10	L-1011
Air Canada (ARR)		18		18	16.5	18		18.5
Alitalia				20				
Allegheny*(FAAR)						18		
American**	17	17		17.5			17.5	
Braniff		13						
Continental		17.42–17.66					17.42–17.96	
Delta		17			18.5	20		15
Eastern (FAAR)		17.25				18.5		
El Al	16–17			16–17				

Airline						
KLM Royal Dutch (ARR)					17–18	17–18
Lufthansa		19.6	19.2	19.2	21.6	19.6
National (FAAR)		17.25				17.5
Ozark*** (ARR)						
Pan American	17.25	17.25			17.625	
PSA		23				
SAS					17.5	17.5
Swissair (ARR)					17.5	17.5
TWA	16.8	16.8		17.9	17	18
United (ARR or FAAR)	16.5–17.5	16.5–17.5	16.5–17.5		18.5	18.5
Western	16.5–17.5	16.5–17.5	16.5–17.5		17.52–17.96	

Note:

1. Seat belt extensions available. Request one or more from the flight attendant.
2. Most aisle and window seats are about 1" smaller in economy class than the middle seats.
3. In the first row of each class there is always more leg room.
4. According to CAB regulations, you must pay for only 1½ seats if you require 2 seats. Should there be an empty seat, ask to be seated next to it and request a refund of the extra ½ seat.
5. When you make your reservations, remember there are smoking and nonsmoking sections.

ARR—Armrests removable
FAAR—Foldaway armrests
*Has no first class; all planes 5-abreast seating
**Armrests not removable except in 3-abreast seating
***Has no first class

Chart prepared by the National Association to Aid Fat Americans, Inc. (NAAFA) from information provided by the airlines. No portion of it may be reproduced without permission in writing from: NAAFA, P.O. Box 745, Westbury, N.Y. 11590.

If You Go by Bus

Preview the bus. Don't spend a week in a cramped seat, endure aisles you must walk down sideways and a bathroom that is a miniature horror chamber. With high travel costs abroad and gasoline shortages at home, bus travel can be smart and fun—if the bus is spacious.

Motor coaches offer many kinds of tours in the United States and Canada ranging in length from a day to a month and in price from $15 to more than $1,500 per person.

Greyhound is the biggest. Trailways only offers charter buses and drivers for private groups. Other big bus names in the industry which your travel agent can tell you more about are Bluebird, California Parlour Car Tours, Maupintour, Percival and Talmage. The local Chamber of Commerce can tell you still more about smaller and very good bus tours. When taking a bus tour, remember that besides going the entire way by bus between home and your destination, you can also combine a bus tour with a flight.

Many people feel that buses, if you don't want the responsibility of driving yourself, are the *only* way to see a country. They thread their way through rural villages as well as bustling cities.

Check to see if your bus company has any special promotional fares in addition to the fixed fares for any one particular trip.

What's a bus like to live in, for a while? Intercity buses have two-abreast reclining seats that are seventeen inches wide, at this writing. Check in your own community to see if a local company has wider seats if seventeen inches is not comfortable for you. *Don't hesitate to ask them to measure!* It's your money. They have heating and air conditioning (make sure they're not "air-freshened" or "air-cooled," which is vastly less comfortable), tinted windows to reduce glare, individual reading lamps (like the airlines) and usually a too-tiny restroom in the back of the bus which you simply must try out before you buy. Aisles are generally fourteen inches wide and many of the newer buses "kneel" to provide an easy step aboard if your weight makes it difficult to climb high steps.

On bus tours your overnight accommodations are usually included in the fare.

If You Go by Train

The glamorous and once ubiquitous train has recently fallen into disfavor because miniature seats, shoddy service and dusty windows took over for a while. But have heart. Amtrak has taken over 95 percent of the nation's trains and things are looking up for those who feel the pull of the rails. The newest Amtrak equipment features certain overnight first-class staterooms, for instance, which are almost as large as a small den in your home. These generally are reserved for handicapped people, but if no handicapped persons reserve them (and it happens quite often that they don't), they are released for general sale to the public. Naturally, because they are built to accommodate wheelchairs, they are truly spacious, stretching across the entire width of the train. They're equipped with upper and lower berths and are marvelous for larger women who find most train compartments unbearable. Tell the passenger agent with whom you speak that although being large is by no means a physical handicap, it does call for special accommodations for comfort. A letter from your doctor might also help to reserve these staterooms. Also remember that if you find the seats in the Amtrak coach cars too narrow, you can pay the premium for the very comfortable club car seats. But be sure to get a reserved seat. Amtrak is very popular in these days of gasoline problems. Standing all the way to Kansas City is not fun.

Some sample train rides in this country which are once again alive with promise and even romance are the Broadway Limited from New York to Chicago, the Silver Meteor from New York to Miami, the Panama Limited to New Orleans, the Southwest Limited and the San Francisco Zephyr. There are even high-speed trains like the all-electric Metroliner from New York to Washington.

Think you can get there much faster by plane? New York to Washington by train is three hours, Chicago to New Orleans takes eighteen hours and San Francisco to Los Angeles takes ten hours.

Day coaches have wide, reclining two-seaters. Longer trips, if you don't go for the roomettes, feature leg-rest seats and deep but not-impossible-to-rise-from cushions.

Prices vary with each trip, of course, but Amtrak offers fourteen-twenty-one or thirty-day fare-discount tickets for unlimited rail travel with unlimited stopovers.

Trains in Europe are generally terrific, cheap and efficient. Scribner's puts out a book called *Enjoy Europe by Train* by William J. Dunn (along with many other books on train travel) which lists up-to-the-minute details about train schedules and tips on cheaper fares. The Eurail Pass is the most famous discount number. After you pay a set fare you can travel in comfort for up to three months (depending on the pass you buy) almost anywhere in thirteen Continental countries without spending any extra on rail transportation. It *must* be purchased here from a travel agent or railroad. And if you lose it, forget it. It's like cash. Unlike Travelers Checks, it can't be replaced.

Great train trips exist abroad. To give you an example: check out the Citizens Exchange Corps, a nonprofit organization at 18 East 41st Street, New York, NY 10017, telephone 212-889-7960. The corps arranges trips with the Soviet Union. This year, among other trips, they are sponsoring a ride of 4,000 miles from Moscow to Khabarovsk. You get to travel through nine time zones on this particular three-week trans-Siberian train trip. It costs $1,725 for the trip, all meals, round-trip fare to Moscow and the flight back to Moscow from Khabarovsk.

If You Are Going by Car

You are free as a bird. Just make sure you get a car with seats that are comfortable for a large-size lady and seat belts that fit and there is nothing, *nothing,* you can't see!

Ten Travel Money Savers

1. If you are a student, contact the Council on International Educational Exchange (CIEE), Charter Department, 777 United Nations Plaza, New York, NY 10017, telephone 212-661-1414, for the *lowest fares anywhere!*

2. Trips off season are always cheaper. Paris is still swell in September. Even sweller. You perspire less in September and that's no small thing for big, beautiful women!

3. "Bed and breakfasts" (usually in lush and local farmhouses) are available throughout Ireland, England and other countries. They offer not only the best local food, the softest feather blankets and the rollingest countrysides but the most wonderful way of meeting the people. It is simply more comfortable for big women, as a rule, to stay in someone's home than in a dwarfed hotel room. Ask a local policeman or shopkeeper about "bed and breakfasts."

4. Choose lodgings somewhere out of the city; hotels ten miles from Rome are ten times cheaper. Even cheaper are accommodations with friends and relatives, whom you should always look up when in a foreign country even if you find them slightly boring at home. Any lodgings that are not with friends should be inspected first: what if the sheets have brown stains on them? What if the room smells of the last twelve occupants? What if the bed is built for Twiggy?

5. Always carry credit cards. Car rental places, for instance, will not give you a car without a card until they can run their own check on you—which could take days and extra dollars. Bank cards, American Express, Diner's Club and Carte Blanche are the most useful cards.

6. Buy discount tickets for trains and museums *before* you leave for Europe. Ask your travel agent for details.

7. A loaf of bread, a jug of wine and a hunk of cheese are more delicious and cheaper than Maxim's for lunch.

8. Check into exchanging houses: you give your house or apartment for a month to a nice English couple who, in turn, give you theirs. No fee to do either. For other interesting travel options, check out Servas at 11 John Street, Room 406, New York, NY 10038, or Traveler's Directory at 6224 Baynton Street, Philadelphia, PA 19144. For a small fee, these organizations have members who put up affiliated travelers in their own homes. Traveler's Directory requires you to be equally willing to host other members in yours. Servas does not.

9. Never go first class on European trains. It's cheaper not to and you don't even get to meet the *real* people that way.

10. Plan ahead. Cars should be reserved in advance so you're not

stuck with the overpriced, skinny jobs. Hotels should be arranged so the largest rooms and beds for the price are your choice. Cruise ships have certain economy rooms which are still quite roomy, but the longer you wait, the less chance of getting them, you have. Talk to people who have been there, while planning, for money-saving tips.

XII Sex and Sensuality

Big can be very beautiful in bed.

Too many women, thwarted and oppressed by society's impli-
cations that they are ugly, turn themselves off as sexual people.
Their desires, their sensuality, seem to them almost obscene,
somehow superfluous. They are afraid that their lust, their sexual
movements, even their expressed affection will be embarrassing to
them and their sexual partners. The best they can do, they feel, is
to be grateful for any attention at all. To demand equal time, equal
pleasure, is not only ungrateful, it's grabby. They think that when
they initiate sexual advances, they seem clumsy. Sex becomes
something graceless, to be gotten through guiltily, if at all, like a
double-fudge ice-cream sundae.

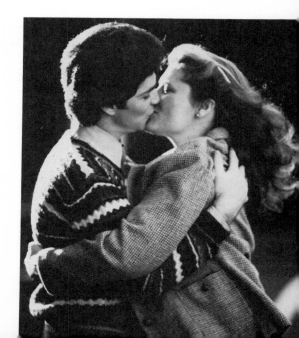

Wrong, wrong, oh, *very* wrong. If you are heavy and any of these feelings strikes a familiar bell with you, it's time to yell *stop* to your own libidinal destruction.

It is true that the current cultural attitudes against pounds have inhibited the heavy woman from expressing herself sexually. Even worse, we suffer from unnecessary plagues of guilt and feelings of inadequacy. Too many of us equate romance and love with thinness à la the current cover photos of *True Romance.* And when we feel unbeautiful and unsexy because we are not thin, what do we do? To compensate for the sexual frustration, we eat. Even when our lovers and mates do not mind our pounds, we still do it. We find ourselves whomping up excuses of tiredness, illness and "the children are up" to avoid sexual participation.

It is really crummy that we are not proud of ourselves in bed, that we find distasteful the thought of our flesh being sexual. It's so crummy that anyone who doesn't do something about her feelings has only herself to blame.

If we can learn to run IBM machines, be successes at parties, be brain surgeons, be mothers, be *all* things we have already proven we can be, we can also build our sexual self-esteem. If you have buried lust in your craw for so long now that you think you're lustless, look again. It's there, waiting to spring free with glorious relief.

How do you do it?

Start with learning to touch, respect and like your own anatomy. Experts tell us that what you say to yourself has a distinct relationship to how you feel. Those who think they are clumsy, sexless and unappealing often carry on internal dialogues loaded with negative references. Change that. Psych yourself up into feeling desirable and lovely. Stare hard for three whole minutes at your naked self in a full-length mirror. Run your hands over your body—you're allowed to, honest! Feels soft, feels good, doesn't it? That's how it feels to someone else, also. Tell yourself, "I am as beautiful as anyone else. Actually, I am delicious. I am wonderfully wise and witty in bed. I am touchable and I react to touching. It feels nice." Turn slowly and observe your naked image. Think of the pounds as voluptuous planes instead of the excess baggage *Vogue* labels it. Look at the changing landscape of your lovely form. Forget about everything else you've been told about hard angles, flat-board stomachs and chickenesque body profiles. Who says that's pretty? People who want to sell diets, that's who. Look at *You!* Appreciate your erotic and full self. Love your own capacity for loving.

Waiting for Prince Charming to come along to give you pleasure? Don't. You are responsible for your own orgasms, let alone your positive psyche. There *is no* Mr. Right in the wings ready to turn you on. In sexuality, a woman must be able to turn herself on first, with her own attitudes and self-knowledge. She must be secure enough to ask for what feels good to her. Before she can accept good feelings and vibrations from others about her sumptuous body, she must center her own attentions on that body. And then, somehow, Mr. Right comes, *not* from the wings where he has been waiting, but from your everyday life.

So self-experiment. You've been walking around with your body for a lot of years: are you totally familiar with it. Do you know where your clitoris is? Do you know what your hair and lips feel like? If you feel uncomfortable with the size of your body, rest assured that discomfort will communicate itself to your lover. A woman who is hesitant to touch even her most private parts, her own breasts, her vagina, will be uncomfortable when her husband or lover touches them. So get to know *you.* Touch yourself, exploratively, gently, as a lover would. When you do that, do you touch sweetness, softness—or something ugly? If *you* think it's ugly, who can think otherwise? But you can train yourself to see beauty in your body, even if you never have before. The more you know yourself—the way your body moves when you dance, the way your eyes look when you're feeling love—the more intimate and desirable you will look to someone who cares.

Only when you recognize and understand what makes you feel good, what there is to cherish and respect about yourself, can you easily transfer this self-cherishing to sharing with someone else. Your rounded and marvelous self is a wondrous thing in bed. Believe it! It is not to be ignored, glossed over, denied. You have a natural capacity for physical pleasure, as natural as your capacity for abating hunger and thirst.

You might be interested in some statistics to help you build your sexual self-esteem. They're on your side. Those who think of the amply endowed woman as a mother image and not as a sexual being will be surprised to learn that researchers at Chicago's Michael Reese Hospital found that fat women have greater and not lesser sexual appetites than their skinny counterparts. Amateur psychologists have been brainwashing us for years with the fiction that we got fat to *avoid* normal sexual relationships—who wants a chubby woman? The *truth* is that in terms of erotic readiness and general sexual excitability, fat outscored thin two to one. In a recent study at Harvard Medical School, it was discovered that women who have the greatest difficulties with weight problems average consistently *higher* scores in femininity on personality tests. So scratch the stereotype that women who are fat are not feminine or sexually interested. In more graphic illustration of the latter, another study—of young thin and young fat lovers—showed about the same frequency of sexual intercourse (about nine times a month). The difference was that the heavy women said even more would be very nice, while the bony, thin women said they'd had quite enough, thank you.

In her enlightened book *Fat and Thin, A Natural History of Obesity*, Anne Scott Beller says that not only do fat women have "heightened sexual readiness" but they probably have "a particular penchant for pair formation"—which means they appreciate one husband or one lover more than fooling around with the multitudes.

What about caring and love? Do they have anything to do with sex? With us, anyway, they surely do. (I cannot speak for the thin, ascetic types.) We are a giving, devoted group. We cherish our partners and we know how to share. Our very bigness connotes warmth and affection. Our sexual unions are usually deep and lasting because we love deeply and because we usually seek more than just temporary stimulation. We are, for the most part, devoted lovers.

How come everybody loves thin? They don't. Twentieth-century America is in a distinct minority in pushing thinness as an erotic ideal. In a historical and worldwide vote, most people still opt for round. It makes sense. Round is warm and lush and grabbable and erotic. Bony is polite and hard.

Beller states that "a strong presumptive case for the general desirability of fat women can be made from the ethnographic evidence; of a total of twenty-six tribes from all over the globe who have ever put on record as expressing a preference in the matter, only five preferred their women slender."

The European, Middle Eastern and South American cultures also admire and desire the rounded curves of a woman who looks like a woman and not like an adolescent boy. American culture stands almost alone in its twentieth-century skinny worship. But knowing that is not much help if America is where you happen to live.

So after you raise your sexual self-esteem by concentrating on admiring your own body, try to raise the consciousness of the people around you. It really can be done by making yourself a model image of neat, chic, pretty, caring and sexually attractive. If you are in the habit of going to the supermarket in curlers and stained jeans, very few people will think of fat as adorable. If you take special care of your image, your hair, your skin, your clothes, as outlined in this book, you can't help but upgrade the image. A sweet-smelling, marvelously dressed, intellectually aware woman who knows in her heart of hearts that she is a sensual creature will invariably attract others sexually.

Here are some things to know about the sexual experience as it applies to the big woman.

Sex is *good* for you. Look at your skin after orgasm. Your complexion absolutely thrives on sex! The orgasmic flush has sent all that blood racing toward your face, spurring on your circulation, lowering the blood cholesterol level and making you look delightfully fresh and renewed.

Dr. Abraham Friedman, an expert in obesity, says that sexual intercourse has the added benefit (not that it needs any added benefits) of using up approximately 200 calories plus whatever you'd have eaten when you weren't making love. Not that you'd care, but it is interesting to note that regular lovemaking can create a weight loss of four or five pounds a month. Dr. Friedman also points out that sexual activity helps get rid of excess fat deposits because it results in an increased production of fat-destroying hormones such as the pituitary growth hormone, epinephrine, and thyroid. "If you reach for your mate instead of your plate," Dr. Friedman says in his book *Fat Can Be Beautiful*, increased sexual activity promotes weight loss because you substitute the emotional need of eating with another, less fattening emotional need. Sexual activity is not to be equated with jogging in terms of exercise, but then again, it's considerably less boring and easier on the feet.

If there is a universal American complaint, it is the common backache. Whether it comes from towering heels, slipped discs, overweight or posture, one thing is for sure: coitus cures it. The arching of the back during sexual activity, the involuntary and voluntary contractions of the pelvis and back muscles, the action of the spasmodic jerks and the relaxations, the tensions and the letting go of the tensions, all seem to miraculously ease the back that's been naggingly aching all day. Heatings pads are nice, whirlpool baths are lovely, massage is delicious—but for instant back relief, make love.

Do you have arthritis? At last, an antidote for pain: Dr. Jessie Potter of the National Institute for Human Relationships in Chicago recently told a meeting of the National Arthritis Foundation that sex can temporarily alleviate the pain of arthritis. It seems that sex stimulates the adrenal glands to produce additional cortisone and "this alone provides from four to six hours of relief from arthritic pain."

Too many orgasms at one time (it should only happen) *can* be tiring, but in general intercourse builds strength and vitality. Sex when practiced regularly rejuvenates interest and capacity for more sex. Masters and Johnson say menstrual cramps, often a problem with large women, are wonderfully eased by intercourse. Dr. Alfred Kinsey says that the pulse rate of a sexually aroused person increases from a normal 70 per minute to as much as 150 per minute: that's great exercise, equal indeed to an athlete's pulse rate at the top level of his exertion! Alfred Meier, a zoologist, concluded in his Louisiana State University studies that people who want to lose weight ought to make love and follow it with a little nap. Can it hurt? No! It's *good* for you.

And finally, some words from Dr. Barbara Edelstein's book *The Woman Doctor's Diet for Women.* "Being overweight does affect a woman's sex life," says Dr. Edelstein, "but not in the way or to the degree you might expect. The women who are the least overweight report the most trouble with their husbands. The women who are less than twenty pounds overweight seem to have more sexual problems with their husbands than women who are more than twenty pounds overweight."

Edelstein also declares that men with thin wives "generally expect them to stay that way and get turned off if their wives become heavy." Men who marry fat women, however, "seem to stay relatively interested in their wives sexually no matter how much they weigh."

Good sex, then, means good physical and good mental health. There is a kind of nonviolent revolution growing in the groins of enlightened big women which says there is nothing ugly or ungainly in weight. Sexual freedom means not locking women into beauty stereotypes and modes of behavior dictated by the amount of pounds you carry. If anyone tries to intimidate you into being less than you are sexually, fight back—with the truth of your great self.

Down to basics: sometimes a stomach, cute as it is, does get in the way. There are a few sexual positions for the very big woman which make intercourse more satisfying. Any position is good if it works and is mutually satisfying. Nothing is wrong or prurient if you are both adult and you both like it. In fact, it is delightful to be inventive with sex. Make sure, as I said, you *both* like it. Do not suddenly pour a Rocky Road malted over your partner's abdomen unless you have mentioned it and received permission first.

Some suggestions for sexual attitudes:

- If he twists his hips slightly to one side he can enter her from behind. They fit like spoons, and his hands will be free to caress her breasts and clitoris.
- She lies on her back with her legs bent at the knees and her thighs spread wide apart. He lies on top and between her thighs. She places a pillow under her buttocks which makes vaginal entry much easier.
- He lies on his back and she squats over him in a backward sitting position. He inserts his penis from the rear, avoiding abdominal contact.
- He can lie comfortably on the bed and she can straddle him on her knees as his penis is inserted into her vagina.
- After attaining insertion in the "missionary" position—man on top—the woman closes her legs and the man moves his body in a 45-degree angle so together they make an X. Again,

abdominal contact is avoided, making sexual pushes and thrusts somewhat easier and more satisfying.

People are enriched when they feel free to experiment sexually. They have a responsibility to provide their partners with pleasure, but they have a right to expect pleasure themselves.

Speaking of partners, of great interest to the heavy woman is the question "Can a slender man ever find me attractive?"

The question is worthy of research.

I started at a dance of The National Association to Aid Fat Americans (NAAFA). Guess what? Many, many young, good-looking, *slim* men attended.

Aha, thought I. *Kinky guys for kinky stuff.* Wrong.

Losers. Wrong again.

They were your average, bright, aggressive, right-thinking kind of guy. Why were they at a dance for fat Americans when they were not in the least fat?

They liked bigger women. Simple as that. And they were tired of being thought peculiar and yes, kinky, for that sexual preference. I interviewed many of them.

Jim (tall, crinkly smiling attorney): "Believe me, I've thought this thing out. I've talked to good friends, analysts and have done an inordinate amount of reading on the subject. I've come to the conclusion that people are individuals who do not always conform in tastes. I am healthy, sane and happy and I like bigger women."

Randolph (bald, sweet and funny): "Do I love a fat woman because I think I can't make it with a thin woman? Nope. Sure, there must be losers in our rank. And men who are driven by a need to be unusual, different. Three-legged women would turn them on also. But me, I'm just a good-natured fellow who definitely would not care for three-leggers but who finds big women tremendously appealing. I married Ruth, here, when she weighed sixty pounds less. Now that the kids are grown and we are freer to concentrate on ourselves, our sex life has grown greater along with Ruth's weight. And I'm happy about it! We both take good care of our appearance and our health. Nothing has changed except Ruth's pounds. We're the same us. We still court each other, and I find her infinitely more desirable with the weight gain. I don't know why. Just lucky, I guess. We are both very involved with this organization because of what we perceive as a real prejudice against heavy people."

Harvey: I'd like to see a *Playboy* centerfold that folds out. Folds out. Folds out. Folds out . . .''

What kind of organization is NAAFA? I spent an evening talking to William Fabrey, the president and founder of the group, which has grown to nationally respectable numbers. We spoke in the living room of the apartment he shares with a terrific big woman.

He's a young and preppy-looking, blond guy with horn-rimmed glasses and a considered, thoughtful way of answering questions. After studying at two of America's finest schools, Cornell and the Rochester Institute of Technology, he became an engineer who spends his days trying to find cures for air pollution. As a citizen and a very human being, he is also spending a good bit of his time trying to wipe out another kind of pollution—prejudice pollution. Why do so many people resent fat and why do fat people themselves think of their bodies as ugly and even weird? He wants to know.

There's nothing weird about Fabrey, nor even remotely kinky, even though he is what he himself calls an F.A.—fat admirer. He has a wry and delightful sense of humor and probably could have his share of size 10s battering down his door, if he so chose. He does not choose. He is sexually attracted to big women although, to paraphrase a cliché, many of his best friends are thin. Here's some of our conversation.

Question: Let's ask the question right out without embarrassment. Isn't it odd and more than a little peculiar to prefer fat women as sexual partners?

Answer: To question the idea of admiration for fat is to completely overlook the generations of humans who feel and felt differently. My own grandfather married my grandmother when she weighed 170. If she were any thinner, he would have thought her a consumptive. Those were the esthetics of the age. One esthetic standard of taste is no better or worse than any other, just different. If I admired slender women, my taste would not be suspect. If I said I was turned on by brunettes, many men would nod in complete understanding. If I said that I was a "leg" man or a "breast" man, I would not cause a flap. Why then am I considered peculiar if I like fat women? Why should your set of esthetic standards be more socially acceptable than mine?

Question: Have you always felt the same way?

Answer: When I was a young adolescent, I noticed that all the girls to whom I was attracted were fat. I had to come to terms with my desires and sexuality as soon as I realized I had uncommon tastes. Maybe I *was* weird, I thought. What kind of conclusion can a kid form when he looks around and there's no mention of his needs anywhere? I began researching art and history and I found out that in every previous era, and in some places in *this* era, fat was considered beautiful. It made me feel that instead of there being something wrong with me, I was merely born in the wrong century. Small comfort for a sixteen-year-old. Actually, when I came to terms with this, I also became somewhat of a rugged individualist. You can't have a minority taste without being a rugged individualist. So I guess, in answer to your question, yes, I seem to have always felt that big women are more desirable than skinny women.

Question: How did your parents and your peers react to your growing sexual tastes?

Answer: There's an old saying (we make up a lot of old sayings in our organization): "Try bringing a fat girl home to mother . . ." My parents, through a lack of understanding, exerted a lot of pressure on me. They truly felt there was only one standard of beauty, at least with regard to weight. It took years for my parents and me to arrive at an understanding about esthetics and personal choice. Meanwhile, I dated fat and slender girls throughout high school and college—but mostly fat. There's no question about it, a slender guy who walks down the street with a very heavy woman gets stared at. I dealt with that by saying to myself, "I have the right to be attracted to whomever I please. To hell with what other people think."

A lot of men can't come to terms with this. I know for a fact that many suppress their true feelings so successfully for so many years, responding to social pressure, that they'll marry the skinny women their parents and friends admire—and never feel comfortable sexually. We estimate that from 5 to 10 percent of American men are closet Fat Admirers. Not a huge number, admittedly, but enough to be counted—and recognized.

Question: What happens if the heavy woman you've come to love loses weight? Is it all over?

Answer: What happens if the thin woman my pal loves gains weight? Is it all over? Love has to do with personality and spiritual qualities. Hopefully, the weight loss or weight gain would not turn either of us off. Still, I want to give you an honest answer. It is conceivable that I'd have a struggle to feel the same sexually. I know it's not the most democratic attitude in the world, but it can't be helped. Anyway, it hasn't happened, so it's an unknown. I'll tell you one thing, though. Statistically, I have a far better chance of the woman I love *not* losing weight than my friend has of his girl friend *not* gaining weight as the years go on. How can anyone guarantee there will never be any changes?

Question: What do you see in a fat woman?

Answer: I see beauty in rounded, voluptuous forms. When other men see a fat woman, they only see a fat face. I see all the differences, which are marvelous. Thin women all look the same to me. It's a matter of what you train your eyes to perceive as beauty, I guess.

Question: How did you come to get so involved that you actually formed an organization? Couldn't you have just been content with dating women whose physical characteristics matched your standard of beauty?

Answer: In the course of looking into the biology, the esthetics, the sociology of fat, I became essentially outraged to see what goes on in this country. Look—there are a lot of injustices in this world and no one can solve all of them. I related very personally, however, to this particular outrage. I felt very angry on behalf of all the heavy people—not just women—out there who had trouble finding chic clothing, good jobs, social acceptance. I wanted to do something about it.

Question: How do you feel about the future of NAAFA?

Answer: How can we lose? Our appeal is an appeal to reason and rights and respect for all. A respect for differences. We've already made great strides. Every day we receive dozens of letters from people who have seen a representative on television, radio or in another medium. I believe it was we who made designers like Gloria Vanderbilt and Evan Picone conscious that we are a buying and interested market. Our membership increases so fast, we can hardly keep up with it. There are literally millions of heavy people out there who are just beginning to insist upon first-class citizens rights—thanks in part, I believe, to us. Look—it is simply unfair to discriminate against anyone because of body build. Would you tell someone he couldn't go to your school, or work in your office, or ride on your airplane for a single fare, because he's too blond or too tall or too skinny? It happens all the time with heavy people.

Fabrey's view is one man's view which represents many men. Whether or not a woman is sexy and appealing depends, according to the experts, not on her pounds but on her attitude.

One of the women who has an excellent attitude about her fat and her sexuality is Melanie Osborne, interviewed in an article published in *Penthouse Forum Magazine.* "I consider myself a beautiful woman," she says. "My face is beautiful, my personality is beautiful—and my body is beautiful. A man likes a curvy woman and I'm just curvier." She goes on to explain how the way a fat admirer makes love to a fat woman is different from the way another man makes love to a thin woman: "He usually takes more time to caress, kiss and pinch her body. He's usually much more into the flesh, into feeling the fat, the weight and the softness of it . . ."

One man interviewed in the same article by author David Haldane says that fat women tend to be much less inhibited in bed. "There's a natural food/sex relationship: eating is an extremely sexual instinct."

Fat admirers like Fabrey and many others, says the *Forum* article, come from virtually all socioeconomic backgrounds. Contrary to popular belief, very few of them have fat mothers. Indeed, says Fabrey, "There's something warm and comforting and pleasant about the curves of a woman's body. To me, that doesn't represent Mother—it represents Woman. I'm not dumping on thin women, mind you, but to me the whole womanly thing is curves. You can't possibly have straight lines on a fat person."

So what does it come down to? Where does the big woman stand when it comes to sex? It seems to me there is only one way to look at it.

Big women own their own bodies. What we do with them, how we feel about them, is our own responsibility. It is certainly possible to enjoy the sweetest sexual life with fat thighs and a mid-waist tire.

XIII An Organized Life

There's a harried, heavy woman on a popular greeting card. Her hair is wild, her clothes are torn, her house looks as if nine college students had spent the weekend. "Tomorrow," she says, "tomorrow, I must get organized."

It's nice for anyone to be organized, but crucial for us. I have already said that we can be sexy, sultry, angry, happy, intellectual, exotic. Almost anything except sloppy. And that goes for our home as well as our person. The large woman must organize her home to make her life easier. She needs accessible shelf space so she doesn't have to bend so much. She needs uncluttered rooms so she can move gracefully and efficiently through her home. There are certain appliances and products that are functional and practical in her personal grooming. Look, let's face it. It is uncomfortable to have to stretch or bend for pots and pans, to retrieve the blouse that's fallen on the floor of an impossibly stuffed closet, to wash one's feet when they seem blocked by one's belly button. It is harder to reach, twist, dry, wipe. Messy kitchens and bathrooms are depressing. Have you ever worn the stained sweater "just one more time" before you invested in a cleaning bill? Bad. Size 6 might get away with it; size 42s, never. Perhaps if you had that classy giant bathroom hamper instead of the puny little pail you use, it *might* remind you that it is totally unacceptable for a large woman to be sloppy—if she wants to give off an image of great and desirable!

So, here's how to organize your home and get your head on straight.

Let's Start with the Bathroom

Buy a bidet. No chic Frenchwoman would be without one. If you've ever traveled in Europe, you've seen one in every fine hotel room. It's not that expensive when you think how useful it is for personal hygiene. It may be indelicate to discuss, but sometimes our extra pounds make it clumsy for us to cleanse ourselves comfortably and thoroughly after we move our bowels or urinate. The bidet is a low-set bowl which provides refreshing and total cleanliness. The user straddles the bowl facing the faucets, which control water temperature and pressure. Jets of warm water spray upward at her touch, cleansing the anal and pelvic areas. Most bidets come with stoppers so they can be used as baths for tired, swollen feet—another constant annoyance to large women. A bidet is such an intelligent, useful appliance that no woman, no matter what she weighs or what her nationality is, ought to ignore its possibilities. If you find it clumsy going, because of pounds, to reach certain body areas, join the company of the most elegant European ladies, classy whores and informed Americans and do yourself a favor. Be the first one on your block to buy a bidet. (Check with any major plumbing supply house for purchase and installation costs.)

Some *toilet seats* come wider than others. Shop around till you find one that fits you.

A built-in *seat in the shower* is great for washing feet. Check with a local carpenter to see if he can make you a hinged seat that folds back against the shower wall when it's not in use. Make very sure it's "through-bolted" onto the wall for total security. If your wallet can't afford built-ins, a rubber-tipped chair, available in any orthopedic appliance house, is also sturdy, steady and fine.

Grab rails on the side of the toilet and in the bathing area double as towel racks and pull-yourself-up aids.

A small Rubbermaid *dish rack,* suspended at shoulder height in the shower, holds all the stuff that always seems to slip out of the dopey little tile openings found in most walls.

Hand showers can be attached to your own shower head: marvelous for reaching hard-to-reach spots.

Big *plastic-coated hooks* for robes and towels forestall bending and come in handy in a lot of other ways.

A wall *magnifying mirror,* mounted at eye level, that tilts and sways for tweezing and close makeup work is neat, always available and bigger than the compact mirror you're in the habit of using.

Who says you have to live with that narrow, cramped *medicine cabinet?* Replace it with two or even three modern, spacious ones that will hold all your bottles, jars, tubes, lipsticks, brushes, etc. *Nothing* should live on the windowsill. Throw out any medication you haven't used in a year—yes, even the antibiotic cream that worked so well on the eye infection you had in 1973. *Out* also with empty prescription bottles because someday you may have a use for them. You won't.

And who says a bathroom can't come equipped with a *full-sized closet* all its own *instead* of a crammed-full medicine cabinet? You can create storage and make bathroom cleanups simple by buying a metal floor cabinet—spray-painting it a color to match your bathroom—and have a place to hold toilet tissue, makeup, towels, soaps, tampons, douches, syringes, whatever. If you don't have room for a full floor cabinet you can buy a full-sized kitchen cabinet, which beats a medicine cabinet by many feet.

Right now, *dump any towel* that is noticeably frayed or built for a midget. There is nothing so demeaning as an ample body drying itself in a measly, stingy, fraying rag. Your towels should be *huge* and gorgeously fluffy. Lose yourself in your towels.

Rubber tile *matting,* available in many colors and at floor-covering stores, is easy on the feet and pretty!

There must be at least one and preferably two *full-length mirrors* in the bathroom. Learn to look at yourself squarely and appreciate your lush and round body. Don't ever look at yourself sideways, hoping to miss the hips. Your hips are inviting, suggestive, womanly. Your newly laundered belly is delightful. Even if you're not thrilled with the size of your thighs, don't try to hide them, even from yourself. Accepting yourself, being comfortable and familiar with your own body, will make you carry it more proudly.

On to the Bedroom

First, the *closet*. It's a mess, right? When was the last time you took everything—even the shoetrees—out? Do it. Now. Don't wait till you redecorate, or have the cash to buy matching hangers. Spray-paint it shocking pink, canary yellow—whatever color turns you on. Don't worry if it's not in your decorating scheme—who looks in your closet? Now's your chance to use the bad-taste color you've secretly admired all your life. If it makes you cheerful, it should color your closet.

Get yourself a large, empty box or five shopping bags. Now, honestly go through every item of clothes you've flung on your bed to see if it's (1) irrevocably stained, (2) hopelessly torn, (3) too small. If it's stained and it hasn't come clean in three cleanings— into the shopping bags (or the box). If it's frayed or torn in a place that's not a seam and not repairable—even if it's the skirt you wore to your first seduction—into the shopping bag. Now the hard part. You are not alone if you have three or four different-sized wardrobes in your closet. Most big women do. There's the dress that fit you when you were twenty-three and at your thinnest and you're saving it (you've been saving it for nine years!) for when you lose some weight—maybe next month. There's the blouse you bought when you were fifty pounds heavier than you are now and it looks as if another person lived in it. Still, the material is so pretty. And there's the evening skirt that never fit you and never will, but your Aunt Sadye (who is close to your size) gave it to you and you hate to throw it out even though you're not so big on silver tassels. *Into the shopping bag. All of them.*

There is nothing so depressing as a closet jammed full of clothes, and none of them wearable. If two or three years have gone by and the article of clothing (including pocketbooks and shoes) hasn't seen the light of day, get rid of it. It is better to have four wearable, stunning outfits hanging in a closet than fourteen useless decorations. Think of yourself as you, a person, *now*—not when you've lost forty pounds. And donate the clothes of the dream person who lives in your closet to a worthy charity, which will be delighted, maybe will even come pick up those bulging shopping bags and give you a substantial tax deduction as well. Figure it this way—anyone who can close the zipper is entitled to it! No one should go through life with an open zipper.

Tip: Don't hang shoes in a bag on your door. They keep falling out and brushing against white skirts. I use a covered shoe box which accommodates about nine pairs of shoes and sits on a shelf at the top of my closet. Shoe racks on the floor are always hard to get to and always spitefully seem to dump at least two shoes on the floor daily. They also collect thick balls of dust.

Tip: When putting things away for the summer, be careful moth-balls don't come in direct contact with clothes. They will discolor. Use a moth disk hung on a hook.

Tip: Hangers that take up the space of one but really have room for six or seven blouses or skirts, are great. They're those graduated jobs which cleverly fit one piece of clothing over another.

Tip: Never hang anything in the back of your closet that smells of perspiration unless you want to infect everything else. Perspiration attracts moth larvae. Professional cleaning will kill them. Also, stains tend to oxidize over a long period of time and become more stubborn; they can even weaken the fabric.

Tip: Never hang anything in the back of your closet that needs a button or a hem.

Tip: Never store anything in plastic; it can create a moist environment and lead to mildew. Polyester garments should be hung to avoid permanent wrinkles: everything else should be boxed.

Tip: You can double your closet space with heavy-duty steel shelves of plastic-coated vinyl, available in any houseware or hardware store and sold by the foot. The shelves can be home to sweaters, linens, shoes, boxes of junk, pocketbooks, you name it. Standing on the floor of the closet should be a *roomy* hamper for everything even slightly soiled that you take off. Stackable baskets on the shelves (made from the same plastic-coated vinyl) are great for storing socks and stockings, bras, anything you can never find in the morning. And don't underestimate the power of *hooks.* They're to the heavy women what a personal valet is to a Rockefeller. Large hooks are space and bending savers, and can be used to store coats, scarves, belts, your hair dryer, brooms, bicycles, even skis.

Consider using *metal pipe* instead of wooden closet poles. The metal will not sag under the weight of the clothes and can be waxed so the hangers glide easily.

Even though you've always felt superorganized with those giant *garment bags,* tell the truth—they *do* take up more room than they're worth, don't they? They're great for seasonal storage, but for year-round protection and space saving, individual garment bags are far less bulky.

If it is always difficult for you to squeeze between the *night table* and the bed, put the night table somewhere else. You *may.* You live here, try to remember. Furniture must be positioned to fit you, not some *Vogue* decorator's idea of where night tables go. Try one table at the foot of your bed and the other on the side you never use for access to the bed.

And another thing, that leopard-skin *throw rug*—you've been skidding on it for years. It's treacherous! Either buy a nonskid liner or tack down the edges with invisible carpet tacks.

Same thing with the *telephone cord* you're always tripping on. Once and for all, hide it behind something! Or call the telephone company, which will be happy to install a retractable long cord for you.

If you feel that you are a big woman trapped in a tiny space with millions of *little hazards*—extend, unroll, expand that space! Trap the hazards in safe places. Give away dressing tables you never use and stools that would never hold your weight. (They probably wouldn't hold Jackie Kennedy.) If your taste runs to tiny Copenhagen figurines, fine, but don't leave them cluttering your dresser just because your mother likes them and she happened to go on a trip to Copenhagen two years ago and bought out the market. God won't punish you if you throw out something your mother loves. Actually, enlightened big women can best organize their homes after they organize the inside of their heads. If you feel like a clumsy, ugly duckling, you'll still bump into the only chair in the room. A good place to start your psyche reorganization is by a physical reorganization of the *things* around you.

For instance: You have all these exquisite heirloom sheets inherited from your Great-Aunt Pat. They're treasures but you hate them. Every morning, you have to remake the bed from scratch because they didn't know about fitted sheets in 1899. Still, how can you buy new sheets until these wear out? *Buy some! Now!*

Give the heirloom ones to your cousin Charlene who will struggle with them dutifully for a generation or so. You get the all-cotton (for comfort) fitted sheets so you don't have to retrace steps or tuck in corners every morning. And think of sleeping without bunched up mountains under you . . .

Now the Kitchen

Put a wall to work. Instead of stacking your pots and pans in low, difficult-to-reach cabinets, buy a plastic-coated steel grid (or any kind of a steel grid). With a few hooks and small baskets, you can hang everything from pots and pans to scissors, ladles and dish towels. Pot covers must be stored elsewhere, as in Rubbermaid's slotted rack. A few magnetic racks, available at your hardware store or places like the Pottery Barn, are great for storing can openers, spatulas, even food-processor blades. The idea is to put as much as possible at, or just above, eye level. It is easier to reach *up* for something than rummage *under*. Of course, whatever you have hanging out in plain view must be spotless, and shining prettily.

Check your *spice cabinet.* Does it take ten minutes to find the onion flakes? Turn your doors or walls into storage spaces with narrow racks to neatly hold small cans and bottles of every description. If you like to keep them in the kitchen cabinet, by all means get a revolving stand for them. And again, *throw out* the cumin and the pickling spice if you haven't used them for six months (and you can't even remember what cumin *is!*).

Rolling service carts: They serve as small, mobile islands, saving trips to the dining area. Use them for distributing laundry, entertaining, as plant or typewriter stands, and garage them under the kitchen table when they're not in use. (A wood top for chopping is a nice addition on any cart.)

Do not put *any signs on your refrigerator* that are demeaning. Why go along with the mentality that says fat is synomymous with ugly or slothful or funny? The "Bridget" calendar showing the fat woman in a series of ignominious poses is meant for ridicule. I have seen it in too many heavy women's homes. Sure, you should have a sense of humor about yourself: being heavy is not grim or serious. But it is self-deprecating to caricature yourself by reminders that "if you open this refrigerator door you will blow up." That's taking dignity away. That's masochistic. If you are big and if you are careful with fashion and makeup and neatness and psyche, you will not want to laugh at yourself or have others laugh at you. If you're a "put-together" person, that self-ridicule has no place in your life. Never again apologize for the wonderful, big woman you are.

If you use *tablecloths*, they don't have to be shoved in a linen closet where they will have to be ironed twice, once before you

A kitchen designed by Allmilmo Corporation is a perfect example of an interior that makes life easy for the big woman. The kitchen is neat, pretty—and organized!

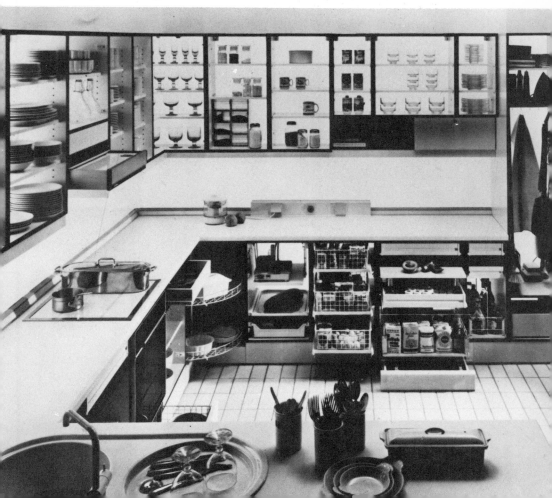

put them away and once before you use them. *Hang* them in an
out-of-the-way closet on round, thick, hollow plastic rods (available in hardware stores) and held in place by tiny chains attached
at each end of the rod and to the ceiling of the closet. They'll be
ready at a moment's notice. Again, this saves bending, rummaging
and ironing for the busy woman who has other, more important
things on her mind.

I hate *ladders,* step stools, whatever you wish to call them. They
are rickety, tippy, they collapse easily, they are not geared to handle extra pounds. If you need to reach overhead storage in your
kitchen, (or anywhere) very often, have a simple, sturdy *wooden
box* constructed by a local carpenter. Surely *anyone* can make a
box—but it *must* be capable of sustaining weight. It can be stained
and finished prettily so it can even be used as a spare stool or
serving table, and its flat surface and sturdy nature make it infinitely safer to use as a ladder than a real ladder. Send for a KIK-
STEP. It's a sturdy, compact, miniature barrel, 14 inches high,
with casters that lock as soon as you step on it. It's a real *find* for
high places.   To order, send a check for $39.95 (which includes
postage) to: Co-ordinated Furniture Systems, 621 Oakhurst Road,
Mamaroneck, N. Y. 10543. Or telephone: (914) 698-0932.

You remember that grab-all *extension arm* your neighborhood
grocer used to take the boxes of cornflakes down from the highest
shelf? You can have one also and eliminate most of the need for a
ladder. Hardware stores and fancy places like Hammacher Schlemmer all carry them. They run thirty inches or longer and are invaluable for retrieving cans, boxes and other objects stored above
a normal reaching span. They should cost no more than ten
dollars.

Redefine your kitchen space to make it fit you. Do you really
need the Mixmaster you haven't used in two years kept out, all
the time? Do you need to keep four chairs around the kitchen table
if you are mostly only two in the kitchen? Give yourself ample
space to maneuver and work comfortably, and sacrifice gadgets
and hardly-ever-used appliances, for space. Big women should
avoid *crowded* at all costs. No matter what kind of a cook you are,
naturalist, grandmotherly, gourmet or indifferent, your kitchen
should be a place that's safe, roomy as possible and, best of all,
happy. Because many big women are marvelous cooks, their kitch-

ens should reflect their creative and lusty appreciation of the delicacies of food. Kitchens are also nice places to kibitz.

Need more space? Put a *flip-up counter* on one wall to provide counter or work space. (Fold out of the way when not in use.) Hang pretty pots or spice racks on walls. Build shelves above your cabinets to store seldom-used articles. Hang a garbage can on a door or inside a broom closet.

If you are redecorating your kitchen, be careful of the *flooring* you choose. Many big women have trouble with feet and ankles, and a hard, nonresilient floor like Spanish tile or marble can be a real back and feet crippler if you stand for too long. If you have *inherited* a very hard kitchen floor that gives your feet and back muscles grief, equip it with nonskid, spongy rubber mats in front of the sink, preparation center and, if you're like me, in front of the refrigerator where I spend a lot of time.

Also stay away from creating narrow, cramped *dinette alcoves* which are torture to maneuver in. Better take a few more steps and eat in the living room or dining room, like a person!

If *too-low counters* are straining your back, you can build them up with butcher blocks.

Brighten kitchen cabinets by adding *new knobs* with spices caught in lucite, knobs in sleek aluminum, knobs in marvelous woods.

If you don't have central *air conditioning,* do yourself a favor and put a small unit in the kitchen. Logically, it's the place that needs it the most with the heat from the stove, dishwasher, etc. With our tendency to perspire so much, a cool kitchen is heaven.

Hang up appliance cords. Screw hooks into handles of mops and brooms, and also hang. Hang toilet brushes and buckets: never put anything smelly into a closet!

Relationships Need Organizing As Much As Closets Do

Okay, you've got your closets in shape, you're no longer tripping over the light cord and you've finally figured out how to reach the top shelf without collapsed-ladder disasters. Spend a little time organizing your relationships. You've just given away the clothes in the closet that don't fit or are soiled and tired with wear. You've replaced them with just a few viable, interesting and new outfits. Do the same with your frayed and worn-out relationships. Heavy women really tend to cling to outdated friends. Do you still have dinner weekly with the silly pal from college because she was kind to you when you were down and out? Does that conversation with your old boyfriend leave you depressed every time he calls? Is the couple down the street boring, but you still hate to hurt their feelings by not inviting them over at least monthly? Do you feel guilty about never calling Evelyn, the person you met at Weight Watchers?

Take stock of people as you did of your clothes. That includes the people you work with, the people of your childhood, the people you met yesterday. If there are any life-destroyers, mood-destroyers, put-you-downers, gently ease them out of your life, at least temporarily. That's the nice thing about reorganizing *people.* Sometimes, you can pick up a relationship when it has a new interest or new life, even years after you've erased it from your life. It is draining to hang around with people who don't meet your needs and whom you can't handle emotionally or any other way. Funny thing: when you clear away the debris of hangers-on and guilt-producing acquaintances and boring second cousins and roommates from college whom you never had much in common with in the *best* of times, you find yourself wide open to making new friends. Simplifying your relationships is like adding a day or so to your week. You have more time for yourself and more time for new, exciting friends. It's *not* mean or ruthless to play it cool with certain people for a while—maybe forever. It is life sustaining and a healthy thing to do. Save your loyalty for the people forces in your life who add to your life, who are indispensable to your emotional and intellectual well-being. Gently, spring-clean the rest.

And, get it all done, starting *now.* We all procrastinate. Here are five ways to stop putting off and start organizing your life and your home and your relationships—today.

1. Set goals. Don't dream of doing all your closets at once even if you feel a mad flurry of energy. You'll get tired in the middle, leave half the stuff on the chair and be in worse shape than before.

So decide before you start: bedroom closet today, kitchen cabinets tomorrow. A huge, terrifying job can be broken down into several manageable parts.

2. Browse through hardware stores and dime stores for a full afternoon. You'll be amazed at how many gadgets and ideas you'll pick up to make your life more compact. Somehow, something like brand-new skirt hangers can incite you to action.

3. Redo your telephone book. Buy a brand-new, beautiful leather telephone book and a pen with an ink color you rarely use: you'll feel innovative and creative as you ruthlessly leave out half the people in the old book you *never* see, from your new beautiful book.

4. Reward yourself for each task. If your medicine cabinet is particularly terrible and you have been avoiding it for months, promise yourself a new blouse if you get it cleaned out *this week.* You do not get the blouse if you miss the week by one day. Make that hard phone call to the interesting woman (and potential new friend) you met last week and ask her to join you for lunch. Reward yourself with that new, expensive book you've wanted for a month.

5. Make daily lists. Go through your house and your life with a pencil and paper. List each chore and result you wish to obtain by the end of the time you've allotted yourself. Write a week's worth of reorganization lists at a time so you'll get a sense of where you're going to end up, ultimately.

XIV The Big Woman and Her Home

Mussolini had his desk placed at the end of a long and grand salon. Those who wished to see him were made to walk the length of the salon, and a magical thing happened. Because of the placement of the desk, as one walked toward the figure pompously waiting, the closer one got—the larger and more imposing the figure grew. Mussolini could have written a book called *Decorate Your Way to Power.*

The Emperor Nero had fortune, power, generals, as well as Rome to burn. It wasn't until he began to furnish his spectacular palace that he really felt terrific about himself, though. "Now, I can begin to live like a gentleman," he said (or the equivalent).

The writer Victor Hugo greatly admired a certain Parisian cemetery. One of his characters in *Les Miserables* says, "To be buried in Père LaChaise is like having mahogany furniture." In other words, a status symbol.

George Washington, also concerned more with status than taste, asked a friend by letter, to "pick up forty yards of the new textile mill's best weave." Not the best blue weave or the best wool weave. Just forty yards of the *best*. So much for Washington's sense of interior decoration.

Why *do* people decorate their homes? We probed the deepest instincts of human nature to find the answer. The way you decorate your home tells other people what kind of person you are and what kind of person you'd like to be. The furniture you choose is a litmus test of how you feel about yourself. If you feel fat, sloppy, clumsy, unattractive and angry with the people who surround you —rest assured that your feelings will show up in your environment. If you have become adept at living and making yourself, regardless of weight, a knockout of a woman, your home will also be a knockout.

The way you live is the most graphic expression of your taste, your needs, the status you wish. Women who wish to be thought of as intellectuals will have their walls lined with books and art objects. Those who wish primarily to be thought of as wealthy will buy furniture that is instantly labeled as expensive.

Our kind of women, the big and wonderful women of the world, have individual tastes like everyone else, of course. And one statement we all should try to make with our homes says: I am heavy but I can live with good taste, grace and safety. Even if I can't always control my outside environment, I surely ought to hand pick everything in my own home that spells elegance, style and comfort for a woman of my size and temperament.

And make no mistake. We *do* have special decorating needs. If you have ignored that truth, you are not living as comfortably and with as much éclat as you should. Your home should be the one place in all the world where you are "at home." That means you should be inordinately proud of how it looks; you should have furniture that is gracefully designed for your particular comfort and safety; you should be able to move with suppleness in, out of and around your furniture when you are alone and when you are entertaining. No more plunges into down pillows from which you cannot recover without perspiring heavily. No more dining room tables that tip into your lap when your extra weight leans on them the wrong way. If every piece of furniture in your house does not fit your own size and style, then it's furniture in bad taste.

Decorating has been around for a while. The first decorator was probably a cave matron who threw a dinosaur skin over her best rock. The paleolithic Joneses, next cave over, added mammoth tusks on the wall. Taste was born.

To help us write this chapter we needed someone with somewhat more modern taste. Someone who could give us specific as well as general tips and ideas on decorating for the larger woman's home. Someone who was a thorough professional and who had vast experience with our particular concerns.

Laurette Arnel was our choice. Her advice constitutes much of these next pages. A decorator for twenty years, she has counted among her clients such organizations and individuals as New York's swank Barclay Hotel, the Kimberly-Clark Corporation, actress Liza Minnelli, television host Dave Garroway, financier Henry Ford, movie producer Martin Bregman and hundreds of other names you'd instantly recognize. What is more important, her clients have also included innumerable people whose names you'd never recognize but who are big, very beautiful in their attitudes and looks and who share your concerns and needs.

"A successful room for a large woman looks easier than it actually is to achieve," says Ms. Arnel. "It is not only vital to buy furniture for comfort but also for scale and graceful proportion. Scale means you don't have all sturdy furniture and plants but a mixture of strong and delicate. Scale means you wouldn't place a massive, square walnut desk in back of a painted and gilded Louis XVI chair. Balance means that if everyone who comes to your home gets an irresistible urge to rearrange the furniture, something is wrong. Novices often make mistakes that shout 'Oh, a *fat*

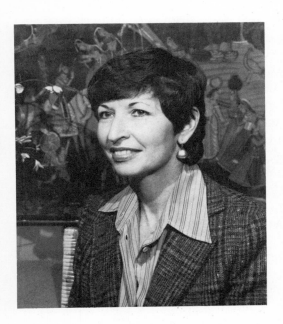

Decorator Laurette Arne

person lives here!' or, even worse, 'Oh, only teeny size fours live here!' The heavy woman who has good taste chooses her clothing so she will look attractive. Her dress does not proclaim, 'This is a fat woman's dress.' Her home should not either. There is a total correlation between your personal look and your home's look. Still, you cannot ignore the fact that your furniture should be sturdy and safe. And that sturdy, safe furniture can be made to look light and fashionable in an easy-to-move-about, pretty environment.''

A list of basic needs in every home is easy to compile. You will need a place to sit, to talk, to read, to sleep, to play, to eat, to put things in or on. All of these places should be able to accommodate you or your possessions comfortably. They should be easy to get into and easy to leave. And, of course, they should be pleasing to the eye.

What follows is a compendium of ideas about those places from Laurette and from many big women who were kind enough to share their ideas and experiences in the home decoration arena.

First, Some General Advice

In a recent magazine cartoon, a man about to leave for work is seen pleading with his wife as he says goodbye, "Promise me you won't be involved in a trend when I come home."

Trends are big these days but trendy furniture is not for big women. That style, aptly named life-styles furniture, is made to last for a year in a college kid's apartment. Trendy furniture, like antimacassars, is destined to lose its popularity with the next fad's arrival. Also, it breaks a lot. Tortured chrome tubing may look attractive in the model room, but wait till it snakes all over your living room.

STRUCTURE

Your furniture should be sturdy so you don't fall off or break through it and you can rise and sit easily. Don't be tempted by the charming little French-legged side chair: it's *your* home and noth-

ing should be bought "just for company." If *you* can't sit on it—
chuck it.

FABRICS AND WEAVES

One-hundred-percent wools and nubby fabrics in pile weaves
retain heat: because we are hot-blooded creatures, we often feel
most unfomfortable with these choices.

Chintz, linen and heavy cotton in a plain weave (with possibly
some nylon as partial content) serve well and are most durable.
Try to get them soil treated.

Cotton, silk and rayon in a satin weave is smooth and elegant
but tends to pull or catch. It's strong, though, and can bear a good
amount of weight without quickly wearing thin.

Silk and wool mixtures last longer and fade less quickly than
cotton and wool. They're also cooler than plain wool.

Brocades and damasks wear badly because threads tend to fray
and pull.

The worst thing you can buy is anything made with a *plastic
fabric.* It makes a poop sound when you plop down. It sticks to
your bottom when you get up. Walking away with a chair or cushion stuck to your bottom is definitely not seductive.

COLORS

Just as we do not have to limit ourselves to dark clothes, we do
not have to choose navy-blue and brown couches simply to camouflage their sturdiness. The dark color will not hide that bulk any
more than it does yours. The navy-blue wing chair that is thrust
into the all-other-small-pale-objects room looks clumsier than it
really is. We are limited in terms of fabric (we need the hardiest)
and in terms of scale of furniture (delicate, fragile stuff is silly) and
in terms of upholstery stuffing (too soft is murder), but *we are
essentially free to experiment with color and design.* Keep in
mind, though, certain elementary basics: Colors can blend, complement, soften and attract all at the same time. Warm colors like
reds, oranges and yellows on the walls make a room look smaller;

red used on a large piece like a couch will make the couch seem much larger. The idea is to make your rooms look larger and, thus, you correspondingly smaller. Therefore, you will not want to close in your rooms by too blatant a use of hot colors. You will not want to make your sturdy, heavier furniture even heavier looking with a hot color. Used sparingly, these colors can be intimate and warming, but they should be limited to touches and not used on a grand scale. The cool colors like light blues, violets and greens on walls and large pieces tend to make a room and furniture look larger (and you, smaller). They give a feeling of restfulness. Break up the cool colors with some warm prints and sunny stuff to avoid too cold and barren a look.

LINES AND SHAPES

Rounded pillars, mirrors and other large circular objects tend to invite comparisons. Vertical lines in your rooms add height, slimness and dignity. Mirrors should be long and high; short, squat mirrors have the effect of making *you* look short and squat. Many large women end up looking at their reflections from the neck up —and mentally and visually blocking out the rest of their bodies —in such mirrors. Tall highboys, four-poster beds, vertically striped wallpapers, tend to distract from your own roundness. Curved lines are graceful and feminine. They're great as accents but not great for whole rooms, because they emphasize your own opulent curvature and balance is what we're looking for.

TRAFFIC FLOW

Just as traffic flows smoothly in a well-lit and laid-out intersection, so it should in your home. You and your guests should be able to move from room to room without having to dodge and sideswipe tables and chairs. Entering a room, one should be aware of a smooth flow of traffic rather than an obstacle course of clumpy, squared-off pieces. When you are entertaining, take a minute to see if the guests can move naturally around and through a room or if they bump into pieces from behind and dodge them from the front. Centers of rooms should be clutter free and minus floating furniture.

TASTE

Someone once asked the late Fats Waller, "What is swing?" He replied, "Boy, is you gotta ask, you ain't got it." The same goes for taste.

But are you born with it? Nonsense. Just as you can learn to develop a "clothes sense" you can develop a "house sense." How? By reading many decorating magazines until you begin to sense what's grotesque and what's elegant. By being observant when you go to friends' homes and to the model rooms of department stores. By choosing a mentor and following her or him around for a while, watching to see what she or he chooses and finding out the reasons why. Trust your own judgment. The same good taste that tells you not to wear purple sequined eyeglasses with muumuus to hide your pounds tells you that the elephant with the flowers growing out of his head would *not* make a darling end table. You will feel the weight of ugly and too much furniture, after a while, more than you feel your own weight. You are allowed to copy shamelessly from other sources if you like their taste, but never put something into your home because your Aunt Florence said it was divine. Even if she tells you that the fabric of the chair she thinks is divine was woven in the waters of the Gulf of Hohokus by left-handed spiritualists who weave for their very souls—you can say, "So what? I still hate that chair."

WILL IT FIT?

Carry a tape measure when shopping. Don't buy until you've measured the piece and measured the space at home where it must fit. Pay attention. Here's a super visual aid: after measuring the circumference, width and length of a major piece of furniture, draw it *life-size*, on a piece of brown wrapping paper. Then place the paper where the piece will go. See if it is in scale with the rest of your furnishings. Walk around it to see if you will have at least six inches of access to the places where you will need access. Drawing a representational model doesn't help much to visualize the actual size. You need a paper replica of the true size. And don't, as some decorators suggest, attempt to draw a floor plan from above, looking down. When you come into a room, you don't see it from the ceiling.

HELP!

"I'd like to try to work with a decorator, but I'm afraid it will be too expensive. What are they like, anyway, and where do I find one?" A good decorator is really a valiant creature. She usually has the creative imagination of a Chagall, the stamina of a workhorse, the agility of a Sherpa mountain guide and the patience of Job. If you are lucky enough to put yourself in the hands of a talented decorator, your life will be made easy. Decorators, like travel agents, usually end up costing you *less* than you would spend on your own. They will charge, usually, a percentage of the amount of money you spend on furniture ordered through them and no other fee. But because they have access, not only to sources unavailable to the retail buying consumer, but to merchandise at wholesale prices, your own end costs are lowered—even counting their percentage. And you're getting the advantage of their flare, expertise and legwork.

There are many ways to find a decorator. Look in the magazines to see which people are responsible for the rooms you admire. Look in the advertisement pages of decorating magazines and of newspapers. Check out the model rooms of a large department store. You can use its own decorator (a catch here—you will have to buy everything the decorator orders from *that* store). Decorating organizations are listed in magazines like *House Beautiful* and *House and Garden.* Call them up for suggestions. And finally, be aware of the new "showcase" phenomenon that's sweeping the country. Showcases are marvelous old mansions that have been turned over to charities. The charities then invite many different interior decorators to design individual rooms to their own tastes. The mansion is then opened to the public and for a small, tax-deductible fee, you can meander through rooms until you find one you love. Get the name of the decorator responsible for the room and call to set up a consultation with that person. Ask your local paper if there's a showcase near you.

If possible, have the decorator you choose come to your house. Make sure she understands everything about your budget, your life-style, your special needs. *A decorator should start off by asking you, not by telling you.* If you see that she is going to be overpowering in terms of imposing only what she likes on you, say you'll be in touch. Then don't be in touch. If, however, you seem to be on the same wave length, without personality or taste conflicts, hire her, trust her and you're off and running. Never trust *anyone* so much that you relegate your own good judgment to last place.

THE GILT COMPLEX

Just because it's been gilded, doesn't mean it's gold. Just because it has a famous name, doesn't mean it's good. Chippendale and Tiffany also had their bad days, and turned out some terrible clunkers.

A LAST GENERALITY: DON'T SKIP IT!
IT'S THE MOST IMPORTANT ONE!

Remember that unless you are very rich, the spaces you inhabit have probably not been custom designed to fit your body. More likely you have to maneuver to fit your body into the spaces that have been provided for you in the apartment you rent or the house you buy. Try as hard as you can to avoid spaces like one-room apartments, three-foot terraces, office cubicles. Sometimes you can expand that space by color and design and lack of clutter. Still, the furniture you buy for those preordained spaces should always be big enough and strong enough to fit you and not your size-8 company. Consider the artist Claes Oldenburg. He makes soft vinyl furniture sculptures and then, when they are completed, he sits in them or lies in them to "set them right." He knows that furniture should conform to one's own body. You can find such furniture, perhaps not as snugly molded as a vinyl, soft, foam-stuffed couch turns out to be after you've sat in it, but certainly chairs, sofas, desks and tables that fit you wonderfully well. You will, I guarantee, be more comfortable, look more beautiful, actually feel more happy in spaces that accommodate you than in spaces that fit the current *Vogue* model's sensibilities and derrière.

Okay: Let's begin with the . . .

Living Room: What's Good and What's Bad

- Chair arms should always be high enough to get the leverage you need for rising gracefully.
- Recliner chairs, especially the push-a-button, automatic kind, are lovely. The ones with the raising levers on the side are much easier than the ones which force you to raise your own weight by yourself. Choose a wide-armed model for greater comfort.
- Watch the pitch of the chairs you select. If the chair back reclines at too great an angle, you will definitely have trouble getting up.
- Gimmick chairs are *out*. That includes canvas sling chairs, director's chairs, beanbag chairs (even the *thought* of a beanbag chair sprouting beans is terrifying) and anything suspended (like a hammock). They are graceless, dangerous and wrong for a woman of your size and presence. Also not recommended is the dear, old, ugly, spindle-legged number which you have been trained since childhood not to sit in, but which your mother, in a burst of sentimentality, has given you for your new apartment. If Grandma, who you hear was also respectfully large, had bad taste in 1892, why on earth must you be saddled with it today?
- Rocking chairs, especially with a solid platform-floor base, are great. They propel you out so you can get a running start.
- Love seats are wonderful: they make you look as if you'd lost weight if you're sitting alone in one.

- Even more wonderful and certainly more subtle than a love seat is a little number called A Chair and a Half, which is exactly that: bigger than a single seat and smaller than a love seat. It usually comes in traditional styles.
- Chair height: chairs should be at least standard height and higher. Low-slung numbers are taboo for the bigger woman. When sitting comfortably erect, the backs of your knees should touch the outer edge of the seat cushion and the bottom of your feet should be flat upon the floor. If your feet are dangling or if the seat cushion hits you in the calf of the leg, it's wrong, wrong, wrong.
- Armless chaise longues are terrible. If the phone rings, forget it. You have no leverage for getting up fast and by the time you squoosh yourself out of the chaise, inch by inch, the casting director has hung up.
- While we're at it, armless anythings are ghastly. A lot of the new modular stuff is armless and, therefore, awful to rise out of. Speaking of modular furniture, if you do go for it, make sure it's high and straight-back, with *attached* seat and back cushions (the loose cushions slip around and so will you). If it's too cushy, pitched back, soft and low, you will regret the moment you sit down. Try getting up from an armless, slanted wonder without getting a slipped disc.
- Unless you have your own hoist in your living room, do not buy anything that calls itself pillow furniture. And don't be misled. Pillow furniture is not just pillows plopped on a floor. It usually consists of a wooden base or a fabric-covered platform topped with a couple of loose pillows resting on spindly pieces of metal. What you do is, you fall into it. Pillow furniture doesn't do a whole lot for backs or the essence of effortless rising.
- Stay away from any furniture on wheels except for serving carts. I have sat down on wheeled chairs only to have them lurch away from me as if they were mounted on banana peels. Before purchasing any wheeled furniture from which you intend to remove the wheels, measure the height of the piece, wheelless. It may be too low and uncomfortable when you remove the wheels.
- S-shaped metal frame chairs with pretty little wicker backs

are lethal: one misdistribution of weight in the cantilevered seat instantly topples the occupant.

- Ditto molded one-piece plastic chairs that look like kindergarten furniture.
- You can camouflage the sturdiness of some of your heavier pieces by decorating them in lovely, gay and light fabrics and prints, color coordinated to give a lighter touch to the living room. A massive dark-green brocaded chair, in the family for years and comfortable and roomy as it should be, was recently redecorated in a colorful crewel fabric: it looks half the size and twice as delicate.
- Teeny plants are kind of silly for large-sized people generally. You can use them as touches, but the large, swaying, elegant, impressive green jobbies are nicest for your room. Never buy an artificial plant. It is the epitome of bad taste.
- Consider the use of a fairly good-sized, glass-topped coffee table. It wonderfully lightens the feeling of a sturdily furnished room, and an Oriental or other interesting rug placed underneath is gorgeous! In the center of a conversation area, a glass-topped table seems to make airy moods and conversations. *Crucial:* Never let anyone talk you into a glass top that is less than three-quarters of an inch thick. The glass must also be tempered for safety and should be set *on* (not in) a sturdy wood or metal frame. Rest assured that glass set *into* a frame is thinner than three-quarters of an inch and fragile.
- Are *you* unmistakably stamped in your room? Are the books you like, the colors that turn you on, the art work that you've chosen, the furniture that fits, in that room? Would your best friend, set loose in the room for the first time, instantly know it was yours?
- Coffee tables should not be lower than a seat height and can easily be four to six inches higher for comfort. They should not be placed closer than twelve inches to a couch to allow yourself comfortable access.
- The use of skirts made of charming fabric on hulky, legged end tables softens and makes them more delicate. A big woman with heavy legs wears a long skirt for the greatest grace—same thing in tables. Seats or couches with sturdy frames or platforms you hate can also be made charming with a skirt.

- You can change the whole look of your living room by having a platform built at one end and covering it in carpeting. But be sure the construction is sturdy: plywood-covered box platforms collapse embarrassingly.
- Pedestal chairs tip. A lot.
- Cushions on seating pieces should never be made of down. Save the down for throw pillows. Sitting and leaning on down couch cushions means sinking endlessly in and never rising without help. It is difficult to carry your end of a conversation when you're worrying about how to get up. Foam-core pillows or (slightly more luxurious) foam core wrapped in dacron batting is what you should look for.
- Never buy furniture without testing for proper height. Your feet must touch the floor when you are sitting and the arms of the piece must be high enough for good leverage.
- Things that look good but are good for nothing ought to be discarded. Flops in function, if kept around long enough, generally cause violence.
- The wrinkle in the Oriental rug will never come out no matter what the salesman tells you.
- Table lamps should match the scale of the furniture on which they stand: no massive oak-tree numbers on French curved side tables. *Hint:* Pink bulbs are great: they don't give pink, just soft, light and are great for flattering complexions. Avoid floor standing lamps: they are cluttering and clumsy and easy to trip over. Make sure that lamp cords run along a wall and not in any traffic flow.
- Think about throwing out those heavy drapes. Windows not only admit light but provide a view of the outside which acts like a moving painting—very much part of the decor.

Dining Room: What's Good and What's Bad

- A dining table might function as an all-purpose table to be used for eating, reading, homework, writing, studying. Make sure it's the right height for all these activities before you buy.

- Low-slung velvet chairs are pretty but terrible for dining. Not only is it difficult to reach your food, but wait until you try to get up!
- *Out* is a pedestal dining room table. Your weight, placed inadvertently on the edge of the table when rising, could easily tip it over. (Also beware of leaning on pedestal tables in restaurants.) Of course, a really solid pedestal table is safe and fine for leg room.
- *In* is a table with four sturdy legs. Heavy glass, three-quarters of an inch thick, set on (not in) a frame, is lovely. Anything well constructed with wooden or heavy metal legs is fine. Plastic is taking a big chance.
- Extension tables: watch them carefully. If you buy a table that can be extended by putting board leaves in the center, beware of its inherent tipping danger when you or a guest leans on it. Before you buy an extension table, test it with a considerable amount of weight *with the leaves in* to see if it's well made and collapse proof.
- Bridge-table types are not to be used as permanent tables. They tip.
- Armed chairs for easy rising are recommended. A good example is the early American captain's chair with the wide-splayed leg, the wide arm and the contoured, supported back. An upholstered version is even more luxurious.
- Wicker and straw seats—*out*. Also webbed seats.
- Rattan furniture is deceptively strong. (Remember Sidney Greenstreet in a thousand superb movies sitting in all those oversize rattan chairs?)
- Glass menagerie collections are dust collectors and besides, miniature anythings make you look bigger. They're not even in fashion any more.
- Leave walking-around space in back of the people seated at the table. It is embarrassing to be wedged into corners as you serve at your own dinner parties.
- Wheeled serving carts are the most useful invention since Saran-Wrap. Leave room to wheel one around when you plan your dining room.
- Less clutter in your dining room makes you look narrower, honestly! You can do without your grandmother's doohickey.

If you must have a tiny, useless table or chair as an accent, put it in a corner.
- Lighting: bad lighting produces extreme anxiety and discomfort. The Nazis knew this when they used glaring-hot bulbs to break down prisoners. Modern lighting often resembles this torture device. Just as bad is the lighting in which you have to squint to see what you're eating. People tend to fall asleep in dark rooms. Experiment to get the right light. If you want to empty out a room in which you are having a cocktail party, turn on *all* the lights. People just don't feel comfortable small-talking in a publicly lit room. Consider recessed lighting or track lighting with dimmers. Browse in lighting stores to see what you like.

The Bedroom: What's Good and What's Bad

- Even if she lives alone, a queen-sized woman does not have to sleep in a measly little single bed. Buy the most expansive and sybaritic bed you can afford and you can fit in your bedroom. It's good for the soul. Get the firmest mattress available. Sturdy wooden platforms are even better than bed frames.
- Water beds—the new wave? A matter of taste. Getting out of them is always tougher for the big woman. Do it slowly. I once left my husband in a hurry and started a whole storm at sea. He was actually seasick. But they are sturdier than they were in the sixties and made of a longer-lasting vinyl. Moreover, they are higher off the floor on a pedestal base to avoid puncturing. For those who prefer less mattress movement, there are "baffled" mattresses which divert the wave action, or even a combination water/foam sleep system which is a water mattress over foam padding. Many bigger women I've spoken to say water beds relax their aching bones better than anything else.
- If you read in bed, choose a firm, sturdy headboard.
- Avoid TV sets and lamps on movable tables or carts the way you'd avoid hepatitis.
- Remember hospital beds? Now you can get a home version of

a hospital bed which, by means of push buttons, raises buttocks, heads, torsos, weight-bearing, tired feet. It's most comfortable and luxurious looking. Also expensive.

- Fabric: be wary of tiny prints in bedspreads, draperies or carpets. They tend to be out of scale with an oppulent occupant.
- *Very important:* Make sure all carpeting and loose rugs have liners or padding for safety, long wear and comfort. Skidding across one's bedroom on a throw rug is not so many chuckles.
- Bedroom end tables should be high enough to reach from the bed without straining. If shelves are too close to the floor, you may fall when you stretch. For the same reason, don't place telephones too low on night table shelves.
- Armchairs with ottomans are the last word in comfort. Our feet tend to hurt at night, and a few minutes with them in an *up* position are magical.
- If you are lucky enough to have a friend in your bedroom and he resents your late-night eating and snacking, get a bed light that just hits your side of the bed and eat ice cream instead of Screaming Yellow Zonkers.
- Think about whether you really want to buy that *set* of bedroom furniture. It might be boring.
- Use air space to create storage or listening space for stereo equipment.
- Keep neat closets (see chapter 13, An Organized Life). If you can't keep them neat, at least close them—it makes for a nicer wake-up.

The Kitchen: What's Good and What's Bad

- If you have any choice in the matter, make sure countertops are at a comfortable height for working. Waist-high is too high and makes for aching shoulders and backs. Somewhere below your belly button is a nice working height.
- Kitchen floors have to be carefully chosen because we usually spend a lot of time standing around the kitchen. Wooden floors are reasonably comfortable and so are the softer vinyls and, of course, carpeting. There is nothing worse for a large woman

whose weight makes her back and feet tire easily than marble or ceramic tile floors. Watch the backaches pile up as you slice the carrots.

- If you have the space in your eat-in kitchen, stationary benches have always been charming. These can be constructed with special supports and wide bench seats to make them particularly strong and comfortable. Upholstered, they are a dream.

Thirty-one Decorating Tips

1. Only one or two items in a room should yell out, *Look at me!* No more, unless you want to make yourself crazy.
2. You're allowed to mix styles, periods, fabrics. Anyone who says, "I only like Modern" is as narrow as if she'd said, "I only go to Trinidad when I travel."
3. Decorator sheets can be used as inexpensive bedroom slip-covers, vanity skirts, curtains and wallpaper.
4. Don't buy anything about which you feel impelled to exclaim, "Isn't it precious?"
5. Never economize on mattresses or shoes. You spend most of your life on one or in the other.
6. Change the feel and size of a room by being daring with paint: you're allowed to have three walls one color and a fourth, another. Apartments don't have to be painted in milk-of-magnesia cream.
7. Wall murals, a painted bordering line, a representation of your home painted on a wall by your child, are all examples of the beauty power in paint.
8. Put just a few colors in a small room: a larger room can carry more color variety.
9. One conversation piece is nice in every room. An ancient fisherman's block and tackle. A painting painted in colors from earth and herbs. Something to make someone say, "What's that interesting thing all about?"
10. You'll get bored very soon with whimsical, vapid nudes dancing around your bathroom wallpaper.

11. Although someone once said, "Good taste means nothing flamboyant, freakish or gimmicky," *one* flamboyant, freakish or gimmicky thing in a room can add humor and passion.
12. Baskets are great for holding dripping bunches of purple grapes, magenta plums, Halloween-orange squash or violets.
13. Muddy colors are never magical.
14. Throw out wilted flowers *when* they begin to droop: nothing is more depressing than dying posies.
15. Before you decide definitely on a bedroom wallpaper, think, Could I be sick for two weeks in a room papered in this?
16. Oriental-type seating about two inches from the floor would not be good for even a heavy Oriental.
17. Clutter is a big woman's worst enemy.
18. Antiques can be ugly. Modern pieces can be clumsy and nonfunctional. Get what you like—not what's in style.
19. Rooms often seem smaller without furniture in them. Your eyes tend to focus on walls which, without distracting furniture, appear closer to you. An important point when you're planning for a new and empty apartment.
20. Cloth tape measures are rotten because they curl and stretch and end up crooked: use a steel measure which retracts in its own little case.
21. When buying carpeting, ask the price *installed*. It makes a great difference.
22. A house without a bookcase is a house that houses a big, boring woman.
23. Look for paintings at neighborhood fairs, village art shows, even (you'd be surprised) in elementary art school shows. A charming primitive is delightful!
24. Cocktail tables can be knee-knockers and couch-blockers. Circular shapes are nice for getting around without getting impaled.
25. Cork walls mask kids' sounds. Felt wallpaper is good also.
26. Don't buy a lampshade without bringing the lamp. Never have more mistakes been made than in this area.
27. Change your furniture around for a fresh feeling. Everything that's planted in your living room doesn't have roots.

28. Slab-type couches (usually Danish modern designs) are hard on your bottom.
29. Wall units on tension-pole mounts are destined to fail and collapse. *Avoid.*
30. If you weigh over 150 and are a second over thirty, don't try sleeping permanently on a convertible couch.
31. If you are a terrific tatter or embroiderer or crewel worker, nothing is nicer for throw pillows and chair seats. Put your personal touch in your home.

Above all, don't be afraid to take chances. Boring, monotonous homes belong to women who stick to the same old things all the time. You *can* re-cover the Dreadful Flowered Mistake. Even if we live in a transient world of three-year leases, one-year jobs, four-week love affairs and endless new diets, we can still live beautifully and creatively. To live with style when your own style is larger than that which the fashion czars dictate is the *only* style, takes guts and a certain amount of healthy egotism. (I *do* like myself. I *do* like my home and my way of life. Valuable people don't always and only come in size 10. I *have* great taste!)

Apartment, castle, rabbit hutch or hotel room—the big woman should love to go home.

XV Relax

6:00 A.M. The first thing you notice is the dread in your stomach. Your upper lip is drenched with sweat and your heart is doing flipflops.

What now?

Oh, God! It's happened. They *told* you to lose weight, over and over, your mother and your best friends and you didn't, you tried, but couldn't, how come they can't understand that, but now it's too late, it's happened, dread heart attack, just as they all said, and . . .

Wait a minute! Just *wait a minute now!*

You had a checkup yesterday, right? And didn't the doctor say you were in perfect health? Of course. And didn't he say that as long as you maintained your weight and didn't yo-yo up and down, and your pressure and everything stayed normal, you didn't have to worry about your weight?

Yes—yes, that's *right!*

So what is it? What's the matter if it isn't my heart?

What it is, is nameless panic. Except there's a name for it: *anxiety.*

But what am I anxious about? Everything seems so good. Shouldn't you always be able to identify the cause of anxiety?

Not always. But don't worry. You're not alone. Nearly one in every three adults in the United States takes antianxiety pills at least sometime during his or her life, according to Dr. Herbert Kleber, professor of psychiatry at the Yale Medical School and Director of the Substance Abuse Treatment Unit of the Connecticut Mental Health Unit.

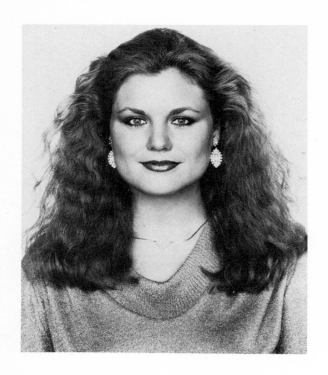

And heavy women who have trouble finding clothes, boyfriends, jobs and self-admiration seem to suffer from anxiety more than the myth that pictures them as "jolly and placid" would ever let you suspect.

And it's getting worse. Thirty years ago, who ever heard of Librium or Valium? Who ever heard of meditation except in a book about the Far East? Who *hasn't* heard of the weapons to fight anxiety, today?

We all suffer from the little, invisible pinpricks of stress that seem to culminate in feelings of depression or nervousness, more and more. Traffic jams, noise, money worries, weight worries—nothing major, but boy, it all builds up. Until one day, you wake up on what should be a golden morning with a sweaty lip and a pounding heart and no real, outstanding, *obvious* reason for either of them.

What do you do?

Relax. You can, you know. And without pills. They have been trying for too many years to pump the heavy woman up with pills: diet pills and metabolism pills and green pills and orange pills and sleeping pills, and anti-anxiety pills and you-name-it pills. Enough with the pills. Out with all of them. Begin to rely on *naturally* relaxing resources.

First thing to consider is sleep. Are you getting enough? What's enough, anyway? To some people, twelve hours is enough. Others need only eight. Others manage on six and an afternoon nap. Some feel dopey if they get more than five. It's not how long you sleep, or even when you sleep, but how thoroughly you sleep. I have a friend who drops off as soon as her head touches the pillow. She loves to quote Mark Twain on sleep: "If you can't sleep, try lying on the end of the bed. Then you might drop off." Very funny. Those of us who toss and turn all night would like to strangle such wise guys.

Try These Strategies to Relax Enough to Drop Off to Sleep

1. Unstretch yourself. First relax your legs, then your stomach, then your chest, then your arms, shoulders and neck. Last, let the muscles of your jaws and your mouth and eyes go. Concentrate on relaxing the tight skin on top of your scalp. Pretend your body is a bag of sand through which is oozing a tiny trickle of sand, slowly, slowly, until the bag is empty.

2. Didn't work? Hmmmmm. Okay. Get out of bed. Do *not* toss and turn for hours in the dark. Change your physical space. The bed should only be associated with sleep. Read a book in the living room. Call a friend, write a letter, clean out your refrigerator, clean a closet. When you start feeling tired, think about going back to bed—not before.

3. Then prepare for the sleep that will come. Have a glass of warm milk, a glass of wine, even a bowl of oatmeal, if that relaxes you. Take a warm (not hot) bath, daydream for a while, free your mind from the day.

4. If you have been having trouble with sleep, no one has to tell you to cut down on coffee, colas and other caffeine-containing drinks. Or do they?

5. Saul Bellow once wrote of a terrific cure for a stiff neck; I find

it works as well for insomnia. Lying in bed, I write the alphabet with my head, slowly and lovingly, tracing each letter from A to Z and, if necessary, through them all once or twice around. I have never finished the routine three times before sleep came.

6. Ever self-hypnotize yourself? You can. "You are getting drowsy, your arm is falling asleep, oh boy do your fingers feel tired, each finger is falling asleep . . ." and so on.

7. Hair brushing. Never fails to send me off. Someone else has to do it for you. Yesssss . . .

8. Buy a "sleep sound." Many large novelty stores like Hammacher Schlemmer carry little boxes which give off the soothing sound of the surf. Or a mother's heartbeat to bring you right back to a womb. You can try it, although I think a loud heart-beat would make *me* more nervous.

9. Breathe in, hold for ten seconds, breathe out. Repeat.

10. Dr. Peter J. Steincrohn, in his book *How to Get a Good Night's Sleep*, suggests the tongue-in-cheek method as pretty close to infallible. He tells you to take inventory, see what's tense on your body. Neck? Legs? Maybe, tongue. Aha, the prime offender —the tongue! Not until your tongue "tires and drops back, relaxed, and your teeth have unlocked will you relax," says the good doctor. Disengage it from pressing hard against the roof of your mouth or along the back ridge of your upper teeth (where most insomniacs' tongues are). Keep it away. "Gently slide your tongue tip between your teeth, against your inner cheek, either side. Relaxation will come immediately.

Okay. You can sleep. Hooray for nothing. You still get anxiety attacks. You're still not relaxed. What now?

Well, *don't* take a whole bunch of pills unless your trusted doctor says you absolutely need them. They don't cure although they do make symptoms disappear. Tranquilizers and, of course, barbiturates can certainly be habit-forming and psychologically addictive. There are lots of other things that can help.

TRY TM

It's no mystery, transcendental meditation. Find a quiet place and sit in a comfortable position. It helps to close your eyes and place your hands palms up, either cradling each other or one on each thigh. Choose a word or a phrase that has a pleasant sound or is meaningful to you. *Ululoo* is one *I* like. That is your "mantra." Repeat it, over and over. Don't worry if irrelevant thoughts and ideas flit through your mind. Just sit passively, repeat your "mantra," relax your body and let go. TM followers say that a daily twenty-minute meditative session is better than Valium and Hershey Bars. The Beatles and Mia Farrow were famous TM devotees. Also any number of Maharishis.

TRY YAWNING

It's the greatest. Let your jaw drop down. Don't force it—let it drop naturally. Oh, let go more than *that*. Now think of other people yawning and feel your own yawn start, deep deep down in your throat, wider now. It feels as if the yawn will never be over —even your eyes may start to tear. What's happened? You've taken an enormous breath and you've filled your lungs. Your jaw has been stretched and relaxed. Ditto your mouth, cheeks and tongue. You've put new energy, new oxygen, into your system. You've relaxed. Try it before important meetings, before sleep, when stopped at a traffic light, when you feel sluggish, when you feel tense.

TRY HEAD ROLLS

Backache? Tension headache? Kids getting you wild? Close your eyes. Drop your head until your chin is almost resting in your chest. Relax. Now breathe deeply and around to the right, all the way, now slowly let it fall back, complete the head roll. Now the other way. Your head weighs fifteen pounds and it's *heavy*. Head rolls do nice things for the shoulder and neck muscles that must support the head. They relax.

TRY YOGA

It looks simple but it's deceptively complicated. You must buy a book or a tape or take a course to learn how to properly relax in yoga fashion. Devotees swear that the comtemplative concentration, the breathing and the various postures, recharge emotional and spiritual batteries and relax like nothing else. It takes about forty minutes a day. You need a cushion and/or some blankets and a quiet place. You learn, particularly, how to breathe deeply to cleanse, give energy and refresh. Yoga is a philosophy, a physical and mental discipline; a way of life that teaches mastery over the body and the senses. No one can be tense and have an anxiety attack in the middle of a yoga session—it's not allowed.

TRY ACTIVITY

When anxiety or tension hits, do something. Don't allow yourself to be paralyzed by a fear you cannot even place. Action provides immediate relief for tension. Go for a bike ride, a brisk walk, go through the exercise routines in chapter 7 of this book, do a *physical* thing. Making love is nice. Thinking doesn't help at all. Eating doesn't either. Well, maybe a little.

TRY DUSK

Stop what you're doing, *right now*, and take account of the tension state your body is in, *this minute*. Does your back hurt? Are you clenching your jaws or your teeth? Do your eyes ache, way back there? Try the simplest thing of all—the absence of light and sound. Close your shades and doors, turn off your telephone. Take ten minutes, in the softly, soothing dusk you've created, to just stop. Everything! Sit back or lie back, and *stop!* Come to a halt! Free-associate—which means let your mind wander all over the place, picking up the sweetest memories it can find. Think of islands and oceans. Think of perfumed night air and fireflies. Think of tender voices. Think of limitless space and miles and miles of desert or sky. Wind down. If you have suffered from a sensory overload of too much noise, light, smells, movement, janglings—disengage. For ten minutes. No light (or a very dim light) and no sound. Just relax.

TRY LETTING GO INTERNALLY

Breathe slowly. Listen to yourself breathe. Slow it down. Focus on it. Feel your heart rate slowing down. Feel your brain slowing down. Shut out the telephone, dog, kid and refrigerator noises. Shut out the thought of the crummy thing your sister-in-law said. Block out your backache and your itches. Block out smells. Feel the blood coursing through your body. Let go of the stomach muscles, the chest muscles. Develop control of your inner landscape by actively slowing down parts of it. Relax.

TRY MASSAGE

Get a friend to do it, or go to a professional. There is nothing in the whole world like massage for relaxation. For the full effect:

- Lie down on a firm surface.
- Take off your clothes, or most of them.
- Turn the lights down very, very low.
- Whip out the mixture of avocado, peanut, olive, mineral, and lime oils you've prepared (or plain old Johnson's baby oil, if you're lazy).
- Let a nice person go to work on you.

This is what a gentle, kneading, stroking, tapping massage, administered with strong, expert, smooth hands, does:

- It works like a sleeping pill with none of the dangerous side effects.
- It increases circulation.
- It soothes nerves.
- It unkinks tired muscles and aching joints.
- It increases oxygen consumption.
- It has been known to turn people on, sexually.
- It loosens muscle spasms.
- And, boy, it relieves anxiety.

The rhythm and tempo are everything in massage. Pummeling is not terrific for frazzled nerves. Neither is erratic pinching. It's stroking and kneading and pressing and tapping and rotating and kneading some more. It's paying attention to toes and spines and backs of knees and backs and, very important, crucial in fact, buttocks. And under eyes (very gently) and around temples and individual fingers and noses and everything except breasts with warming, loving, vibrating motions.

The best thing you can do for yourself is to send your partner out for a professional massage so he/she gets a good idea of what's great. Warmed-up creams are nice to use as a change from oils. If you have no partner, you can give yourself a massage, but I'd be lying if I said it was just as good. Still, it's better than nothing, and a real aid to relaxation. A bathtub is a good place for a self-massage because soapy hands move more smoothly. Knead your temples, thighs, underthighs, the balls of your feet, your neck muscles, your ankles, firmly and gently. Use both hands to give your abdomen a soapy, circular massage. With the balls of your fingers and with the flat of your hands, don't miss a reachable spot.

Here's who and what *shouldn't* get massages:

- Anyone who has ever had a blood clot.
- Any area that is swollen or inflamed.
- The abdomen of a pregnant woman.
- Your breasts.

TRY BIOFEEDBACK

This is the newest of all the methods aimed at inner relaxation. Biofeedback has been used, rather successfully, for cure of headaches, certain cardiac irregularities, stroke patients' residuals, and hypertension. Through a delicate electronic device, patients are taught to recognize and modify or alter their own body functions and psychological responses—until they can recognize and modify without the machine. Clearly, this could be marvelous as an aid to relaxation. The tense, heavy woman can *learn* to depend on her own, nonelectronic, easily portable machinery of her own biological system through biofeedback. She eventually won't need electronics or pills to know when and how she should "turn herself off." Although it is still in the experimental stage, biofeedback promises to be a true weapon against anxiety and stress. Check in your local hospital or with your doctor to find out about biofeedback programs in your community.

TRY ACUPUNCTURE

It sounds crazy, but it works too often to ignore it. Sometimes, by inserting needles in various parts of the body (a painless procedure somewhat like bug bites), tension, migraine headaches, stress, pain, even menstrual cramps can be relieved. Consult your local county medical organization for the names of practitioners *officially licensed* to practice acupuncture. Pregnant women should *never* have acupuncture since it can induce miscarriages. Do *not* fall for the line that staples in the ear are like acupuncture and will help you lose weight along with tenseness. It won't. You'll just look dumb with staples in your ear.

TRY FIGURING IT OUT

Try to find out what's behind your anxiety. It may be very abstract, very submerged, but there *is* a reason, rest assured of that. You will recognize it when you dredge it out and then you're on your way to relief. Talking to someone who is supportive and who cares is always an enormous help. Start anywhere. Explore your psyche, your needs, your doubts. Don't worry: talk long enough and you'll hit on the cause of your stomach-dreads. What *are* you afraid of?

Is it that you've always wanted to do something, *accomplish* something, and time is going so fast and your birthday is coming up and—aha! So that's it!

It's tenth reunion time at school and how great, *everyone* will be there, and so what if you've put on all this weight, this year, you're still—aha! So that's it!

Your job has become a bummer. Dullsville. The time is coming to make a move, but how can you possibly go for interviews until after the diet and—aha! So *that's* it!

Your parents are growing older, and your father had that crying jag the other day and you felt so helpless, so angry at having to be the parent instead of—aha! That's it!

You're bored. You have nothing to do. Aha!

Your best friend's husband has just announced he is having an affair, and you know you have nothing to worry about from your husband, but still you've been having these stupid dreams and—aha!

TRY STOPPING THE DIET

You're walking along a wooded path. Everywhere are flowers blooming and tiny creatures of nature doing their natural things. In the distance looms a wild and wonderful mountain. The air is warm and sweet as the exotic frangipani flower.

But it is not frangipani you actually smell. It is a fried egg sandwich. You are on a diet and you crave it and it crowds out all other thoughts, all other smells. Fried egg is what you smell—in your head.

By all rights you should be calm and relaxed. You should be able to slow down, take it easy, in this place. You should be able to be serene by this bubbling stream with jumping, lyrical trout.

But nothing works. You are only relaxed when you are able to eat naturally. You are interested in lyrical trout when they are poached with plenty of butter. And what would really relax you is that damned fried egg sandwich you cannot have.

Your diet makes you consumed, obsessed with the food you have forbidden yourself to eat. You smell the flowers but what you are really smelling is the bacon that is not on the diet list. You see the wild and wonderful mountain but you are really seeing only the Big Rock Candy Mountain. Or even Big Chocolate Nougat Mountain. And you hear that gurgling stream, you really do, but you can't concentrate on streams when the only thing in the world that would make you happy is a fried egg sandwich.

Go off the diet. Relax. Not having a fried egg sandwich can ruin a beautiful landscape and make you very tense.

TRY NOT FEELING GUILTY

One of the biggest impediments to relaxing is that good old twentieth-century condition—guilt. Although certain nationalities claim to have invented it, guilt strikes all races, creeds and colors. (Well, maybe Jewish sons and daughters do feel slightly more guilt than anyone else.) But rest assured you're not alone. Guilt strikes kings and common citizens and even Shakespearean characters. Lady Macbeth spent a lot of time washing her hands because she felt guilty. Oedipus, the legendary king of Thebes, blinded himself and gave up his kingdom from guilt. My cousin used to get twice the allowance the rest of us got because her mother felt guilty about leaving her so often. We feel more guilt than anyone else, I think, because we've been made to think it's our fault we're so fat and if only we used a little willpower, we could stop aggravating everyone with our size.

It's bad for you to feel guilty. Aside from making you feel tense, it does nasty things to your stomach and your libido. Here are four things you don't have to feel guilty about any more. After you read them, make your own list.

1. *Stop feeling guilty about bingeing on food.*

Listen to what the Fat Liberation Front (FLF) has to say about bingeing: "Relax. It's okay to binge. You've been repressed about food a lot, and you deserve as much as you want. There's nothing to be ashamed of; eating isn't a crime and doesn't have to be 'rational.' . . . Food is a natural tranquilizer. Society approves of Valium, Milltown, etc., but frowns upon food intake as a 'neurotic' solution. . . . Keep plenty of binge foods around the house. It's okay to make mistakes and eat more or less than you want."

What happens when you give yourself "permission" to binge and stop feeling guilty about it? No one says you'll lose weight; but what will happen is that as you gradually relax around food, stop feeling the guilt of starving, then bingeing when the hunger becomes unbearable, then starving again to make up for the binge —*you will lose the urge to binge.* The FLF says that panic bingeing and starvation cycles must be like "a sledgehammer to the body's blood sugar regulation mechanisms. In just a few moments, the body takes in thousands of calories, usually from candy and other quick-energy foods. This is not neurotic. It is an absolutely natural reaction to intense, prolonged hunger."

2. *Stop feeling guilty because your mother, father, husband or child is depressed and unhappy about your weight.*

You are you. You have enormous value and self-worth. If someone else is depressed and you think it is your fault, listen—*It is not.* Dr. Ari Kiev, Director of the Social Psychiatry Research Center in New York, says, "Feeling guilty or blaming yourself (for other people's depressions) is a waste of emotional energy. Being preoccupied with guilt and self-blame is unproductive, if not counterproductive."

If someone you love is desperately unhappy with your looks, don't let it bother you. You are a viable and beautiful human being and the person you love will have to work out his own problems, because, make no mistake, they are his problems—not yours. Your friends and relatives will have to struggle with their own embarrassments and fears for you and not burden you with them. Your job is to make yourself a terrific person and increase your self-worth daily: *you are not responsible if others can't accept your body.*

3. *Stop feeling guilty about flying the coop.*

- Your six-year-old is in nursery school and doesn't like it when he finds the baby-sitter waiting for him at noon, instead of you.
- Your husband doesn't like getting his own dinner the two nights a week you go back to school for a degree.
- Your boss would like to have you attend his almost-daily lunchtime meeting but you need some time during the day to yourself.
- Your mother is alone and wishes you'd take her shopping and out to dinner more often, but you simply can't afford the time she expects.

Part of finding out that you have enormous self-worth, no matter how much you weigh, is the immediate cessation of self-sacrifice. Others don't really benefit that much when you sacrifice your time, energy, and emotional well-being for them—and *you* have your whole life to lose. Certainly, you must be a giving person to those you love but not at the cost of your own individuality. The husband, kid, mother and boss will all survive without your constant ministrations and support. If you submerge yourself in someone else's needs, all the time, you lose the essence of *you.* Be selfish. You count. You have to do what will make you a person.

You have to go where your life takes you. *They* don't feel guilty about making you feel guilty.

4. *Stop feeling guilty about being neurotic.*

You're allowed to feel depressed, saddened, not answer the telephone, be rude, be greedy, envy someone else's money and figure, tell tales on your best friend, lie about your health, weight or salary, feel paranoid, feel furious at someone who means well, say four-letter words, be uncomfortable alone in restaurants, hate your kid, gossip, say you took the day off because you had the flu when all you really have is a need to lie in bed all day, eat Hershey Bars and read a trashy book.

You're allowed to do these things sometimes, a reasonable amount of times. Who doesn't? Perfectly steady and unneurotic people are not to be trusted. They are unlovable.

If you find yourself being neurotic *all* the time, you've got problems. Get some help from your neighborhood professional (therapist or psychiatrist—not beautician).

Above all, *try.* There are *so many* techniques that twentieth-century America has invented or adopted to help us relax. Among others, there's Rolfing, and Zen, and hypnosis, and deep knee bends, and any of a myriad of techniques that erase the stress of thinking, breathing, being alive! But the real secret to relaxation, I've discovered, is getting in touch with yourself—no matter what method you use. When you increase your self-understanding, you rule out self-deception and you simply find it easier to live and make decisions. Increasing self-understanding means finding out what colors, noises, situations and threats most irritate you—and then staying clear of them, if possible. It means living a busy, changing life which is filled with experiences rather than fruitless searches to lose weight. It means finding ways to soothe over the fears and the frustrations, even temporarily, to give yourself needed respites. A warm glass of milk never solved anything, really. It sure can *ease* the flipflopping heart and the sweaty upper lip syndrome, though.

And be patient with yourself. Relaxation can't be delivered up to you like a Big Mac. You have to work at it until it comes naturally.

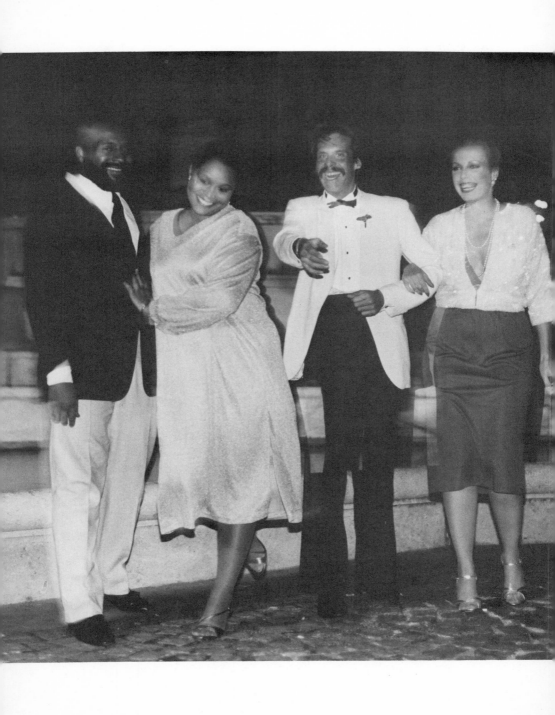

XVI How to Develop a Great Social Life

So you hate the singles bars.

You'd rather not go out at all than be fixed up with the losers your kind but misguided friends have chosen for you.

You shun the resorts' singles weekends because you feel just like another piece of meat (a large piece) being looked over by men who seem like butchers.

You're even tired of the same old women friends who haven't come up with an original conversation since school days.

Do you really think you're unusual? Think. When was the last time you ever heard *anyone,* fat or thin, say she *loved* the rat race to meet new people? It's a universal problem.

Listen—it's hard to be alone, at any age, any size. And there's no getting around the fact that there seems to be, lately, a real dearth of terrific people around—in your life. And the older you get, the more difficult it seems. Whomever you meet seems to be taken or terrible. And you haven't even met *anyone* for the last few months.

Like everything else, there is a right way and a wrong way to attack the problem.

The wrong way is to sit in your kitchen, mope, write poetry, cry a lot, eat solitary sundaes, wait until you lose weight to meet the world.

The right way is to be aggressive. That's the secret. *You* have to move. *Do something* about it. If you're looking for an interesting man, don't limit yourself to plans or places where only men are involved. Some of the best ways to meet men are through new and exciting women! And, conversely, if you are looking for new women friends, don't concentrate just on women. Men have wives, girl friends, women business associates who may end up, after you get to know them, being your closest and dearest friends. If you're lonely, get out and meet some *people.* People lead to new life activities, new options, new relationships, new futures.

One of the Best Ways of Meeting People Is to . . . Have a Party

Obviously, you're not going to meet too many new faces if you invite only the tried and true regulars of your life. Now is the moment to sit down and make a list of "possibles":

- The writer you meet at your sister-in-law's luncheon.
- The nextdoor neighbors who look interesting (even though you're all always too rushed for more than a smile of greeting).
- The pleasant-looking guy you meet every morning in the elevator at work.
- Your cousin whose political views are nuts but who has those interesting friends from Canada visiting.
- The periodontist who has been treating your gums. (You *think* he's not married.)
- The guy at the last business meeting who was telling you about his sailboat.
- The wine expert you met at the gourmet club dinner.
- The young woman who just opened that new boutique in town.
- The couple at Lucy's dinner party who made you fall down laughing.
- Your boss.
- Your old boyfriend.
- Your grammar school enemy.

• The teacher at the course you've been taking.
• Someone from the class.

Ask each person to bring a friend.

You're going to end up with a fabulously eclectic crowd who are bound to be interesting simply by dint of the different backgrounds they do *not* share. This will be a party to end all parties, to open your horizons, widen your life-style.

You know, it's a funny thing. Loneliness is not limited to fat people. The people who look most successful, socially, may be desperate for a touch of new life. And when you get to know people better, a very strange phenomenon occurs. You lose weight. Not the pounds you'd see on a scale, but the *illusion* of weight. Your personality replaces your fat image when someone comes to like you. I can't count how many new friends have said to me, after I've known them for a few months, "Jean, have you lost weight?" I haven't, I've gained spirit and fun and character, in their eyes; they no longer see my size first. Getting closer to people is the greatest diet in the world.

A little nervous? Ask someone to share the hostessing with you.

Still a little nervous about asking all those new people to your home? Too bad. You'll get over it as soon as you see what a ball everyone is having—including you. Life is too short to stick to the invite-only-your-old-pals-once-a-month-to-dinner syndrome. What's the *worst* thing that can happen? Someone will say he can't make it. So what? He has still been flattered by your invitation—you can bet on it. You've lost nothing. You've made a friendly gesture.

Okay. You've done it. Invitations have been sent out or delivered verbally. Now plan the party.

This is a chance for us to be at our most glamorous in the most comfortable of circumstances—our own home.

First—what to wear? The ubiquitous caftan is the dream answer, but the most gorgeous one you can find. A little job from India or Russia with many colors and iridescent threads. You can even wear a pair of pretty bedroom slippers with it. No one will see them and you'll be able to glide through the evening. Let the others wear the polyester slack suits, the girdles, the miserable binding straps. You be the star in the most dramatic loose, long caftan.

This is your home. The furniture is geared to you, you know where the bathroom is for the quick touch-up jobs; the chairs won't buckle under your weight; there are no tiny glass cocktail tables placed in obstacle courses. You can relax. Elude the hammock even if it's yours. This is no time for sinking down, down, down which necessitates a clumsy get-up.

Is your house ready? Hall closet cleaned out with enough hangers for the coats? Soap and towels in the bathrooms? Doorman alerted, or, if you have a private house, outside lights on? Fresh and different flowers *everywhere!* Beds made even if you don't plan for people to go into the bedroom? (There's nothing worse than a sloppy unmade bed and junk on the floor for a party.)

Have you told people how you want them to dress? The wine expert is going to feel like a jerk in a suit and tie if everyone else is wearing jeans.

Do you have kids? They're nice for serving drinks or hors d'oeuvres; they're not nice for socializing or performing unless the kid's name is Mariel Hemingway. Even then, I'm not so sure. When the kid gets to be thirty-two, he or she can come to the party as a guest. Not until then.

Enough seats? You don't have to plan one for everybody because people tend to stand around, but have a reasonable amount of seating available.

Do you have a wheeled cart? Can you borrow one? They're great for a movable feast or bar. Do you have small nests of tables? Buy or borrow some. They're handy for buffets and for the odd ashtray.

Party games? Yecch. That's for kids and unimaginative souls. If you invite terrific people, rely on the conversation to be stimulating, maybe even unforgettable. Stunts, decorations, people who read palms, are generally silly and unnecessary. Music, live or canned, is nice though, but background stuff. *Not* The Grateful Dead or Kiss.

You don't need:

- A fortune of money.
- Three in help (one would be nice—not necessary).

- A huge room.
- Crystal, silver or caviar.

You do need:

- An effective corkscrew (try it out first).
- Good wine (it can be inexpensive, too—make friends with the liquor store man, he'll tout you onto a mellow number).
- Good liquor. Splurge here. It spells class.
- Cook-ahead foods. Sweating over a hot stove during the party is not terrific for making new friends.

FOODS

No diet stuff to prove you're not a glutton. It proves nothing.

Hors d'oeuvres: Oh, you can have a plate of stuffed celery and raw cauliflower around for the purists, but check to find some more interesting, conversation-provoking hors d'oeuvres that you can prepare the night before. Guacamole is nice for a dip. Quiche is easy to make, elegant to serve and can be frozen even if it is prepared even a week before the party.

The main courses: Try a classy casserole for a great buffet help-yourself. Beef, chicken or shrimp curry can be prepared and frozen beforehand and served with a mind-boggling array of condiments like raisins, coconut, peppers, chutney, egg white—whatever is imaginative and pretty. Served with rice, curry never fails to please. Particularly elegant is a crown roast of lamb all done up in tiny booties and maybe set aflame with brandy. But food doesn't have to be expensive to be imaginative. American cheese arranged creatively on a pretty platter, with parsley and Greek olives and maybe some real oak leaves bordering the plate, is much more appetizing than a plate of fancy French cheese running unappealingly all over a paper plate. I know a woman who couldn't afford to serve expensive liquor. She made a fruit-ade punch, nothing spectacular really—unless you looked at it. In each ice cube was imprisoned a whole strawberry, blueberries, some gorgeous chunk of real fruit so that the effect as the ice floated in the punch was of ice-fruit flowers splendidly wreathing the punch bowl. There wasn't a guest who could stay away from it. Vegetables should always be fresh and everything hot should be hot. Ditto for cold being cold.

Desserts: They must be plentiful and astounding. All the whipped-cream stuff, the cheesiest cheesecakes, the flashiest chocolate numbers, the sweetest, ripest, most colorful fruits should be available for guests to gorge on and stare at and gossip about. There's nothing like succulent desserts to put everyone in a good mood.

In other words, if you have always entertained a passion for good foods—trot them out! Spread the good stuff around. Be *proud* of your good taste and your lusty selections. Happy eaters make good conversation.

Okay. You're past the food planning. Now get ready for the guests.

PLAN TO INTRODUCE THEM WITH CLUES

"Betty, I want you to meet Sandy who teaches the most erotic course at The New School." (You've given them something with which to start small talking—Betty's dying to find out what Sandy teaches!)

"Bob, if you play your cards right, my friend Anne here will give you the inside dope on her new novel."

"Sanford, your back hurt lately? Lew, whose hand I am conveniently holding, performs the meanest spinal fusion in town. And an orthopedist and a guy who has ESP ought to have plenty in common."

"Janet, this is my cousin Les who thinks Watergate is nothing to what's coming in the energy crisis. Janet has been playing politics for years, Lester—see if you can convince her of your ideas!"

Forgot the name of your best friend, just as you are about to introduce him? Don't panic. Try this:

"Guess what! It's happened. I forgot my best friend's name. I also am having trouble with my own. Introduce yourselves, you two!"

Or, talk fast, fake it, no one will notice:

"Lloyd, this character hits the fastest tennis ball in town—even if he does cheat. Lloyd, tell another tennis buff about the game last week when Pancho Gonzales stopped by."

DON'T GET SO INVOLVED IN YOUR OWN PARTY, YOU DON'T MAKE BROWNIE POINTS FOR LATER

Remember, what's the point of this party? Why did you bring these disparate people together? To have a good time, yes, to acquit some social obligations, yes, but most of all, to make new friends, *to strengthen your own social life.* Don't forget it for a moment. Walk around from group to group and get to know people. *Stay* with someone who looks promising. Use conversational self-disclosure, which does not mean that you dump your most intimate secrets on the cute wine expert in the first five minutes of conversation, but you do tell him something important, something *personal,* something interesting about yourself. Avoid clichés. Ask him about *him* by using *you* questions. They go like this:

"What do *you* think is the most dynamic American wine?"

"Do *you* know how wine is really made? I've always wanted to know what happens beyond the stomping of the grapes with the feet."

"How does a dummy pick a great wine? Can *you* tell me?"

"How did *you* get involved in wine?"

Tell him who you really are: not just the person whose house it is but the real you and why you would be interesting to know. You might start out like this:

"Hi. You have reminded me all night of a guru I interviewed for a magazine article. You look so controlled, so relaxed. Am I right?"

"I'm not so terrific playing Perle Mesta: I feel so clumsy at hostessing, sometimes. For instance, how would you go about bringing *those* two people together for a conversation? They would be dynamite together, but I can't figure out how to manage the introduction."

"Could you come look at the wines I've chosen? Which should I serve first and which ones should be cold and which ones room temperature? You can't imagine how I'd appreciate some advice!"

"I'm doing a survey. If you could come back to life in another time, when would it be?"

Listen to your guests. Respond, *really* respond by making appropriate comments and nonverbal gestures. Squeezing someone's hand is good if he's just told you something poignant, for instance.

Memorable food, drink, conversation, settings, produce extraordinary effects on guests. You look and sound appealing, gorgeous. You are a fun person—a delicious hostess. You have probably made yourself some good friends: you have started a social ball rolling. And not one person has thought of you in terms of weight but only in terms of *great!* Actually, I don't mind if someone calls me a big woman if they say I'm a marvelous big woman.

Other Ways of Meeting People

Okay—you're tired of giving parties and your air conditioner is on the blink anyway. What *else* can you do to spice up your social life?

Linda Kline, President of Maxima Search Ltd. (and interviewed in chapter 10, How to Get a Job), says this:

"The traditional ways of meeting men are not for me. I've been to a couple of singles bars and they are disgusting. If you are heavy, bars are particularly difficult to deal with because every man at a singles bar is looking for an airline stewardess. You have to remember, I think, that men are not a different species from *people*. If you are an interesting person and if you go to places where interesting people gather—you'll surely meet people."

Start there. The best place to meet men is through other interesting friends. Be frank and open. Let acquaintances know you'd like to enlarge your social life. Ask them to invite you over the next time they have other piquant personalities over.

Another great meeting place is schools. Take a course that is not "female" oriented—*if* your purpose is to meet a mixed crowd. Assertiveness courses, often art history courses, psychology courses, tend to attract more women than men. Politics, economics, film courses attract as many men as women. Studying with people in a relaxed atmosphere makes making friends quite easy.

Organizations shouldn't be ignored—political, professional and social. Join the local bridge club, the chess club. If you have a degree in marketing, for instance, you should join the American Marketing Association. Writers should belong to the American Society of Journalists and Authors. There are organizations for rose growers, businesswomen, civil liberties enthusiasts, history buffs, gourmet chefs. Be careful with political organizations because often, women tend to be treated as "gofers" (go for coffee, stamps, etc.). Be assertive and do whatever you feel capable of doing. Introduce yourself to as many new people as you can—don't wait for someone to find you.

Community groups that try to raise the consciousness of neighborhoods are fine places to raise different kinds of social consciousness. Deciding who gets to be president of the block association takes place over innumerable cups of coffee and experience-sharing sessions. A good way to meet people.

Become an expert at something. Photography. Antiques. Silversmithing. Fund raising. Egyptian hieroglyphics. Not only is the learning fun, but you can offer yourself out to speak to groups and clubs on your newfound expertise. In my neighborhood, one man has made a lifetime hobby of traveling pay off: he makes travelogs with humorous and fascinating commentary, and is in great demand to show these slides and movies. He tells me women are constantly calling him with proposals for dinner, theater and trip advice over romantic candlelight dinners.

The National Association to Aid Fat Americans, Box 745, Westbury, NY 11590, has a pen pal program that was created to give NAAFA members an opportunity to correspond and exchange ideas with other NAAFAns. There are many reasons to have a pen pal: you might discuss mutual problems, receive and offer needed encouragement, make friends who share your problems with dating, clothing, medical care, etc. This is *not* a dating service, although it is true that a few pen pals have wound up marrying each other. It is one more way to increase your social life and reach out to others if you feel shy or if you already know everybody who lives within fifty miles of you.

Be adventuresome. Modify your old behavior. For instance:

You hail a cab at the precise moment a busy-looking guy hails the same cab. Do you fight it out? Jump in quickly? No. Offer to share the ride. You may end up sharing everything else.

Do favors for people. You never know how they repay themselves. A friend of mine offered to temporarily "hostess" in a restaurant newly bought by her next-door neighbor. She would not accept any pay, said she was doing it as a friend and ended up, a year later, owning half the restaurant as the new wife and business partner of the neighbor.

Your mother told you not to talk to strangers on the bus. Or in the supermarket. Ignore that advice. If the risks are small (how dangerous can talking to someone at the checkout counter be?), take them and open up your life to new faces, new experiences!

Believe it or not, therapy groups are great places to meet people. The atmosphere is conducive to sharing and supportive kindness. Rap sessions at groups for the newly widowed or divorced have also been known to start new lives for participants. Of course you shouldn't go to a therapy group just to meet people. One attends these sessions because she is looking for help. Still, it *has* happened that people find themselves with lifetime rap partners. The idea is, that if you open yourself up to *any* kind of new experience, serendipities may follow!

In short, make yourself the best person you know how to be, and your social life will zoom. By trying new things, taking chances, being adventuresome—you will find the *other* best people in the world. Believe—there are millions of heavy women who lead exciting and romantic and inspiring lives. Nothing is closed to you because of your weight—if you only ask. Your social life is directly responsive to all the new places you go, the new things you try, the new people with whom you touch antennas. Throw out the stale, old canards of behavior and create new life experiences. You *can* make it, big!

XVII Women Who Have Made It Big

Sybil: I don't care what you say, I hate being fat and I can never be happy or good at anything while I am fat.

My husband can stop eating, even in the middle of a mousse. I think of that as Mousse Interruptus—there is nothing more impossible for me to do than stop in the middle of a mousse. It's easier to stop in the middle of an orgasm. I have to finish. I can eat half a gallon of ice cream at one sitting. My mouth never stops. It hurts me even to talk about it. My small boys never even mention my weight because they know how desperately I feel about it. Once, when I lost a hundred pounds, I think my youngest was very happy. It's true he complained that I wasn't as soft any more, but I think he preferred the thinner me. I know he preferred the personality of the thinner me.

My husband, who loves me, I know, also never mentions my weight. I know he wishes I'd lose, but when I go down even a pound or so and he congratulates me, he says he feels he "jinxes it," because I just start gaining again. He was a serious drinker for a while. When he saw that alcohol was beginning to hurt him, us, he quit. Just like that. Cold. How come I can't do that? I must be so weak. When we make love, I feel so sad that his arms can't get all around me, that there's a roll of fat between him and me. Although he never says anything, I feel that it hurts the quality of our lovemaking.

And all of this makes me feel damaged, sad. I see nothing about myself to be proud of. The funny thing is that I know, somewhere very deep, if I liked myself and the things I'm doing, the fat wouldn't matter quite so much. I know that I'd always wish I was thin. Still, if I didn't feel quite so useless, so sloppy, so *unkempt*, I could handle the fat. I wish someone would teach me how to do that. I'd give anything if someone could teach me to admire or respect or even like myself, *as I am now.*

Jean: Okay, I'll try. Listen, Sybil, listen.

It would be patronizing to tell you that you have chosen fat because you prefer it. Show me a woman who says that and I'll show you a liar. You have not chosen fat. Nevertheless, fat you are. And you have tried, so hard, to do something about

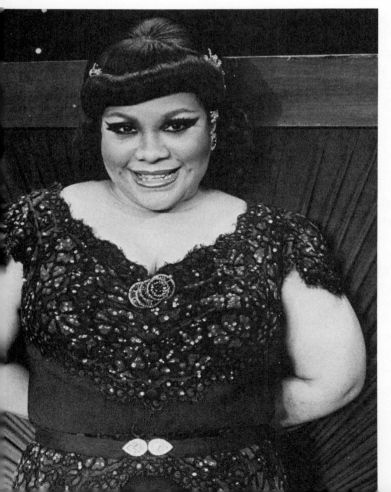

Armelia McQueen.

it. You have dieted and lost and gained and lost and gained again. You spend about 70 percent of your life thinking about food and how not to want it. You've wasted a lot of time, Sybil, thinking about pounds. Enough!

Assume for one moment that you knew for sure you would never be able to lose another pound. That's the way it is. That's the way you are. What would you do? Cry? Go crazy? Give up? Hate yourself forever? Join a convent?

No. Maybe, just maybe, then you would go about making yourself be as terrific as you could be—which would include looking terrific, too. Not thin, you understand, but great. And feeling very nice. How? That's what this chapter is all about.

There *are* many women who have managed magnificently despite and sometimes, you better believe it, *because of* their weight. Here are a few of them. They are in show business, communications, regular business. They are housewives and they are stockbrokers and journalists and photographers.

Perhaps they will inspire you, Sybil, to be yourself. Which *could* be big and very special. Read their stories carefully. They have had as much pain as you have had and they have survived, and more —they have created interesting and attractive and worthwhile people of themselves. They are *women who have made it big.*

Ellen

All business, ink-stained fingers, long wheat hair floating behind her, cerulean blue eyes that know how to hold contact—the interviewer being interviewed. She's used to being on the other side of the tape recorder, but she settles down to the new role, cozily, candidly. She's Ellen Crean, Lifestyles Editor of the Gannett Newspaper, *The Daily Times.*

"It's a question of having your priorities straight—that's what helped me to become what you call a successful big woman. I don't want to come across as some kind of loony evangelist, but I must tell you that a belief in God comes first in my life, then a belief in my career, then a concern with my body. So maybe I'm not your average fat woman, if there is such a thing. I don't think you can

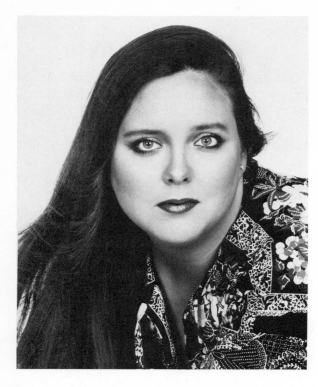

Ellen Crean.

be 'together' physically unless you are settled in your head spiritually and mentally.

"I was a cute chubby kid, then a large adolescent, then I got to be, in fast order, a fat teenager, an obese young adult, and now I'm on my way back down, I hope, to the chubby (although not cute) stage. I'll be honest with you. I would rather, infinitely rather, be thinner. It's easier that way. But even if I don't get to that chubby stage again, it's okay. I've finally gotten the priorities straight. Look—I have to eat potatoes and bread. If I don't eat them, I dream about them—all those ghostly potatoes. So I get on with my life, making my fatness incidental and not primary to it.

"I think I first became fat because it was a way of saying 'Hey, look at me, I'm different, I'm special!' Fat was the way I chose to draw attention. It was essential that I succeed in a career to prove to myself that it is not fat that makes me special, but talent. Now if I stay fat, I won't be thrilled, but I sure won't kill myself. The idea is not to make your fatness your central point of reference. The trick, for me, was to force myself into the world.

"It sounds funny to say, but there's a definite advantage to going through a fat adolescence. I couldn't depend on acceptance for my looks so I had to work on my sense of humor. Some of the world's funniest people have been fat—Steve Martin, for instance. I don't think I would be as generous, as *nice* as I am if I weren't fat. I worked at that. And I understand men very well now, because of the forced 'friend' relationship I had with guys. If I couldn't be romantically attached to them, I was determined to be their best friend, and all those confidences, all those consolations I handed out, prepared me for the grownup romantic relationships. I believe that I understand the male ego a lot better than a thin woman does. I want to be honest about this. At the time, it was miserable. I spent many hours crying in my room, many quiet, desperate hours. But—and this is the point—it wasn't wasted. It helped. It made me whole.

"I must say that I believe that a lot of fat female adolescents grew up with a great hostility toward men because they were rejected so much at a very vulnerable age. A great pity. Now, in retrospect, I can see where that teenage boy was coming from and I say to myself, 'Of course, of course, he couldn't have been interested in me.' Look how insecure his own ego was—what would it have done to his already fragile image if he took out a fat girl? I really was quite optimistic, even in those terrible times. I always thought I had a chance. I still do, always think I have a chance, in anything, even if it looks hopeless. I used to write anonymous love poetry to this one fellow and have it delivered to him. Years later, when he went on to become an actor, I interviewed him and he told me that, even knowing who the letters were from, he'd kept them all these years. Think of that! If only I'd known then that my words would bolster his ego so much he'd save them forever. Maybe I did know.

"I went to college. I got accepted wherever I applied. I know that the statistics for fat girls getting into college are low, but I had a bravado born from fear. I'd tell the admissions officer, 'Look, if you're looking for an athlete, obviously, I'm not her. But if you're looking for someone who will be something someday, and a credit to this school, you'd better take me.' They did. I never admitted this to anyone before, but I went to college following a fantasy. There was this boy, who didn't know I existed, but I was determined to marry him, so I followed him to Syracuse. Naturally, it didn't work. My grades were lousy. I didn't give anyone else a chance. So I left school and got a job in a factory, but somehow I knew I was capable of much more.

"Then one day I walked into the office of the daily newspaper here. I always liked to write but never even thought of doing it professionally. To my amazement, they hired me. At first I just clerked, then wrote obituaries, then worked on the religion page, and now, after many promotions, here I am. I cover people and social and cultural news. I love to interview actors because they are so expansive with their personalities—they're always 'on.' Omar Shariff hugged me and said, 'We all need affection, don't we?' Lovely, sensitive man. I created the job I have now. Someday I'll be a big Liz Smith. Watch me!

"We do need affection—from our family and from our friends also. It helps to psyche ourselves up all day before the Big Date. 'I am gorgeous. I *am* Marilyn Monroe inside, I am *wonderful!*' I don't know—maybe thin women do the same thing. But your sexiness is where your head is, not where your body is. The thinnest models are sometimes frigid, uninterested. I'm interested in men—of course I am. And I'll confide something terrible to you—I won't date a fat man. I know that's reverse prejudice but I can't help it. I can just see other people looking at the *two* fatties out on a date. I hate that look. It's unfortunate, but I'm trying to be scrupulously honest with you. The men I date have to be thin and very attractive.

"I've been lucky. My family has always been most supportive. And I have the Bible for direction. I know it sounds old-fashioned, but everything good in my life comes from that book—all direction, all strength. I'm not a believer in any one religion, although I was brought up as a Catholic, but I believe in that book. Give you an example:

"Take *believing.* Somewhere in the Gospels it says (I can't remember the exact words) that Jesus said, 'If one of you should say to this mountain, be thou moved, and believe it with no doubt in thy heart, the mountain is going to move.' I apply that principle to my life: if I believe that my night date will be a disaster because I'm fat, it will be. If I believe I'm desirable, I will be.

"*Giving equals receiving:* the Bible touted that long before Dale Carnegie did. Say I need some sort of emotional support. I keep my eyes open for someone who needs me. When I've listened to her problems, believe me, my own support comes winging to me, either from her or from somewhere else. It's never failed.

"There are problems. I love to dance and I worry about how I look on a dance floor. I can't wear halters. I can't wear wraparound skirts because my hips are the largest part of me. I worry that people are watching the amount of food I take at a buffet luncheon. But I also know that a lot of women would like to be a newspaper reporter like me even though I don't look like Lois Lane, girl reporter. I still have power and talent and fun in my life, even though I'm heavy.

"A suggestion: pick the thing you like best about yourself. Start with one thing. Enhance it. Capitalize on it. Psyche yourself up. How you feel about yourself is the image you present to others.

"Then go out and do the thing you want to do. Don't wait until you lose ten pounds. The time is now and you are ripe to start. Get your priorities straight!"

Armelia

Broadway—the big time.

I'm sitting in the back row of a darkened theater, every seat filled. The air is thick with anticipation. The show is a Tony Award-winning smash hit and has been for many months now.

When the curtain goes up, the stage is empty except for an old player piano at stage left, and a piano player.

And then she comes on. Five foot three and a half and 190 pounds of woman, dressed in royal blue and dazzling. "Ain't misbehavin', savin' all my love for you," she sings, but no one believes it. Somehow we know that she *is* misbehavin', having a ball, being adorable and not minding at all that she isn't size 10. Reveling in it, glorying in it, absolutely digging her size! She's doing some coy, graceful, delicious thing with her foot, on stage, that has the audience mesmerized. Many things are going on now, on stage, and the dainty, provocative ankle of this huge and marvelous woman is stealing the show!

Armelia McQueen says it for all fat women: "The audience expects a heavy woman to be a heavy-duty woman, a big, bold,

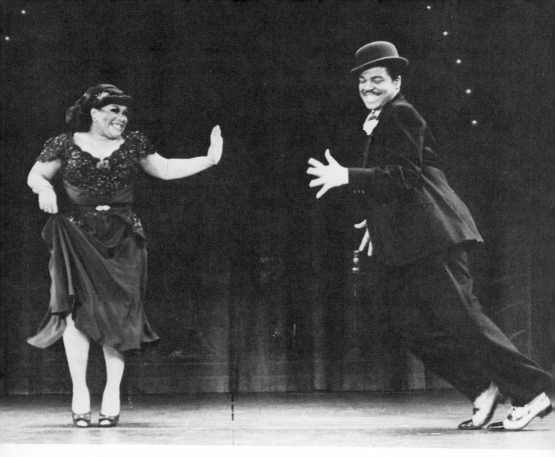

Armelia McQueen and Ken Page in a scene from Ain't Misbehavin'.

push-people-around, knock-down-the-house type, but when I sing 'Squeeze Me,' the number is played to show that fat women can be sweet, seductive and sexy. That's why it's softly warbled instead of belted.

"I was big from size one. Being a preteenager was murder mainly because of the clothes. I was stuck with burgundy or navy-blue jumpers with elasticized bands called Chubbies. I had my little bikini pants and my little bra, like most preteenagers, but I also had my little girdle at the age of ten. So I built up a coat of armor throughout those adolescent years. I didn't allow too many people though to hurt me. I decided to be a fashion designer, and I went to college nights at the Fashion Institute of Technology while I worked during the day.

"And then I realized I just didn't want to be a designer. I wanted to perform. So I took lessons to learn my craft. I studied with

Herbert Berghof for two years and I never allowed my weight to stop me from trying anything.

"Sure, I must have lost some parts because I was fat. Society expects a young black woman to look different from me. One time that I remember, I auditioned for the job of a back-up singer but when the director decided the other girls were to wear hot pants, he also decided I was out. But, so what—lose some, win some.

"Look at me. I wear fabulous clothes in marvelous colors. Sure, sometimes black, but never to hide *me.* How much does a black dress hide anyway? One inch? Two inches? Forget it. When I can't find what I want in the stores, I make it. Learning to sew is one of the most important things I ever did. When I can't find what I want in my size, I make it or alter a smaller size.

"I view myself as a new face on the theater horizon who is fighting to make people aware that heavy people are *here!* Before me, most black, big women were cast as someone's aunt, mother or maid. But in this show I create many characters—a sleepy, sweet lady, a heavy blues lady, a crazy ditz of a lady, a sexy, seductive lady, a patriotic diva lady. I can do anything. My size shouldn't typecast me. Why can't a fat woman play Juliet, play an ingenue, play *anybody?* It's the acting that counts. Big can be transformed into anything if you play it right. If you walk gracefully, feel assured and confident, people just don't see fat any more."

Whatever she's doing, she's doing something right. Armelia is a glamorous woman who knows how to move as if she were carrying only 100 instead of 190 pounds.

"Look, the point is to keep busy. I'm an actress, a religious woman studying to be a practitioner in the Science of Mind movement, and I'm also planning, one day, to open a dress shop for the larger woman—a chic, great, highly styled dress shop! The busier you are, the more time there is. Get out of the house. No one knows you're in there eating. Eat out! Dress up. Vary your life. Try Japanese food instead of roast beef on Wednesday night.

"I guess it's somewhat easier for the black woman. A white woman over size twelve has to drop dead before a white man will look at her. But our men have it in their heritage from generations back to appreciate *sturdy* women. Their sisters, their wives, their mothers all had big hips, big rear ends, big arms. That was what a woman *should* look like. Now, black men still like their women to have some meat on their bones. Look, America has struck, and lately, some black men like their buddies to see them out with the small sizes. But they fall in love with and marry the big women. My current boyfriend is six foot four and very thin. I'm not timid about my body when I'm with thin men and because of that, they're not timid with me.

"Sure, I want to get married and have a child some day. I want it all. I do. And I feel that my size can only help me. *I wear my weight with conviction.* You see, I believe in myself. I've never backed down because of pounds. I am positive. I won't take no for an answer. I may have to travel different routes to get there, but I'll get there—anywhere. Look, I'm a Broadway star, aren't I?"

She's soft and sweet and strong and stunning all at the same time. When she sings, you listen. When she walks, she moves wonderfully. She's fat. And energetic. She runs up the five flights to her dressing room every day and twice a day on Wednesdays and Saturdays.

But then, there's a big silver star on the dressing room door.

Linda

Linda Kline's office is Oriental rugs and plush couches and her own art photographs of iguanas from the Galapagos and shining-eyed children from Mexico. Bookcases are lined with books of advice for women on how to make it. Other bookcases are stacked with biographies of women who *have* made it. And here and there, a button is perched jauntily: "Maybe the Man for the Job Is a Woman," "Women Mean Business."

Linda Kline is a woman who means big business. She is tall, and no mistake about it—*big*. Dressed in a stunning, sharply tailored black suit, her blond, shoulder-length hair lends just the right touch of femininity. Femininity, yes; weakness, no. In fact, she is totally in control, willing, smiling, but firm and self-confident, all at once.

"I'm a headhunter," she says, improbably, "which is another name for a person who does executive search. I work for major corporations and I help them find executives, mostly in the fields of finance, marketing and engineering. I'm known for placing women and minorities, although, as one of my clients puts it, I also place 'regular people.' In that capacity, I'm the president of Maxima Search Ltd. I also have two other businesses, Maximus Consulting and Majority Money. They are in-house training programs for corporations and educational workshops for women. These firms specialize in resource planning, corporate communications and personal financial counseling. Because women have only recently entered the job market in full force, they desperately need more sophisticated knowledge of available benefits, insurance and savings plans. Until recently, the thought in so many women's minds has been that 'somehow, someone, somewhere, will take care of me.' We are teaching them to take care of themselves.''

Among Linda's accounts are Avon, Citibank, Exxon and Irving Trust. Big business, as I said.

Linda Kline.

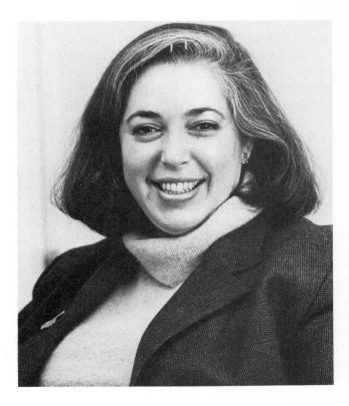

She lights a cigarette, leans back in her leather executive's chair and continues:

"I was always thin. My friends' parents would tease my parents, saying, 'Why don't you feed her?'

"I grew up an independent, competitive, popular adolescent. And it wasn't long before I realized that a serious career meant more to me than any home in the suburbs, than any marriage. I broke two engagements on two wedding eves to understand that I *really* wanted a full-time and successful business life. So I never sacrificed marriage—I *opted* for business. And I am well satisfied. Sure, I have romantic relationships—and one in particular, right now—but although marriage is always a possibility, somehow I doubt it will happen. What I really need is a wife instead of a husband. I'd love someone to give me back-up support, cook and clean and do the laundry—as so many wives uncomplainingly do. But since I can't have that, I'll settle for a lover and do the other stuff myself in my spare time. Look, I'm here once. I'm not guaranteed a return trip. I'm going to be dead for a long time. I might as well do what I want to do.

"I'll tell you something. It wasn't until I began to make real money that I started putting on weight. I have a good idea why. First of all, my life-style changed when I came to New York. Part of my responsibility lies in entertaining clients and I find myself eating lunch at "21," drinking cocktails, having fancy dinners several times a week—when I *used* to grab a cup of soup on the run. The other reason is deeper but just as valid: ever since I can remember I have literally been the only woman in any of the companies I've worked for. Which meant that no matter how bright I was (and I was always a top business woman), I'd be treated as a sex object, because I had a good figure. Men tended to deal with me from the neck down rather than from the neck up. 'Sure, Linda, your advice is sound, we appreciate your help, and what are you doing for dinner?' I think, to a large extent, I allowed myself to get heavy so I would not be hit on as a sex object—so I would simply be a powerful businessperson.

"Which is not to say I wouldn't like to wake up a size twelve again. I don't love being fat, being almost seventy pounds overweight. But I don't dislike it enough to do what I'd have to do to get rid of it. I haven't the *time* to worry about diets and weight and self-denial. And I know medically, if my health is good, I am much better off maintaining this weight than rollercoasting up and down, as I'd surely do.

"Being a fat adolescent definitely shapes your self-image, I think. I was not one. And I feel pretty good about myself. I ride horses, I walk, I can go anywhere and not be self-conscious about my weight—except maybe on the Riviera in a bikini.

"Sometimes when I look in the mirror I think I look like a Mayan fertility symbol! It's fat. Not plump or well rounded. *Fat!* But I figure that any man who comes home with me is neither stupid nor blind and does not expect that I will look like an eighteen-year-old love goddess when I get undressed. Yes, I always make love with the lights on. I am a winner, not a loser, successful, happy and self-satisfied. I am my own boss. I have been ever since I suggested to a boss that he do a cash flow projection.

" 'What's that?' he asked.

"I figured that if this turkey could run his own business without even knowing basic financial procedures, I could do better.

"And I have. No one I do business with has ever fallen over in a dead faint when fat me walked into his office. That's because I always look good—shined, neat and chic.

"Fat has nothing to do with failure or success. Any woman who wants to can make it, and if she waits until she loses thirty pounds before she goes out to find a job, she's fooling herself. It'll never happen. It's true that it's harder to get a job being fat. The lean and hungry look seems to move right in. But you go out and spend a couple of hundred dollars for one *good* interviewing suit. *Never* pants. And you don't anticipate rejection. Women have been taught to wait until they're picked. That notion has to be shredded. No one will gratuitously pick a heavy woman. No one will say, 'You've done a great job darling, and here's the gold star for your forehead. Congratulations, you're promoted.' It's time to start saying, 'I want!' And 'I can!' "

The interview is over. Kline gets up gracefully from her desk, shakes the visitor's hand and, unexpectedly, giggles impulsively and warmly.

"I'm committed to this, you know," she says. "Making a good, professional way of life for me and for as many women who I can reach. Good luck with the book. It's time big women were told how big the possibilities are for them. It's our turn for a piece of the action."

Anne

"Out, out—get out of that house and grab a chunk of the world! It's the only way. Shrinking violet stuff doesn't get you past your parents' front door," says E. Anne Denning, model, actress and host of her own talk-variety cable TV show.

"There's almost no excuse good enough for *not* doing that. I've always been painfully shy and nervous—talking to strangers still terrifies me. I know it sounds funny, being a host of a talk show and being nervous about talking, but believe me, I am. Everything is always not the way it looks. You have to push. There were *millions* of things wrong with me as a child that I could have just used as an excuse to hide. I was not healthy, I had operations, internal problems—I still do. But so what? No one is going to say about me, 'Poor Anne, she's not well, it's okay if she sits home all day.'

"I even hated school. It was a private school and you had to be a doctor's daughter, an athlete and brilliant to succeed there. I was short, dumpy and unhealthy. And I never succeeded. There, anyway. I had one boyfriend—not a happy situation—and I'm still carrying a torch for him. I guess I always will.

"I was always a romantic, a lot older for my age. I was a teenager when I was ten. I was a loner. I read history books in my room. Endlessly. And cried a lot. And wrote poetry. I still do all those things—even cry. But not so much any more. Not nearly so much. You have to fight.

"I knew I'd never make it in calculus but I also knew one thing as sure as my name. I wanted to be in show business. It seemed to me the most *shining* thing I could do. But I never confessed that to anyone. Remember, I was dumpy, short and unhealthy. Theater people are not dumpy, short and unhealthy. So I kept the dream inside and told everyone I'd probably be a history teacher.

"When I got out of high school I started hanging around Broadway. All the other girls were chasing college guys, but I'd spend

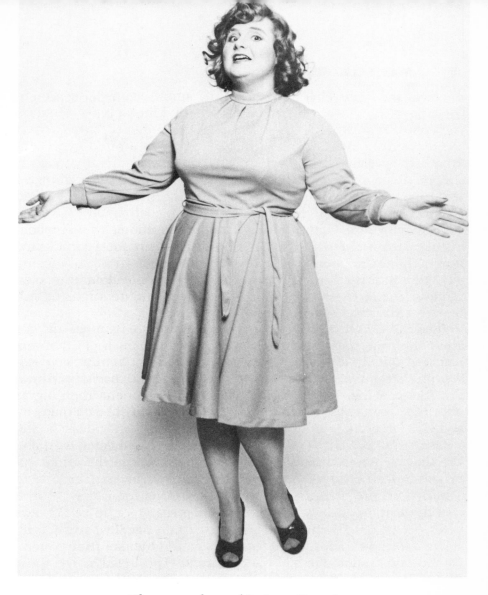

Character shots of E. Anne Denning.

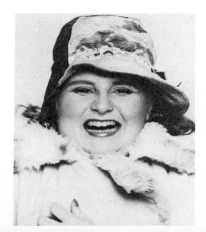
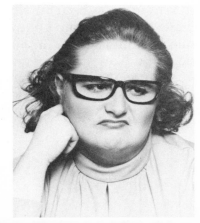

my days and nights watching plays and auditions, hanging around backstage, trying to *ingest* the atmosphere. I met a lot of people. I was *there.* Even when I was just part of the audience, I was part of the play. Oh, it was for me. I knew it. What's more, I even convinced my parents. By the way, my parents, especially my mother, see me as being very beautiful, the cat's pajamas. Even though I will never feel beautiful, her support has been terrific. Sure she'd like me to lose weight, but she never nags.

I began to enroll in theater workshops, take courses. I met teachers like Jose Quintero and Elaine Shore. To be honest, I don't know how helpful the courses were because there's nothing like being *out there* to learn. Still, it kept me in touch. We learned how to do monologues, correct our pacing, mount a production—but not how to go out and get a job.

"So I did that part on my own. I went to a photographer and got a bunch of pictures showing me in different characters. I wrote a resume, putting down any experience I had at the time—which was pretty slim. And naturally, I got turned down, countless times. But I kept going. And I began to get small parts and then bigger ones. Between jobs, I haunted theatrical agencies, off-Broadway auditions, repertory groups. I mean, it was *work*. And all the while, I wasn't sure my size would not handicap me. I modeled (still do). I'm the woman on the Exquisite Form Bra box and the milkmaid in the Selig Furniture ad. You can find my picture in a *True Confessions* magazine or on a movie poster.

"I decided, because I couldn't afford a press agent, to be my own press person. Everytime I had a small role in a play, I called up radio, TV and newspapers to try to tout it. One day I met a man named Eddie Rane. He had his own cable TV show. At the time, cable TV was a baby, a fledgling. There were no rules—it was just a kind of soapbox to advertise yourself. I went on his show to push the play I was working in, and he suggested I try to get my own show. Why not? I thought. I talked to the people at the studio, asked around, and before I knew it, I had my own show. Poof! The E. Anne Denning Show. Simple as that. Of course, I got in on the ground floor. Now it would be harder because cable TV's such a growing, gorgeous thing. But the point is, you have to get out, talk, push. Be *there.* One of the places you'll be in will be the right place at the right time. So at twenty-five, I'm still short, dumpy and unhealthy, but I'm a working actress and cable TV's Johnny Carson. Not bad! And I'm not so dumpy any more, astoundingly enough. When you feel good, you all of a sudden *look* a whole lot better.

"I'm in love with show business. I thought a full-figured woman could never be inside that world. I was wrong. But boy, you have to keep plugging. A lot of people do you wrong. You'll go home, cry, have stomach attacks. But so what? You're *moving, being!* I don't want to sound like Pollyanna, but I'll give you a hint—there's magic in being polite. I've gone a long way on a 'thank you.' Sure, you have to be aggressive, but if they yell at you for asking stupid questions, instead of being rude, you gently and gracefully apologize for bothering them—but *you get the answer to the question.* People respect you for softness combined with drive. No one has a market on happiness—not thin women, not full-figured women. The world expects you to be pushy, loud and sloppy. But you surprise them. You smash the stereotypes and you become *someone!"*

Phyllis

Walk up two flights in an unremarkable-looking building that's smack in the middle of a bustling New York, and what greets you behind the door marked Cuington Studio takes your breath away:

Sky-high ceilings, a block long and a block wide of pristinely white walls, cameras, tripods, photographic essays on the walls, negatives, *Vogue* magazine covers—and a softly beautiful, roundly feminine, dazzlingly smiling woman draws you into her life.

Phyllis is the photographer who took the pictures for this book. She was chosen for her consummate skill, yes, and chosen also because she is what this book is all about: Women. Bigness. Success.

"I was born in Houston and I grew up in Dallas, Texas. A heavy kid, always. The teachers never chose me to give the correct answer, although my hand was always raised. Fat was dull and stupid, then. At least everybody thought so. My mother didn't. She gave me voice, viola, violin, accordion and piano lessons to make

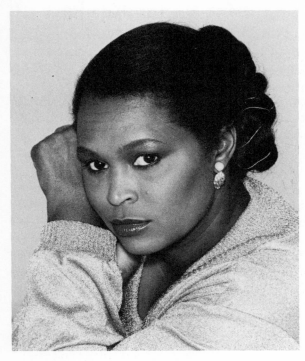

Phyllis Cuington.

sure I'd be an accomplished person. She shopped with me every week, sometimes heartbreakingly, because I never could wear children's clothes in my size. She had to hem women's clothing for me, and dressing older tended to be just another separation from the kids who didn't ask me to their parties anyway. And my mother had a passion—perfect skin. My skin was impeccable. There was no such thing as a blemish. My mother would tolerate no pimples. If a bit of redness appeared, she'd whip out her medication kit and go to work on me. My mother taught me the value of taking pride in my looks—no matter how fat I was.

"I was a pretty, little black, fat girl in Texas and once when a white woman on a bus asked me to go to the back where I belonged, I began to be acquainted with the world and knew I'd have to fight hard to get somewhere. So I tasted everything—music, art, whatever I could find that was creative.

"It was when I was a young woman and working in a department store as a salesperson that I touched on the world of high fashion and modeling. I was entranced with the life on, and backstage of, the fashion show runways. It seemed so glamorous—all those clothes, all that excitement. And one day a fashion coordinator came over to me and said, 'You know, if you lost about fifty pounds, Phyllis, you'd make a fabulous model.' I couldn't get the idea out of my system. It turned my whole life around. I went to a weight doctor, exercised myself to a frazzle, ate almost nothing and lost the weight. Before I knew it, I was on the runway, and two years later I was the highest-paid model in Texas and the leading black model in the entire Southwest. I married, had two children and my career bloomed.

"But I was tense and nervous every day. *Keeping* the weight off was a constant, daily nightmare. I never could relax and eat like the other models because a piece of chocolate cake meant two weeks of near starvation for compensation. My body wasn't meant to be thin. It was torture.

"And one day, the world fell in. I was on my way in a train, with my mother, to Kansas City, and I feel asleep. When I woke from the nap, I was sitting in a puddle of blood. My shoes, my legs, my coat were soaked. The doctors had been ignoring warning signals for years and now I had what turned out to be an advanced case of cancer of the uterus. Needless to say, I was rushed in for an emergency hysterectomy. At the same time, my father was dying of cancer and I had never really told him how much I loved him. And my marriage was breaking up. Life was turning grim.

"I started eating. My dress size went from a seven to a ten to a twelve and on up, inexorably. I felt I had failed to take care of my own health and my personal relationships. Everybody made sure to remind me of the weight I was gaining back. I didn't need the observations. I was hurting, terribly. Several years passed and I was down and depressed because I thought I was fat and ugly beyond redemption.

"And then, one day, I took stock. 'I've got to come alive, I've got to live, even though I'm fat,' I said. So I started again.

"This time, as a makeup stylist. And then as a fashion stylist. And the more I fought, the more it came together again. I was demanding top dollar for my talents, again, but this time I didn't go on a killing diet. I stayed myself. And I kept my eyes open for new fields, new experiences.

"And then I met Terry. He was a young and wonderful photographer and he came to be my closest advisor, my best friend. I found myself telling him how to take his pictures. 'Try it this way, aim her that way,' until he finally put the camera in my hand and said, 'Shoot it yourself, then. The way you think it should be done.' I did, and I found out I was good. Really, very good.

"Terry wanted to come to New York, the big time, and I took a chance, I followed him. Photography had become my life, but I really didn't give myself much hope. Look, I was fat, and I was black, and I was a woman. Three strikes before I started. But I was motivated to succeed and I fought back, and I think maybe that being fat turned it around for me. I fought harder because I *had* to.

"And here I am. Pretty damn successful. How do I see my future? I would like to be a female Avedon. Actually, I feel there's no mountain I can't move. My children and my friends are all proud of me. I must say this—sure, I wish I were naturally thin, but it wasn't until I became a bigger woman that I felt powerful. I am strong. I feel sure. My voice, even, has changed. When I talk, people listen. When I sing, it's with vibrancy. My heaviness has been, in many ways, a gift of power. I do feel confident about my appearance. My mother told me that dressing smartly and neatly makes a person take on a new elegance, a defined clarity. She's right. When I dress up, I find I want to stand straighter, walk more gracefully, even sit more beautifully.

"For a long time, I had great periods of depression. Even now, there are some almost unbearable moments of self-anger because of my size. But I know I have beauty. And I know I'm good in my work—I can't count the number of famous people and magazines I've worked for. And I know I am blessed. I am still a woman, still black, still quite big, and *I have made it!*"

"While researching this book," I tell Phyllis, "I have met many big women who are trying to reconstitute their lives, like you. Could you give them some hints on how to have a picture taken for the resumes, the albums, the applications and for their lovers and friends? Suppose someone lives in Tallahassee and she has never had a satisfactory picture taken, not since she's been heavy, anyway, and she needs one now. As a photographer who has photographed probably more heavy women than anyone else in the world, because you work for several 'big model' agencies, can you give this Tallahassee woman some pointers on how to put her best foot (and face and body) forward in front of the camera?"

Here are eleven Cuington camera cues.

1. Check yourself out in front of a full-length mirror before you even get to the reputable photographer you've chosen. Put on the clothes you plan to wear for your photographs. Turn slowly and look at all your angles. See which ones make you look most graceful, prettiest. See which ones emphasize the parts of you with which you are least pleased.

2. Now sit down and have a chat with the photographer. *Don't* tell the professional how to shoot you, technically. But you can, gently and without giving orders, share your thoughts on what kinds of shots *you* feel best flatter you.

3. Now, prepare the skin canvas. Make up your face with the care a *Vogue* model takes, with soft and muted colors of nature. A round, fat face should never wear dark or bright-red lipsticks. Bright lips will come out too bold, too big, and dark lips will make your mouth smaller and your face look even larger, in contrast. There is more to your face than a double chin and jowls. Your eyes should capture a photograph. Use an eyelash curler, mascara and a soft, *smudged* line under the eye. (Never put eyeliner on in a sharp outline, always smudge for softness.) Don't contour as much as you're used to—just kiss the cheeks lightly with a soft peach or rose.

4. *Hair:* Long hair should always be swept off a round face or, if you must, softly layered around the face. It should never *hang*, long and limp. It should also never stop at the jawline. A photograph of a heavy face with jawline-cut hair looks as if the hair were sheared off bluntly while the fat just continues through. Short hair is fine, of course.

5. *Crucial to remember:* Almost every photographer who knows his or her business will tell a heavy woman to pull her head up to lengthen her neck. We who photograph heavy fashion models all the time have learned something else: It is not enough to hold the head up and the chin high—one must also *pull her face forward* to avoid showing more chin than personality. It incredibly erases any jowly bulk of your underface. Remember, head up and high—and *face forward!*

6. Bare necklines and bare upper chests are not great for heavy women unless they have superb bustlines and lineless necks. The best clothing neckline is the simple shirt-blouse or shirt-dress col-

lar. Cowl necks are sometimes too busy; their bulk emphasizes your bulk. Long neck scarves photograph wonderfully, also.

7. Be careful of partial profiles. Often the eye away from the camera gets tucked into the fleshy part of the nose and face and almost disappears in the photo.

8. Make sure your photographer places your legs and feet gracefully for full body shots. Big women tend to look bottom heavy, and that's not esthetically pretty in a picture. Balance is the key word.

9. Ask your photographer to allow you to move, even just a drop, for your photographs. I often photograph big women moving, even when all I'm aiming for is a head shot. When you're not posing and when you're concentrating on anything else—running, jumping, walking—your face's personality is released from a stiff pose to natural *being*. Even though many photographers doubt it, big women can move as gracefully, as effortlessly and as appealingly as anyone else.

10. Remember, the idea is not to look thin in the picture—that wouldn't be you—but to look fabulous. And fabulous can be glamorous, sexy, natural, *pretty* you.

11. *A special tip:* A couple of drops of Visine in each eye will make them sparkle wonderfully.

Yvonne

Yvonne Hammond Roome is tall, big, smiling and very, very blond. She's a housewife but looks no more like the stereotyped housewife than Anita Ekberg. "Naturally, I'm blond. I was born in Sweden, where I spent the early years of my womanhood as a journalist for Radio Free Europe in Stockholm. I love my size, don't you? I think it gives me *presence.* In Europe, I *never* had a complex about fatness! The only person who ever objected to my weight was my mother, who kept reminding me to 'cover your legs—they're so big, darling.' Funny about mothers. Legs are the only part of me I'm still self-conscious about today. Harping about them never made my legs thinner and damaged some of my confidence.

"Actually, I never wanted to be a mother myself. Is that a terri-

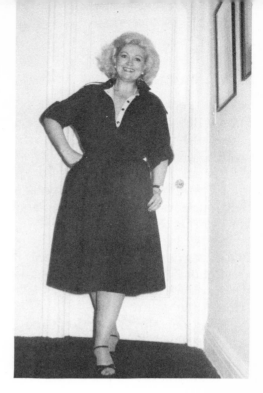

Yvonne Hammond Roome.

ble thing to say? I like all my husband's attention for me. I have stepchildren from my husband's other marriage, and I can't say it's very easy all the time, but we work it out. So now I am a housewife —full time—and I love it. I love to cook. I love to care for a pretty home and for our son. I love to travel, also. If you are a large woman, make sure you check out any hotel room they give you, before you say you'll take it. The bed has to be wide enough, the bathroom roomy enough. You're allowed to say, 'No, this won't do.' Be assertive and not embarrassed.

"That's the clue, I think anyway, assertiveness. You have to have a sense of yourself as a large woman and not as a thin woman who has put on some weight. You have to know what looks good and feels good on you and reject everything else. When we were first married, my husband gave me one of those little dolly night-gowns with feathers all over it! Can you imagine? I said, 'Oh, no, not me, I won't wear this damned thing, Norman. Impossible!' Clearly, *he* thought my thighs were not too fat and my stomach not too big if he thought I'd look good in that ridiculous thing— but I knew better. It's how *I* see myself anyway and how comfortable I am. So I got myself what *I* think is one hell of a sexy night-gown and, rest assured, when I feel like it, I keep it on—even when we make love. You're allowed. You don't have to do what the marriage counselors say is right. Damn it, if it's right for you to keep your nightgown on when you're making love—it's right! It's natural! It's comfortable! Be your own judge. Write your own love scenes.

"I dress to look stunning. I wear a lot of white. I always wear a bra. (Everyone should, don't you think, big bosom or not?) I wear a light support stocking in the largest size (I know Hanes and Givenchy put them out for $5.95). If you hate girdles as I do, support stockings kind of hold you all together. Bathing suits? Can't say I'm thrilled with myself in them, but that doesn't stop me. I never wear those two-piece numbers and I make damn sure I get a good tan first. Also, I wear high heels—they're dynamite with bathing suits when you're big.

"Romance, love? My husband loves me just as I am. I think that's because I'm proud of myself as I am and I always make sure I look neat and attractive. In Venice, we once went into five restaurants, one after another, stuffing ourselves with pasta because it was so *good*. That's part of the quality of life, don't you think? And it's more important than an obsession with dieting.

"I can't think of anything my weight has stopped me from doing except maybe scuba diving. Fat floats, you know, and it's hard to dive deep. Also, I wouldn't be thrilled about being taken out for the day on a small boat where everyone else is in a bikini, size eight. The contrast would make me feel awkward. So I avoid those situations. There *are* certain restrictions. We can't wear bikini underpants. We can't wear those midriff shirts that expose your waist. Not that it's a shame to be fat, but there's a certain dignity that should go along with it. Rolls of fat bursting out of midriffs are not dignified. Same thing with too-tight bras that make fat bulge out and around. Common sense, that's what large women need. More than their share, actually.

"We arrange our lives and even our furniture to make our bigness feel comfortable. (My husband is slim but six feet five.) We sleep in a huge bed. We took an apartment with high ceilings so we wouldn't feel too big for our environment. Our furniture is solid and European—comfortable. If I could change anything in this apartment, it would be the counter tops in the kitchen. They're too low and when I have to chop for a long time, it gives me a backache.

"I love to walk, you know—and I'm not afraid of being mugged. Men tend to think twice before they attack someone my size—so there's a plus! Big women are not meek and teeny targets for attack —they're actually safer than thin women would be in a big city.

"One point I'd like to make is this: I am supercareful not to ever eat or act like a slob. I think heavy women have to be more *aware* of potentially graceless situations so they don't spread the stereotype that *fat is clumsy.* I try to move carefully and with grace through my days. I wouldn't be caught dead looking like a slob.

"Advice? Dark furs, if you possibly can! Long minks are heaven. I adore bulky white fox furs, but they're much too bulky for me.

"You ask me if my image of myself is as a 'cute' woman. Good heavens, no! I'm *striking!* don't you think?"

Rosilyn

I've never before been in a stockbroker's office, but here I am now—she who had to be tutored in elementary algebra— surrounded by numbers and symbols and clickings of statistics in the famous offices of Merrill Lynch Pierce Fenner and Smith. It's awesome and a little scary: the tapping of typewriters, the sliding of teletapes, the buzzing of little "quotrons" which spell out the newest, latest stock market doings.

In the very center of this world, which until just recently used to be peopled exclusively by powerful gray-flanneled men, is Rosilyn H. Overton. Twenty-two voices call out quotes to her; she's in charge, in control and she announces that she will be busy for a while. With me. Into a small, private conference room she marches me to tell me how a woman, a no-bones-about-it, substantial, size-18 woman got to be where she is. Which is a top account executive at the very hub of the business action—in fact, Businesswoman of the Year in New York City, 1976. What does she do? She very effectively handles retail accounts in stocks, bonds, tax shelters, options—the entire spectrum of finances and services that Merrill Lynch offers. Her clients swear by her acumen.

It didn't happen all at once. Nothing is *that* easy for a very big woman, as Rosilyn explains.

"I was a housewife from Beaver Creek, Ohio. I did the right

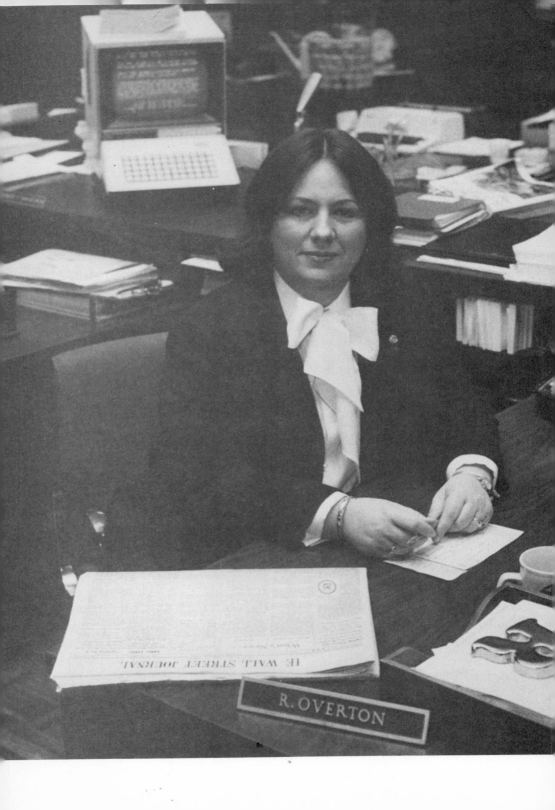

THE WALL STREET JOURNAL.

R. OVERTON

things, took care of my husband and children, crocheted, embroidered—the whole trip—and secretly I knew I needed much more.

"My father weighs over three hundred pounds. I grew up at a time when there were only two modes of dress: either the straight skirt with the angora sweater or the Villager shirtwaist dress. Both styles didn't do much for very heavy arms. I'm thirty-seven now and I was born in a small oil town in Texas. At the age of six I remember the kids taunting cruelly, 'Fatty, fatty, two by four, can't get through the kitchen door.' I was aggressive and competitive and bright, but I had a fragile self-image because I was fatter than the other kids. Puberty came early—I got my period when I was only nine—and I think I was subject to too many adolescent stresses before I even became an adolescent. I performed the Mozart Bassoon Concerto with the Houston Symphony when I was sixteen and graduated from high school at sixteen also. A year later, I'd found a brilliant, also heavy, young man to eat with me, and we were married when he was only nineteen—I was 17.

"We moved and we moved as he changed jobs and finished school. Our focus was him, *his* education, *his* career. I didn't think to question it. I just gained more weight. I worked too, and wherever I worked, I got promoted as fast as they'd allow. I was smart, good in math, good in anything they gave me to do.

"In the sixties it was considered somewhat sinful to be married for five or six years without having children. What was wrong with you if you didn't or couldn't have a baby? So, even though I wasn't sure I wanted kids yet, I got pregnant. And miscarried. And got pregnant again. And miscarried again. The doctor told me to stop working and stop the part-time schooling I had recently started (and very successfully). How I hated that! But I did, because now I was determined to have a baby, to show I was a true woman. Finally, after yet another move to Minnesota, I had my first son. I managed to keep busy with volunteer work and volleyball, but I yearned for something else—*what*, I couldn't say, yet. Another move, California this time, and I entered my 'hippie stage.' I learned how to dye wool from herbs and roots. I was weaning my son and wasn't chained to him by my breast any more, so I had lots of spare time. I was beginning to get bored—my intellect had nowhere to go.

"Every now and then Lou and I would go on agonizing self-appraisal trips and say, 'We've *got* to lose weight,' but then we were each secretly grateful when one or the other of us went off the diet wagon. I think I clung desperately to Lou because I thought he loved me, fat or not.

"For all of my marriage, I'd been feeling self-conscious that Lou had finished school and I hadn't. My God, if anything happened to him, what would happen to us? So I went back to school. I was never so happy. I did brilliantly. And immediately became pregnant again. Still, now nothing could stop me and I continued with school. With the pains coming four minutes apart in the middle of a Numerical Analysis class, and in a snowstorm, I drove the thirty miles to the hospital myself, to have my cherished second son. *But I was committed now* —to finish. And a wonderful professor (who was himself over five hundred pounds) became my mentor—he understood what it was to be fat and bright and have problems with prejudice, and he guided me toward a Masters in economics.

"In the meantime, back at the ranch, my marriage wasn't going too well. My husband had always played the pedagogical role—he was the student, and he taught me. He was the sports car racer, and he taught me. But I got the M.B.A. first, and I raced so well I held the woman's track record, and I had to get *him* a job when he'd lost one, and this brilliant, lovely man became unhappy. One Christmas he announced he simply didn't want to live with me anymore. I was taking charge of my own life, and he didn't like it. Both of us were brought up in Texas fundamentalist families where fathers were bosses and expected constant respect and total authority. Old, fat me was breaking role-model expectations. I was being a little too assertive.

"I never believed he meant it. Still, I started writing resumes and began getting affirmative responses. Lou really wanted out, and I got a good job offer in New York. We talked at great length and finally decided mutually that the kids were better off, initially at first, with him. Their lives would not be disrupted—their friends and background would remain constant.

"I struck off on my own. The rest is simple.

"I became someone of whom I could be proud—despite my weight. Maybe even because of my weight. You'd think there would have been a lot of stress and in a strange, new city I would have responded by stroking myself—eating—as I was used to doing. On the contrary. As soon as I changed my life-style to one of an active, busy person, as soon as I *affirmed* myself, I went down from 230 pounds to 190—*without dieting!* Instead of eating, I walked. I loved all the new things that were happening.

"It wasn't all great. The job I took was not challenging enough and I switched to another which required a company physical. I was in *astounding* good health—blood pressure and all—but still the company doctor gave me a C rating, simply because I was big. What blatant discrimination! I was angry and I felt so helpless. The vice president who hired me had to sign a form saying my weight would not be a hazard on the job. Ignominious moment!

"Still, I was finding my way. I must say *Ms.* magazine helped me a lot in those years. I learned to like myself better because of the feminist movement. A lot of the stuff about being skinny and fashionable is foisted on women by men who don't know any better. Not that being a feminist means rejecting men. I enjoy men enormously and I feel that I am very feminine and warm. I love to dance, even though Gloria Steinem says, "We walk backward all the time when we're dancing." But being heavy means also to me that all things feminine are possible—just as all things business are possible. I'm not bad because I'm fat any more than I'd be bad if I had blue eyes. Being heavy is a physical fact of life and it has about as much to do with self-worth as having blue eyes—which is to say, nothing.

"One of the things that has made me heavy has also contributed to my success in business—my sense of perfectionism. I do make mistakes and when I'm dissatisfied or when I don't get the praise I need, I tend to eat again to stroke myself. Perfectionism has also made me a crack account executive at Merrill Lynch—and one of the first women in the field, as well.

"Sure there's prejudice against fat, but I try to deal with it as a fact of life, just as it's a fact of life that people don't trust strangers. It's not *personal!* And on that level, you can ignore it or fight it and learn to live with yourself the way you are. I am a person with a bundle of attributes, and being short or tall or fat doesn't have anything to do with being jolly or sloppy or dumb—the stereotypes people tend to attribute to fat. I think that when we can stop worrying about crazy and false myths, then we can go on to make our lives the best our lives can be."

Lisbeth

She was the cover girl on the prestigious *Washington Post Magazine* last year. Perfect white teeth, long brown hair cascading down the shoulders of the rainbow print dress, thick eyelashes framing soft hazel eyes. In other words, a knockout.

A knockout in excess of 200 pounds.

Fat pride! blazoned the *Washington Post* cover and Lisbeth Fisher became the emblem of fat pride to hundreds of overweight women.

"There was a time," says Liz, "when I sat in a double seat on the Long Island Railroad, and if no one sat near me because they were obviously avoiding a 'fat girl,' I'd be mortified. There was a time when I was sure everyone was staring at me, making fun of me in

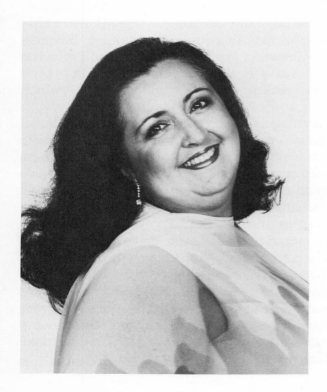

Liz Fisher.

their minds. A time when I thought I was just the grossest, ugliest thing in the world. But look at me now. Do you think I'm gross looking?"

She was wearing a marvelous caftan that was alive with color. Her grin, her freshly washed hair, her whole self was exuding a sense of sweetness, of excitement and of self-confidence. Gross? Liz Fisher was a doll! Rounder than a Barbie doll, for sure, but also a lot more vital.

"My teenage years were horrendous," she continued. "The only way I could make it was to be a clown and make fun of myself. If I was invited to a party, I felt I'd make a faux pas out of every sentence and I always felt people would say behind my back, 'Is she *kidding*? Such a fat slob can't have an opinion about *anything!*'

"My parents were worried but they didn't know how to help me find myself. In fact, they gave me double messages all the time. If I took a piece of cake for dessert, my mother would say gently, 'Are you sure you really need that?' If I didn't take the piece of the cake she'd just baked, she'd coax, 'Oh come on, one little piece won't hurt you.'

"I'd cry at the drop of a hat. Guilt-ridden, unhappy, I snuck candy bars into my room and made myself literally sick with them. It was murder.

"To me, the be-all and the end-all of life was to be a wife and have a family. I cared for nothing else but being cherished. Education, creative work—nothing counted, next to that. The urge to be loved is *so* overwhelming. It outweighs everything else. You want to read a book or hook a rug, but you can't concentrate. All you can think about is, 'Oh, I wish someone was with me. I wish someone wanted me.' I didn't know, then, that I had to love myself before anyone else could love me.

"College was an unmitigated disaster and I left in the middle. I distrusted anyone who showed an interest in me. Something must be wrong with anyone who thought me attractive, I reasoned.

"I came home. My parents made me go to business school. I got my own apartment and began to work. The boss liked me because he thought I was always so cheerful, but inside, boy, I was not cheerful. I was becoming increasingly unhappy. And desperate. I kept this security drawer in my desk filled with licorice and Chunkys and Baby Ruths. As long as I wasn't actively dieting, I never touched it—never thought of it. It was just there—like a fix, if I got in trouble. But when I went on one of my periodic diets which never lasted, and cleaned out that drawer, I could think of *nothing else* but the candy I'd thrown out. Whenever I dieted, I never lost weight permanently anyway, and the idea of food drowned out all other ideas. When I *wasn't* dieting, I was in control of the rest of my life.

"Finally, I met a man. By the second date, I was madly in love with him. We married, and had a son, and finally I was a wife and I had a family. But it was all no good. I still thought I was ugly. I was still dieting hungrily and angrily. The marriage failed—it had to. There was no place lower I could go in my head.

"And then, things began to look up. They had to because they couldn't get any worse. Because of my son, I got involved with PTA, Cub Scouts, Little League and Parents Without Partners. I found that I was running things, that I had great organizational ability. Parents Without Partners, at that time, used to hold formal dances at public places. They were really cold and not much fun, so I decided to throw a few parties in my own home for the group. They were an immediate success and soon became *the* place to go for all the single men and women of the neighborhood. I saw a way to become an entrepreneur and began to charge money, first just to cover expenses and then as a business arrangement. It worked! People were delighted to pay for the parties and I'd found a way to supplement my income. Even more, I'd found a social life. As soon as I began to get busy, not concentrate on my loneliness or unhappiness, naturally I began to meet men. For the first time in my life, my phone began to ring regularly.

"One of the men I met, a brilliant young, slender lawyer, told me he preferred heavy women to thin ones. I thought he was sick or was trying to con me. But he was determined to prove that caring, nonweirdo, desirable and lovely men with a preference for rounded women, did really exist. He gave me an article about an organization called NAAFA (National Association to Aid Fat Americans), which I promptly stuffed in a drawer. It was to change my life.

"One day, I was rummaging through the drawer and I found the article. Somewhat interested, I wrote away for some literature, and that was the beginning. NAAFA showed me that big women can learn to feel better about themselves. I began to work for the organization, just a few hours a week in the beginning, hoping it would make me feel better about myself.

"It did. I became involved, totally. I met heavy and thin people, all dedicated to wiping out the insidious prejudice against pounds. It was harder even than a religious or gay group working to combat prejudice, because fat, unlike the other two, is immediately visible. If my body was enclosed in fat, others' minds were enclosed with the idea that fat meant sloppiness, weakness, even moral decay. It was hard to break through.

"But marvelous things were happening to me personally. I never thought I'd see the day when I could pick and choose among desirable men. I never thought I'd be able to walk into a room and have all heads turn—with *admiration!* I felt once, at a dance, as if I were having my junior prom at age thirty. And I found out something else, too—*Why* it had always been so impossible for me to lose weight. Dr. Neil Solomon, who writes a syndicated and very respected column, examined me and told me that because of my metabolism I only burned 750 calories a day while a thinner woman might use up almost three times as much. I would have to eat only 750 calories a day to lose weight—*impossible!*

"My job as executive secretary at NAAFA is my full-time occupation now. My psyche has changed as my exposure to people who are active, busy, fat and beautiful has grown. My live-in boyfriend (he happens to be a thin and beautiful person) will measure seats in a theater to see which would be more comfortable for me before I sit down. I do not hesitate to ask a manager for a larger restaurant chair if I need one. A funny thing has happened—remember I told you I used to feel constantly *stared* at? Well, it doesn't happen any more. I'm *convinced* it's because of the new confidence I carry in myself. I changed from the inside out and I don't mind if you call me fat. *Fat is not a four-letter word.* Society has made it a word of derogation, but it is nothing more than an adjective like blue-eyed, short, thin or blond.

"You want me to be honest? If you gave me a magic potion and told me that by drinking it, I'd become thin tomorrow, *fantastic!* I'd drink it in a minute. There's no doubt I'd be more comfortable in a world of skinny chairs. But if you don't give me the potion and I have to spend the rest of my life working compulsively at not eating, thinking of food as the primary mover in my life—forget it! I'll take me as I am!"

Suzanne

Down in the, as she puts it, "mean, clean, right-wing Bible Belt" of Raleigh, North Carolina, lives Suzanne Britt Jordan, a teacher at North Carolina State University. She is, also as she puts it, "stately," which in anyone else's language reads downright plump. She is a joy, a fresh, irreverent wit. As a free-lance journalist for the *Raleigh News and Observer*, she writes columns that invigorate and free from guilt countless other "stately" persons, let alone a whole lot of skinny ones. She has a husband and a family who delight in her. In her letters to me and in her columns, she's offered some priceless comments on the subject of fatness and life, which I share with you. Her ideas on fat, as a matter of fact, were marvelously put forth in an article that was originally published in *Newsweek* magazine in a section called "My Turn." With *Newsweek*'s permission, we reprint the whole article here for you.*

That Lean and Hungry Look

Caesar was right. Thin people need watching. I've been watching them for most of my adult life, and I don't like what I see. When these narrow fellows spring at me, I quiver to my toes. Thin people come in all personalities, most of them menacing. You've got your "together" thin person, your mechanical thin person, your condescending thin person, your tsk-tsk thin person, your efficiency-expert thin person. All of them are dangerous.

In the first place, thin people aren't fun. They don't know how to goof off, at least in the best, fat sense of the word. They've always got to be a-doing. Give them a coffee break, and they'll jog around the block. Supply them with a quiet evening at home, and they'll fix the screen door and lick S & H green stamps. They say things like "There aren't enough hours in the day." Fat people never say that. Fat people think the day is too damn long already.

Thin people make me tired. They've got speedy little metabolisms that cause them to bustle briskly. They're forever rubbing their bony hands together and eyeing new problems to "tackle." I like to surround myself with sluggish, inert, easygoing fat people, the kind who believe that if you clean it up today, it'll just get dirty again tomorrow.

Gooey vs. Crunchy

Some people say the business about the jolly fat person is a myth, that all of us chubbies are neurotic, sick, sad people. I disagree. Fat people may not be chortling all day long, but they're a hell of a lot *nicer* than the wizened and shriveled. Thin people turn surly, mean and hard at a young age because they never learn the value of a hot-fudge sundae for easing tension. Thin people don't like gooey, soft things because they themselves are neither gooey nor soft. They are crunchy and dull, like carrots. They go straight to the heart of the matter, while fat people let

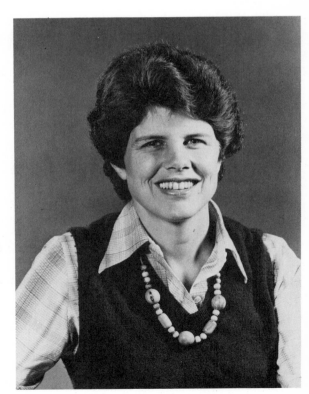

Suzanne Britt Jordan.

things stay all blurry and hazy and vague, the way things actually are. Thin people want to face the truth. Fat people know there is no truth. One of my thin friends is always staring at complex, unsolvable problems and saying, "The key thing is . . ." Fat people never say that. They know there isn't any such thing as the key thing about anything.

Thin people believe in logic. Fat people see all sides. The sides fat people see are rounded blobs, usually gray, always nebulous and truly not worth worrying about. But the thin person persists. "If you consume more calories than you burn," says one of my thin friends, "you will gain weight. It's that simple." Fat people always grin when they hear statements like that. They know better.

Fat people realize that life is illogical and unfair. They know very well that God is not in his heaven and all is not right with the world. If God was up there, fat people could have two doughnuts and a big orange drink anytime they wanted it.

Thin people have a long list of logical things they are always spouting off to me. They hold up one finger at a time as they reel off these things, so I won't lose track. They speak slowly as if to a young child. The list is long and full of holes. It contains tidbits like "get a grip on yourself," "cigarettes kill," "cholesterol clogs," "fit as a fiddle," "ducks in a row," "organize" and "sound fiscal management." Phrases like that.

They think these 2,000-point plans lead to happiness. Fat people know happiness is elusive at best and even if they could get the kind thin people talk about, they wouldn't want it. Wisely, fat people see that such programs are too dull, too hard, too off the mark. They are never better than a whole cheesecake.

Fat people know all about the mystery of life. They are the ones acquainted with the night, with luck, with fate, with playing it by ear. One thin person I know once suggested that we arrange all the parts of a jigsaw puzzle into groups according to size, shape and color. He figured this would cut the time needed to complete the puzzle by at least 50 percent. I said I wouldn't do it. One, I like to muddle through. Two, what good would it do to finish early? Three, the jigsaw puzzle isn't the important thing. The important thing is the fun of four people (one thin person included) sitting around a card table, working a jigsaw puzzle. My thin friend had no use for my list. Instead of joining us, he went outside and mulched the boxwoods. The three remaining fat people finished the puzzle and made chocolate, double-fudged brownies to celebrate.

Pat Solutions

The main problem with thin people is they oppress. Their good intentions, bony torsos, tight ships, neat corners, cerebral machinations and pat solutions loom like dark clouds over the loose, comfortable, spread-out, soft world of the fat. Long after fat people have removed their coats and shoes and put their feet up on the coffee table, thin people are still sitting on the edge of the sofa, looking neat as a pin, discussing rutabagas. Fat people are heavily into fits of laughter, slapping their thighs and whooping it up, while thin people are still politely waiting for the punch line.

Thin people are downers. They like math and morality and reasoned evaluation of the limitations of human beings. They have their skinny little acts together. They expound, prognose, probe and prick.

Fat people are convivial. They will like you even if you're irregular and have acne. They will come up with a good reason why you never wrote the great American novel. They will cry in your beer with you. They will put your name in the pot. They will let you off the hook. Fat people will gab, giggle, guffaw, gallumph, gyrate and gossip. They are generous, giving and gallant. They are gluttonous and goodly and great. What you want when you're down is soft and jiggly, not muscled and stable. Fat people know this. Fat people have plenty of room. Fat people will take you in.

XVIII Straight Talk for the Teenager

Maybe it's strange to start off a chapter for teenagers with a message you should read to your parents, but too bad. It's my book and I get to start where I want.

This is the message. Gather your parents up, place them on the couch, right now, and read it to them. Loudly.

Bug off!

Oddly enough, the message comes from a book which is not my cup of tea because it tells young people how to concentrate on losing weight. Still, Dr. Alvin N. Eden is no fool, not by any means. With his co-author, Joan Rattner Heilman, he writes in *Growing Up Thin*,

> How to cope with an overweight adolescent—don't! I have two words for parents of overweight adolescents: *Bug off.* I've worked many years with fat teenagers and I've found through bitter experience that the less said or done by you about your adolescent youngster's need to lose weight, the better. . . . The truth is that parents who push and pressure, pester, restrict, embarrass, punish and nag, even parents who merely remind, usually have the worst results . . . so cool it!

Those are wise words. You know it. Tell *them*.

I have more wise words for *you*. In my opinion, they are the wisest, truest words you will ever read.

363

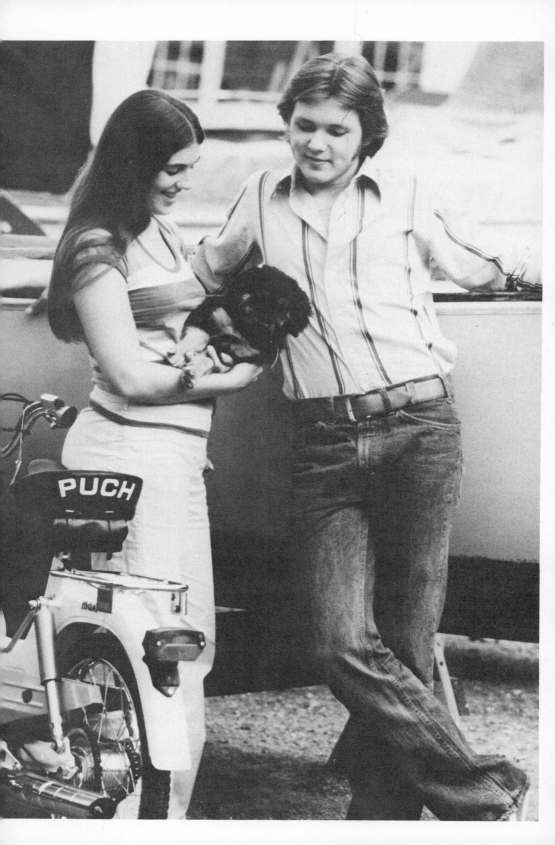

To start with, *no* teenagers, even thin ones, get along perfectly with their parents. You think thin kids and mothers agree on life, sexual appetites and regular appetites? They don't. Listen, if they weren't bothering you to lose weight, rest assured they'd be telling you to stop biting your nails, washing your hair so often, and what *were* you doing in the back of Tommy's car last night, for forty-five minutes?

Still, no one is trying to tell you it's not tougher to be fat than thin. It is. I know it and you surely know it.

Some teenagers like disco. Some like Donny and Marie. Some like to square-dance. But all American teenagers seem to agree on two things: (1) Jeans and sneakers are your national outfit. (2) You don't like being fat.

The way I see it, if you are fat, you have three options. Naturally, there are pros and cons for each.

Option one: You can move to Central Africa where the girls are secluded in "fatting" houses until they achieve a much-admired plumpness.

Pro: Everyone in Central Africa will desire and admire plump you.

Con: You may not like having your teeth blackened and your head put in the elongation press.

Option two: You can resolve to spend *all* of the rest of your life dieting.

Pro: Your Aunt Fay will say, "I'm proud of your self-control, darling." (You can't stand your Aunt Fay.) You will be thinner at times, but you probably will gain back as much as you lose, many times. (In a *New York Times* article of August 5, 1979, it was pointed out that programs to cure overweight have a 3 percent chance of succeeding in keeping the weight off. Even Alcoholics Anonymous has a 33 percent chance of lasting success. The odds are greatly against your being very thin for very long.)

Con: You will go bananas dieting. You can't even *have* a banana. You can't even have a Raisinet.

Option three: You can relax. Don't go crazy eating everything in sight, of course, but don't go crazy *not* eating *anything*. Be *you*. And if you see that being thin is just too heavy a burden to carry for the rest of your life, be gorgeous, happy and interesting, anyway!

Pro: You will learn to be a *doer.* You will develop yourself as a person, and not merely as a thin person. You can revel in a hot-fudge sundae occasionally without tearing your hair out with guilt. You will try your best to use restraint with the Raisinets but you will not punish yourself with feelings of unworthiness if you *must* eat two boxes in the movies. You may become president of the high school because you are such a splendid and active young woman—you've worked at it! And you will find you are pretty, but you'll have to work at that also (who doesn't?).

Con: Face it—you will definitely be chunkier than many of your friends. People who care a lot about "thin fashion" won't admire you or probably be your best friends. You will have to learn how to deal with discrimination against pounds.

In all seriousness, you *should* make a choice even though it may not have to be as black and white as the ones I've laid out. If you have had a terrible time losing weight (and you are not grossly obese, which may create medical problems), you do have the option of remaining big and *still* being a beautiful young woman. I know you've read and heard that you can't relax the fight for a moment. If "ugly fat" takes hold, you must be ever self-punishing. Nuts to that. Heaviness does not have to be ugly, and your efforts now should go toward making yourself a terrific and good-looking person. You don't have to be thin to do that.

Did you know that 20 percent of all teenagers are overweight and those numbers are increasing daily? I have met so many of these wonderful young people who are positively crippled by their self-images if they are plump. They don't indulge in sports, they don't go to the theater, they don't initiate socialization efforts—all their "teenness" stops, comes to a roaring halt, because they are trying to lose weight. They don't experiment, they don't take chances, they hide in their rooms. What a mistake.

Because the thing to do is just the opposite. When you are busy and active and happy—you're great to be with. Fat doesn't loom so large, either, in your eyes or in the eyes of your friends, if you are interesting!

So join everything to which you are drawn, and make no mistake: political influence gives power and power makes you an interesting person to know. Say you manage to become editor of the school newspaper: you are able to dispense assignments, create editorials, do any number of things in which other people are interested. You find yourself at the hub of excitement, at decision-making levels—and also in the swing socially. But it doesn't happen by itself. You have to work for it—prove your mettle, so to speak. If you are going to be a heavy person, be the finest heavy person around and make heaviness synonymous with *great!* And guess what? It may be possible that you are not even destined to be heavy all your life. You may just find out that when you are busy and active and caught up with life, the pounds come off—by themselves, and much faster than if you'd spent the time being obsessed with dieting. Don't misunderstand me: if the weight stays, and you stay healthy, that's fine too! That's you. Big, splendid you. Someone to be admired and cherished because you have made yourself an admirable, lovely person!

So don't search for even one neat little calorie chart in these pages. Or a ten-day-wonder-magic-diet. You can find those elsewhere and you know what you can do with them. Because ten-day-wonder-magic-diets never, never work more than ten days.

What you will find in this chapter are concrete suggestions on how to make yourself terrific—even if you are not thrilled with your weight.

First things first. Face the thing out and find out . . .

What Kind of Fat Am I?

Is it honest fat? Or is it weapon fat? Only you can tell. Neither is terrible. There are reasons for both. Good reasons.

Honest fat is the kind of fat you are when your mother, father, Aunt Elizabeth, Grandmother and maybe another relative or so have all been chunky. Your *whole* family album is filled with people who look like Tubby the Tuba. You can never remember the last malted, but unlike your friend Pam, you just *think* malted and there it is—on your hips. You sense, in your heart of hearts, that you are genetically and physically programed toward heftiness. That's honest fat.

Weapon fat is quite different. It is not the *opposite* of honest fat, which would be dishonest fat. (What *that* is, I can't imagine.) No, it is quite honest and real but it is the kind of fat you put on to protect yourself.

There are many kinds of weapon fat.

There's a "get-off-my-back" weapon fat. Mary-Jo, eighteen, expressed her experiences with that kind of fat: "When I was fifteen, I was thin and very afraid of boys who would touch me and make advances I couldn't deal with. So I gained weight, as a weapon, I think. Fat, I could be their best pal. Thin, I couldn't handle my own emotions."

When you are a teenager, you are living through a period of rapid growth and sexual development that is revolutionizing your body faster than Castro revolutionized Cuba. You may overeat or even undereat for reasons having nothing to do with hunger and everything to do with emotions. Many teenagers gain weight, at this time, to ward off threatening and strange challenges of the opposite sex.

Another kind of weapon fat is cuddle-weapon fat. When you were little and you hurt, what did your parents give you? Sure, a zwieback! And if you were sad, you got the box of animal crackers with its own little handle—remember? And the lollipops and the chocolate pudding to take your mind off your tears. What was the message? The message was that soothing equals food. Talk about comforting. Perhaps now, when you eat a lot, you are trying to get that cuddling, comforting, nurturing feeling that enveloped you when you were little. So food is a cuddle weapon against the world.

Other people use their fat (or food) as an attack weapon. Do you find yourself eating when you feel angry, hostile or anxious? Remember how you used to bite when you were three years old and furious? Eating is also biting and can act as an attack or retaliative weapon on the world that is not being so marvelous to you, at the moment.

And the last kind of weapon fat can be, is a penalty weapon, used to punish yourself. It's kind of like saying, "Damn them. I try so hard and I still can't be worthy of my parents' or friends' love so I'll just punish myself—and maybe them too—by making me fat. That'll fix me!"

If *some* or all of this rings true to you and you feel you are weapon fat, you might want to get help working things out by talking to a professional counselor or a very wise, objective parent or friend. (Objectivity actually counts more than wisdom. Just because a parent loves you or is wise is not proof he or she will be able to help you with this kind of problem. You may need to unwind to an unbiased ear.) Fat is fine if it's honest and natural and *you*, but if fat signifies that you're unhappy, you'll need to deal with the causes. If you live with a feeling of fury or resentment, you must try to find out why that ball of anger inside exists.

On the other hand, if you are sure your fat is honest fat, then you have to decide whether to spend the rest of your life trying to lose it or the rest of your life trying to become marvelous. It's possible, of course, for *some* teenagers to be slimmer than parents and grandparents who were all constitutionally fat if they work at it much harder than friends who have naturally thin jogger-parents —and it may or may not work. But that's up to you. Let me assure you that there *have* been many teenagers who, determined not to fight that perpetual battle of the bulge, have still turned out romantically, professionally, and emotionally fulfilled people. They *like* themselves, heavy or thin.

The whole thing is pretty heavy, literally and figuratively. You'll be interested to know that a brilliant Yale researcher named Judith Rodin evolved, from extensive studies, the belief that heavy people don't gain weight *because* they have problems or are unhappy, for the most part. They have gained weight simply because eating feels so damn good, with *no* underlying connotation. And the problems come only *after* the weight gain, because they cannot deal with society's down-putting attitudes.

Take Responsibility, Now

Don't blame Mom for her genes or yourself for your compulsion to eat. Talk about *responsibility* instead of *blame*. It is *your* responsibility to make sure you don't hide in your room and lead a wasted life because of a few Mallomars. Even a million Mallomars. I am not telling you to walk around singing, "Ho, ho, ho, I *love* my 189 pounds." Singing on the outside may mean screaming on the inside. But if you don't have to love your pounds, you *do* have the responsibility of building up the person they encompass so you can respect her. Get passionately involved with *life.* It's a trip you shouldn't miss even if you make the scale shoot higher than you'd like. Your genetic makeup, outside influences and pressures, all contribute to the physical shape of your body: you can't claim total responsibility for that. But you also can't dump the responsibility for having a super life on any mother, husband or outside influence. It's your responsibility and your future. Claim it and live.

Spot the Enemy and Put Him Down

Sometimes it's a well-meaning enemy who comes from strange quarters—like your own home. Sometimes the enemy is not so well meaning, like a supposed friend who actually needs a scapegoat on whom to take out her own problems. The enemy is *anyone* who says you are "weak" or "lack willpower" or are "morally or emotionally insecure" because you weigh more than the enemy wishes you to weigh. Understand one thing—enemies can love you and really wish for your best. The reason they are enemies is because they do not understand about individuality. And choice. And the right to be different. And the difficulty of trying to be who *they* want you to be. Try to figure out what *you* really want. Do you really want the Yankee Doodle? Then *eat it,* by God. Do you reach for the Yankee Doodle to spite *them* or to show how strong you are? You don't want that cute little chocolate cupcake, my friend. *Don't* eat it.

Do *they* tell you how to act with boys, with makeup, with your schoolwork? Well, if everyone told you the same thing, it'd be pretty easy and you'd probably listen. But the messages you get are all different: your best friend tells you that Earth Brown is the best color for your lips; Revlon tells you Earth Brown is out and Plum Wine is in; your mother tells you that Earth Brown makes you look as if you had dirty lips. To whom should you listen? Listen to them all, then allow *yourself* to make a decision that is right for you. Take in all the considerations. Do you really like brown lips? Do you have the money to buy a new lipstick? Is your friend really looking out for you? Is the hassle with your mother worth the color? If you can truly say yes, *this* is what *I* love and what *I* choose then paint your lips Earth Brown. Also the rest of your face, if you like.

Suppose the enemy comes in the guise of a respected counselor who tells you that you should consider being a home economics major because it is hard to get into medical school when you are fat. You really know you want to be a brain surgeon: you also really know that home economics would make you a crazy person. Say thanks, but no thanks, to the kindly enemy who is not doing you a favor at all and set your sights on Frog Dissection 101.

Finally, be gentle, be firm, be reasonable—but be true to yourself. And listen to no friend or enemy if you're sure that you are doing and being what *you* want to do or be.

Move

Over and around and up and down and horizontally and anything, as long as you *move!* You may have heard that exercise increases your appetite. It's a lie. In fact, as Dr. Jules Hirsch of Rockefeller University says, "Exercise even has a 'euphoriant effect' that cuts down the need to eat for emotional satisfaction." Teenagers should move as much as possible. Do you know that it has been shown that teenage obese girls are only about one-third as active as thin ones? And that *inactivity*, rather than overeating, in many cases tends to put those pounds on?

It is true that being heavy makes you want to sit around reading, watching TV and talking a lot. Why? For a lot of reasons. You may feel sluggish, you may feel that you should move slowly. *Rubbish!* Let's face it—you may also not like the way you look on a tennis court or horseback riding or swimming. NAAFA (the National Association to Aid Fat Americans) has a fine suggestion about the latter: "If you are self-conscious about how you look, practice by yourself until you learn. Then people will notice your performance, not your size." Boy, are they right. If you can hit a tennis ball like Billie Jean King, do you think the team captain gives a hoot how many pounds are behind the backhand? If you are the sleekest swimmer in the pool, they'll admire you at the beach for your style and not your stomach.

Being active makes you feel alive. Moving does marvels: try jogging to let off steam, if you're fuming at something. Try bicycle riding to release your anger or frustration. Try walking briskly to feel *alive, alert*. Exercise makes you firm: it's not fat that most people object to, it's flab—and *there's no reason on earth that a teenager should be flabby*. You can tone up muscles, make yourself feel vital and alive, burn up a few calories on the side and become a physical person—no matter how much you weigh. (See chapter 17 of this book for some marvelous home exercises to bone up on before you get out on the tennis court in earnest!) Join a dance or exercise class. Don't worry about how you *look* dancing: everyone there is interested in her own progress and doesn't even notice you. Really. You are more invisible than you think.

Don't drive to school—walk. Don't bargain with your dad to take the dog out—you do that and let him do something else. Stretch in front of a mirror as long and as hard as you can. Grab your hair on the top of the head and pull up—you'll find your body follows and you are standing straighter than you ever did. Take the stairs instead of the escalator. *Stand instead of sit, walk instead of ride, run instead of walk! Move!* You're a young, strong woman. Show it! Look it! Don't be an ornament with teased hair that can't be tousled, or starched clothes that can't be *used*.

Boys, Men, Males, Guys, the Opposite Sex, Them

I must tell the truth. Sometimes it's murder. One, only one, teenage girl I spoke with, out of hundreds over size 16, told me she had an active and easy social life. The rest of you have problems. Why?

Teenage boys are battling their own problems. They have to feel tough and look tough. They are told by their mothers who are feminists that it's okay to cry, but their fathers (sometimes) and their peers label them queer if they're different. They can't even touch each other in warmth and friendship for fear of being labeled gay. So they don't have it easy, either. And when it comes to girls, they generally are not looking for trouble. Give them the ninety-eight-pound cheerleader who flirts and flits and giggles, every time. (Until they get older, that is.) They may be drawn to the more womanly, more *zaftig* girl, but boy, they're letting themselves in for a ribbing if they take anyone over ninety-eight pounds to the prom. And most of them don't have the strength, the temperament or the wisdom to put up with peer censure. *Yet.*

And another thing: never forget that boys mature later than girls. When you feel all womanly and ready to share your most intimate secrets with someone who *looks* like the sensitive and loving type, keep in mind that if he's close to your own age, he's probably still mostly interested in soccer and how far anything will go if he kicks it.

It *does* happen occasionally that a young man who is secure and steady and knows what he wants, comes along. Watch for that guy. (He won't be the one clowning around with the lampshade on his head. He also probably will not be on the football team.)

You must know this: as you get older, it will definitely get better. You will hopefully travel in circles of people who prize individuality and depth and you will find many men who admire and lust for and look for *real* women, no matter what their size. What can you do in the meantime? Two things. Prepare yourself to be that *real* woman of the future by touching as much of life as you can. And for now, in the meantime, steel yourself to *reach out.* It's not easy but you have to try to be more assertive. Seize the moment now, not when you're thirty-two. This is how to reach out.

AT A PARTY

When you go to a party, don't wait to be discovered in the corner. Come prepared with piquant conversation and ideas so that guys feel comfortable and interested in chatting with you. You'd be surprised how many "friendships" turn out to be something more. Listen to what people are saying. Be available for friendships and confidences. Don't make yourself a damp pillow for someone else to cry on, but be a friend. You may turn out to be the girl friend.

Wear a conversation piece like a tiny pink stone glued onto your cheekbone. (Make up lies about what the stone is. It was given to me by Mick Jagger? It was on me when I woke up this morning?)

Come to the party with a prop: a camera, a guitar, a notebook. Use it. (For the notebook, say you're writing a magazine story about favorite gripes. Interview people; everyone loves to be interviewed! *Really write* the story. Send it in to a local magazine or school publication.)

Learn how to tell fortunes. You'll find a lineup for "Me next!"

No one should feel sorry for you at a party. You're the greatest —you always have a new thing to talk about or try out! (Even if you have to work on it very, very hard before the party.)

What if you're not invited to the party? Give one! Ask the very best people in the school—the winners, not the losers. Don't get a reputation of hanging around with dullards. (Dullards have *their* problems, too. I'm not telling you to be mean to them—just work on your own popularity for a while.)

WRITE HIM TO INVITE HIM

It's easier than saying it face to face, for many people. Try the following:

> Dear Jeff,
> The junior prom is this weekend. I've been too busy to think about it [make sure that's true—be a busy person], but here we are and I'd like to go. With you would be nice. Check one:
> _____ Sure, great, I'll talk to you in chemistry.
> _____ Can't, already going with Sue, Joan, Barbara, etc.
> _____ Can't, I have a club foot.

> Dear Jeff,
> I'm having some kids over this weekend to discuss starting a hosteling club. [A poetry magazine, an SAT review group, a camping-out trip, a teacher evaluation program, a house of prostitution—whatever!] Care to join us? Let me know!

> Dear Jeff,
> I understand you've been involved in door-to-door politics during Senator Kennedy's last campaign. I need to know more about

how that works, where I start, advice on whom to speak with, etc. Can I call you tonight for some information?

Dear Jeff,
My Uncle who works for CBS just willed me two free tickets for a Rolling Stones concert. Interested? See me in Biology.

Dear Jeff,
Help! Being editor is fun but *too much!* Can you help me out with a column on school sports? If yes, let's make a date to discuss content and what ideas you have. My house at 8 tonight? If no, don't worry. Someone else has expressed great interest in doing it. I'd rather have you.

Dear Jeff,
Betty is having a bowling party . . . like to go with me? I warn you, I'm a brilliant bowler.

Jeff may be flattered to death at your interest. If he's not, you've lost nothing but have shown a friendly interest. Try it! Write him a note. *But be cautious about one crucial thing:*
Do not write anything in the note that can't be passed around to 300 other guys without embarrassing you. It is possible that your note will circulate: don't ever write anything of a confidential or embarrassing nature on paper.

PSYCH YOURSELF UP

It shows when you think you are attractive, desirable. It actually is convincing if *you* believe it. Learn to small-talk (see chapter 9, Life Situations). Learn to dance, learn to put makeup on and dress beautifully. Don't settle for being a sloppy mess if you're fat. You can be seductive and appealing and delightful if you work at believing it. Be honest. If you feel scared or doubtful about something, say so. It's very appealing to men to be able to give advice and be strong. Not stronger—never fake weakness, or dumbness or lack of skill, because you think that will make you more appealing as a woman. It doesn't. It just makes you dumber and klutzier and weaker. The days when you had to lose the checkers game so you wouldn't make him feel bad are over. Women are allowed to be strong and smart today. Thank God for Gloria Steinem.

Don't choose boys who are "losers" just because you think you'll have a better chance with them. The brighter a young man is, the more successful he is at his own life and the more he'll be able to see you as an attractive girl and not as a threat to his macho image.

You may feel you're the only girl in the world who doesn't have dates. You aren't. Plenty of thin girls are sitting home too, believe me. You may find that talking to other girls about your feelings gives you ideas on how to open up and expand your social relationships more. And it's also easier with two to do something. Maybe you can both give a wine and cheese party. Maybe you can ask two guys to start a small business with you, like entertaining at children's parties. Remember—romance often grows from friendship.

MAKE A MOVE ON THE TELEPHONE

Size your subject up well. He may be the type who is very shy and would love to be asked out on a date, so he won't have to take the initiative. On the other hand, he may be the kind who is turned off by a girl making the first move. Be prepared for being turned down. It won't, or shouldn't, kill you. Boys have prepared *themselves* for no's since the beginning of dating.

Me, a Photographer? Are You Crazy?

Young women who are overweight are generally unhappy about the fact. Therefore, they should do something that is going to make them *very* happy with themselves to compensate. Become an expert at something. Not only will it give you scads of self-esteem, it will also open the doors to meeting new friends. Just suppose you never thought of photography in your life as something that is (a) interesting, (b) a remote possibility, (c) a distinct possibility for you. So what? Take a photography course (usually given for free or for a modest amount at local high school and adult education centers). *Try it.* Go out on your own being Amy Wilson, girl photographer. Take pictures of your brother, his little finger, a lilac, a blade of grass, a boat, an eye. Learn to develop your pictures yourself. Join a photography club. Give your own lessons. And so it goes: you've become a pro, a person to whom other people come for advice.

It doesn't have to be photography. Try writing children's books. Try pot luck with a pottery course. Learn an instrument, like guitar, or take singing lessons (this opens up all kinds of possibilities of putting together your own musical group to perform at dances, parties, etc.). Ask your local newspaper if they would like a column written by a high school girl (you could write advice to the lovelorn or you could be a liaison between school and community).

For too many heavy young women, the teenage years are a period of marking time, of waiting to grow up and away from the cruelty of young boys, nagging parents, pitying looks. *Don't let it happen to you!* Don't wait for life to begin. It has begun already—don't waste a second. Become an expert at something and that will be a way of not only preparing for a full future but of making a vital life *now*. Not when you grow up. And another thing. Just don't read these words the way you read a thousand other words and say, uh huh, yup, she's right, I ought to, that's right—and then go on to read another thousand words. *Stop right now. Go to the library. Look in the card catalog, under* Hobbies, Spare-Time Options, Career Choices. Do some reading. Find one thing that sounds appealing and follow it up. Who, me, a photographer? Why the hell not?

The Dope on Diets

Be wary of anyone, even a doctor, who wants to give you gobs of reducing pills. Sometimes, under special circumstances, they are called for, but these circumstances are few and far between. Diet pills can be lethal, it has sadly been proven, over and over again.

There are no Metrecal miracles, either. Vegetarian diets, macrobiotic binges, health-food spartan sieges have been proven to be useless and, worse, dangerous, especially during these, your maximum growth years. Meditation and osmosis rarely work, either. I don't want to say you can't, or even discourage you from trying to, lose weight. But the absolutely only way to lose weight is to eat less. Sometimes much, much less. Anyone who tries to sell you miracles should be ashamed. Too many teenagers have been duped into believing there's an easy way. And too many kids your age, wheedled, embarrassed, coaxed and shamed into dieting, have found themselves going the other route, entirely and horrifyingly. Anorexia nervosa is a condition where women in their teenage years, predominately, literally starve themselves—sometimes to death. The disease, Dr. Jean Mayer, the eminent authority on weight, says, "is a grave disturbance of body image in which the adolescent young girl or woman continues to see herself as obese even though she has become miserably thin. She shares with the obese subjects the obsession with body (and contempt for its fatness)."

Do you think you are a unique failure because the diets haven't helped you lose weight? Are you kidding? Thirty million American women are in the same boat!

The thing that bothers you most, is it that you don't eat all that much more than your thin friend? Dr. Mayer says that "often obese girls differ from nonobese girls not by their average intake of food, but by their extreme inactivity." It may be your hanging around rather than your eating which is piling on the pounds. Another reason to start getting active in life! And so many professional people agree on this one. Dr. Barbara Edelstein, in her book *The Woman Doctor's Diet for Women*, says that "the overweight teenager may eat significantly fewer calories than girls of normal weight. Though I feel her basic weight problem is her inborn inefficiency in converting food to energy, studies have shown she is usually less physically active than her thinner peers. . . . Exercise would seem, therefore, to be the great equalizer."

You think you can try any old diet your mother cuts out of the newspaper? Wrong. Dr. Mayer says, "Diets for adolescents should be individual, adapted to the rate of growth and development of the person and to his or her energy expenditure. Weight loss, as in other groups, should be slow to avoid excessive fatigue. This factor is especially important with adolescents." He goes on to make a great suggestion. Since the usual diets fail because they leave you hungry, Mayer recommends something that he finds works especially well for adolescents: have smaller and more frequent meals, rather than three meals a day without snacks.

I've already said that you will not find a diet in this book. You won't. I never found one that worked yet—except to change one's pattern of eating for the rest of a lifetime. But here are a couple of interesting tricks on how to fool your brain into thinking you're full. Scientist Anne Scott Beller, in her book *Fat and Thin—A Natural History of Obesity*, offers these "artful dodges" or ways to beat the system—and even to deal with those eating binges you can't avoid!

1. Eat a lot of nonfattening foods like salads and vegetables.

2. Hot foods leave the stomach and enter the gut more quickly; therefore the gut sends back the message "I'm full" much faster if you snack on hot things rather than cold.

3. Drink gallons of water: it tends to make you feel full and seems to have a close relationship to fat loss.

4. Stay far away from zero- or low-carbohydrate diets and starvation diets; they *never* work permanently and they are dangerous, even for the short run, especially for adolescents.

5. If you are anticipating a food binge shortly—a wedding or a brunch coming up—cut back on your calories a day or so *before* the binge, not afterward, to atone. Ms. Beller says, "Predieting, not postdieting works best for binges. If you must overeat, do it on an empty stomach."

Do Something, Passionately, in School

Write for the school paper, run for the school presidency, try out for the debating club! Do it passionately. You will find that you are more involved in life. And doing things passionately has other benefits: working late with another male reporter over a front-page breaking school story on the newspaper can be very involving—in more ways than one.

Get a Job

There are an infinite number of jobs to be had where you will meet people, expand your horizons and have fun—besides making money. Here are some suggestions:

- Waitress in a coffee house. (You can even set up your own coffee house if you feel like playing entrepreneur.)
- Work in a kennel. A veterinarian's office. Ask if anyone needs help.
- Work at the ASPCA. The zoo.
- Work as a hostess helper (an assistant at parties).
- Give kids' parties.
- Work as a silversmith. (See if the local jewelry stores need help.)
- An usher.
- Start a "Rent a Teenager" business. Get your friends to join you and offer lawn services, cleaning services, baby-sitting services, etc.
- Write a column for a local paper. (You suggest it—perhaps they'll go for the idea.)
- Be a sign painter.
- Design greeting cards and sell them to local stores.
- Model large-size clothes for teenagers (see if you can sell the local "large-size" stores on this one).
- Work in a library.
- Work in a boutique.

Last Word, Kids—Not to Get Preachy, But . . .

Please, please, in your darkest moments, remember—*fat* and *ugly* are not the same, Virginia. Where is it written that it really is so awful to be heavy? In your mother's book? Your doctor's book? Your best friend's book? Are their own books such best sellers because they are thin? Does thinness guarantee a perfect life, acceptable to all society? Are the thin ones really so happy? If you think about it hard, you will see that even if you love all these people who are judging you, they may not be correct! No one has the right to judge your life-style. It may be time to gently begin ignoring the "experts," not only on weight but on your life, and to accept yourself for what you are, no matter what you weigh.

If you feel well, if your extra pounds don't create any medical problems, if you are strong and healthy—take control of your own days. Not when you're thirty. *Now!* Use your weight to compete in the big leagues.

Dr. Hilde Bruch is one of the world's leading authorities on obesity. She says, "Weight excess in adolescence is commonly blamed for interfering with sexual adjustment . . . but from my observations, it is not the weight excess itself but the attitude toward it, or more correctly, toward oneself, that interferes with any personal relationships."

In the final analysis, it is your own attitudes that will make you a big and beautiful young woman, not a big and defeated one.

XIX Facts and Myths/ Truth and Lies

This is the saga of Jody White who is not real.

Actually, maybe she's too real because Jody is the composite picture of five very real, different women. You will recognize Jody because many heavy women seem to share the same parents, the same childhood ordeals, the same pressures, even though they grew up thousands of miles apart. The diet devices that tortured her are also real, and can be bought in a variety of stores.

She was born cute and round. Her grandmother's first words on seeing Jody were, "She's gorgeous because she's fat! They don't look so wrinkled and scrawny when they have a little meat on them, you know! God bless her!"

She grew up loved, squeezed, pinched and hugged. Her darling chubby cheeks and her cute little waddle were delicious!

Jody's mom was much admired by all the other moms whose kids spit out their pablum.

"How do you do it?" asked Mrs. Tiegs. "My Cheryl is so skinny that I worry about her. What's your secret in feeding up that healthy-looking Jody?"

Jody's mom would smile in secret pride. She felt like a real *mom*. The truth was, she wasn't doing much of anything. Jody seemed to thrive and grow rounder and cuter every day. Of course, Jody's mom and her husband were substantially built, but everyone knew that had nothing to do with it.

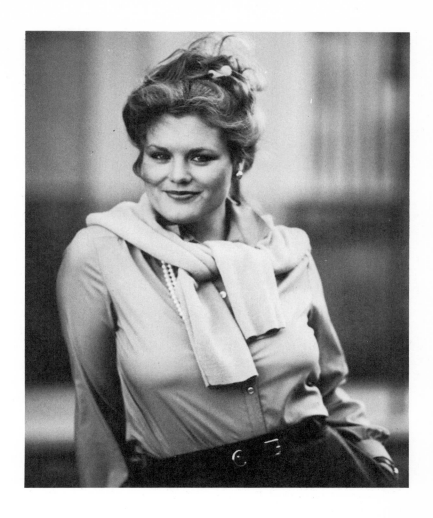

"If you clean your plate, I'll love you," Jody's mother used to say to her.

"But I'm full," Jody would sometimes complain.

"What do you mean full? *Full?* Are your arms full, are your legs full? Don't be crazy. Eat up. The children in Europe are starving."

So Jody ate up because she was a good girl.

Jody grew. And learned to talk, And she grew rounder. And she learned to charm. And she grew rounder. And happier and healthier. And rounder.

Until she was six.

"Jody's getting a little, uh, *chunky*, don't you think?" mentioned the grandmother one day. "Maybe you ought to cut down on the muffins."

"I was thinking that just this morning," Jody's mother guiltily blurted. "Another kid called her 'Tubsy' in kindergarten."

Jody's life changed almost overnight. Her mother still insisted that before meals she bow and pray, "Give us this day our daily bread," but no one gave her bread anymore. Or muffins. Or the mashed potatoes she was weaned on with the darling little square of butter—yum—melting in the middle of the creamy mound. She couldn't understand it. What was encouraged, was now discouraged. She was a good girl and had always finished her milk and cleaned her plate—and now they frowned when she cleaned that same plate. Oh, boy, was she getting double messages. One said *You're good if you eat*; the other, *You're bad if you eat.*

She grew up confused and, of course, fat. She had trouble sorting out the messages. Of course, she understood in her head that most people did not think fat was so terrific any more, but she would always remember the love and adoration poured on her for being baby-fat. It still always made her feel comforted when she ate. And somehow, even though no one believed her anymore, she wasn't even eating all that much more than anyone else. She just seemed to gain weight if she *looked* at an ice-cream cone.

She hid in her room during her teenage years. The television set wasn't much help. The messages *it* gave were very clear—and downright cruel.

"Nobody loves a fat pen," screamed Parker Pen. The new, slimmer Parker pen said smugly, "It's changed my whole life. People want me near them. I feel needed."

"Get in on *thin*," called Silva cigarettes, "the one that's *in* . . ."

Her Detecto talking scale, a blabbermouth, announced her weight out loud, in sonorous, disapproving tones.

And so it went on.

She got more and more depressed. Even games didn't help. Her friend Lucy got a game called Fat Chance that all the kids were playing. You got to play with "fat man" pawns and if you were lucky, you might challenge another to a "weigh-in." It was important to avoid the spaces like "mozzarella mess, sundae driver and cube steak special." The fewer "pounds" you gained in the game, the better chance you had of winning Fat Chance.

Jody felt demeaned from every angle. Worse yet, she felt ugly and stupid and weak-willed, because *weren't* fat people ugly, stupid, and weak-willed?

When she was eighteen, the *buying of the pills and the gadgets* began. She bought Sauna Suits. She bought Ayds. She bought Twisters and Pounders and Things That Twisted You and Things That Pummeled You and nothing, not one thing ever worked.

And then she became a grownup. She got into college although at first she was turned down all over the place (for her weight, she rightly suspected, not her grades, which were excellent). It was difficult getting a job. She felt that her pounds made her look terrible so she slouched around trying to hide some of it. The navy-blue, baggy muumuus and the shoulder slouch didn't seem to work. Although she had executive qualities, she ended up filing papers in a back office.

Her social life was nothing less than disaster. She hid from new contacts and she never thought anyone would want to love her—not the way she looked.

Her mom and grandmother never gave up. They sent her the latest diets in the mail. Hardly a day passed when the Rockefeller Diet, the Grapefruit Diet, the Watermelon Diet, the Last Chance Diet, the Scarsdale Diet, the Doctors' Quick Inches-Off Diet, the Total Starvation Diet, the Bananas Diet, the Eat All You Want Diet, the Drinking Man's Diet, The Mayo Clinic Diet, the Atkins Diet, didn't come winging its way to her. She counted 197 diets that friends and relatives suggested. None of them worked.

Once, a well-meaning friend gave her Slender Fork, an electronic bully with a traffic light on it which would help her time her chewing. "If you chew more slowly, you'll eat less, Jody," the friend explained.

Her mother put the Diet Conscious Box on the refrigerator. Every time Jody opened the refrigerator door, the little box coarsely and obscenely derided her. "Ha, ha, ha. No wonder you look the way you do. Shame on you. Eating *again*? You'll be sorry, Fatty! Ha, ha, ha," snickered the box.

Her uncle thought it would be fun to buy her Diet Soap which lost weight as she bathed instead of snacked. And her cousin Estelle thought it was a riot to give Jody, for her birthday, a place setting of diet silver. The fork tines and knife blades were sawed off and the soup poured out through a hole in the soup spoon.

Jody despaired.

Her guilt grew and every time she reached for a spoonful of peanut butter, she was sure she'd get a leprous rash on her fingertips.

And one day she was forty-two. And she weighed exactly what she had weighed when she was nineteen. (After all those diets.) And she looked in the mirror and she said,

"Enough. It's time to begin living."

You can write the rest of Jody's story.

Did she really begin living? Did she overdose on Baby Ruths? Did she go on another diet? Did she smash the laughing refrigerator box?

If you decide to write a downbeat ending, a *cinéma vérité* number, you can do it right now. You already have all the information at your fingertips that you'll need. There'll be more diets. More frustration. More hating herself. More hiding. More boredom. If it is really clear to you that Jody will fail and will live all the rest of her life condemned to a body she hates and which she cannot conquer—the ending is simple and sad and really an ending.

But if you are determined to write an upbeat, a positive, a realistic ending which, in truth, is a beginning—you will have to have more facts. You need to know what the researchers and the finest medical minds say about the problem. You'll have to know about the places which offer Jody useful and supportive help. You will have to find out the best way she can learn to live with her body —and end up actually liking it. (Well, maybe not loving it, but so what? Liking herself will be enough to open marvelous doors of opportunity.)

The rest of this chapter will arm you with the facts, should you choose the second ending, the ending which is the beginning.

Facts About Fat

They don't let us live.

One year they tell us that sugar substitutes will save our lives because the sweet stuff's awful for everything. The next year they tell us that sugar substitutes give you cancer. In the 1950s, every movie star reached for a cigarette instead of an O'Henry bar. Smoking was chic, cool and not fattening. Now, the American Cancer Society would rather we be overweight than dying of lung cancer from the same cigarettes. Twenty years ago, every red-blooded American mother gave her kid red-blooded meat in great quantities. Also lots of milk and ice cream for calcium. Now they tell us that steak and cream cause cholesterol clogs.

We can't win. They've got us frightened of nuclear energy, hair dryers, even the good old American maraschino cherry. With good reason. Always with good reason.

I guess it's wise to believe that nothing is sacred and that everything bears rethinking. What was Dr. Spock and Common Knowledge in one generation is Haim Ginott and Dangerous Ignorance in another. That's the way it has been. That's the way it will always be. Think for a moment. Is there *anything* that is not subject to revision, different minds, different advertising campaigns? Vegetables? I would not stake my life on it that next year's headlines won't shout that vegetables give you gout. Jogging cuts down heart disease? I wouldn't fall down if next week the tabloids yell that jogging *gives you* heart disease. Also piles. And if the new wave of child psychiatrists comes out chanting that hugging, kissing and kindnesses of other natures gives kids insecurity, you won't find me gasping with shock. In this world, nothing is an absolute, nothing is a sure bet.

Take fatness. Tomorrow, when some brilliant, public-relations-conscious doctor finally says that gluttony wasn't what made all those fat ladies fat and that weak moral fiber and lack of self-control have nothing to do with gaining weight, I won't throw my hands up in amazement. One must expect contradictions in style.

Big women used to be thought marvelous. Really. Rubens, Botticelli, and Cleopatra's lovers thought so. The Greek and Roman gods thought their hefty goddesses were the last word. The Gibson girls, Madame de Pompadour, Lillian Russell, were all sex idols.

Still we live *now*, and now says that Fat Is Not Where It's At. Almost by itself in a time when many questionable conditions have been accepted, obesity still remains *bad*—morally wrong and weak. If you have the bad fortune to be an alcoholic, it's not so terrible—the scientific world says pressures and God knows what else are responsible. If you are a sexual deviate, your bad home life did you in. If you are mentally ill, society did you in and it's a health problem. If you are underweight, it is also a health problem in the eyes of America, says a recent *New York Times* article. But if you are overweight, corpulent, full blown, fat, big or bountiful —call it what you will—according to the *New York Times,* Americans see you as having an "emotional weakness." You are a glutton and a pig and you have done it to yourself. If you fail to lose weight from the myriad therapies, diets and reams of advice that doctors and your Aunt Shirley have to offer, only you are to blame. There must be something wrong with your self-control. You must have a Freudian fixation on your mother. You must have an infantile need for oral gratification. In a few words, you are a spineless chump. You should feel guilty and self-responsible. Better you should be a sexual deviate.

Take heart. The pendulum is swinging. There is a growing group of doctors, nutritionists, psychologists and psychiatrists who are attempting to set the record straight. There is, as we have learned from history, another side of the coin, and thanks to strong and responsible individuals and organizations, the problem is being coaxed out of the closet. The tide is turning. No longer does everybody who counts look upon being fat as a liability or a weakness. Nor do the majority of responsible researchers see it as a moral problem; indeed, the facts are beginning to show that fat is often not a condition of your own making. Sometimes, no matter what you do, you just can't lose weight.

Volumes have been written on the subject. You owe it to your self-esteem to do some good reading on the subject. Being a big woman is not lethal. If fact, it can be decidedly good.

Here are some interesting facts about being fat that you might want to pass on to people who are in ignorance of the whole story.

DUMB-BELLES?

For every doctor and rumormonger who says that fat women are slower, dumber, less persevering, there is a scientific study which says *exactly* the opposite. In Ann Scott Beller's brilliant book *Fat and Thin,* (Farrar, Straus and Giroux, Inc.), she points out that researchers I. P. Bronstein and his associates determined that obese children have *higher* I.Q.'s than thinner ones.

Dr. Hilde Bruch, an enormously respected authority in the field, also found that fat grade-school children were significantly brighter than nonfat children.

Rodin, Herman and Schachter, three other researchers, concluded that obese college students were better "information processors" than other people because they "take in more information than their normal and skinny peers in the first place, code it more efficiently in the second, and store it more securely in the third."

MENTAL WRECKS?

A resounding no! Beller meticulously analyzed the work of many, many respected authorities in the field, among them Maher, Wollersheim, Penick, Filion and Stunkard. She summarizes as follows: "How crazy are they [heavy people]? Not very—and if anything, perhaps on the whole, just a little less crazy than the population at large. More depressed, possibly, yes: but less overtly psychotic, even so. More placid and socially compliant, yes: but less impulsive and less excitable under stress as well. Immature, yes; passive and dependent, no."

One English researcher, R. F. Suczek, gave some very interesting tests in which he determined that not mental disturbance, but almost a super kind of normality and ability to function socially was characteristic of the very heavy. It appeared that the fatter women were, the more competent and resourceful they became. Thus, scientists *scientifically* scotch many false assumptions made about the fat. In fact, as Beller says, the only real and safe generalization you can make about big women as a whole is that they are a universally and constantly hungry group.

So what else is new?

HEAVY STATISTICS

Guess who's fatter—Jews, Catholics or Protestants? According to research by Dr. Albert Stunkard, Professor of Psychiatry at the

University of Pennsylvania School of Medicine, Jews are on the average fatter than Catholics or Protestants. But no one said whether they were weighed before or after the Sabbath. If it was after, it's quite understandable, with all that good chicken soup.

IS IT REALLY DANGEROUS FOR HEAVY WOMEN TO BECOME PREGNANT?

Absolutely not, according to obstetrician-gynecologist, Dr. Sidney Druce of the Mount Sinai and Doctors hospitals in New York City. He says: "It's not a question of fat at all—we don't care how fat prospective mothers are. It's a question of water retention. Preeclampsia is a toxemic condition characterized by water retention, a rise in blood pressure, convulsions, coma and other nasty symptoms. It is the only big reason, really, for making sure you have excellent prenatal care. It is very dangerous for the fetus and for the prospective mother, and although we can't adequately treat the condition, we can prevent its occurring. We like to keep weight down so we can properly monitor any water retention going on in the body, but it's the water and not the fat that's dangerous. *Of course* heavy women can safely have babies."

WE ALL HEAR THAT FAT PEOPLE DIE EARLIER THAN THIN ONES—TRUE?

No. In fact, say many experts, you will no doubt live longer if you are substantially heavier than the Metropolitan Life Insurance Charts say is the correct weight for your height and age. Dr. Reubin Andres, clinical director of the famous National Institute on Aging in Bethesda, Maryland, has said, "There's something about being obese that's funny, that's good for you." In discussing a comprehensive analysis of seventeen long-term health studies, Dr. Andres said: "Several of the studies show that people who were at or slightly below their ideal weight [as portrayed on the Metropolitan tables] had a higher mortality rate at every age than those who were moderately overweight.

"None of the studies shows a shortened life expectancy for persons who are up to 20 percent overweight. Some show no shortened life expectancy for those up to 30 percent overweight. This may be because overweight people are protected against certain diseases or can withstand illness better.

"We have to question what we're doing when we advise people to lose ten pounds—unless they have some clear-cut medical problem such as diabetes, high blood pressure or heart disease."

Dr. Neil Solomon, formerly assistant professor of psychiatry at Johns Hopkins Medical School and the author of a daily syndicated health column, told the *Enquirer* newspaper that "the Metropolitan height-weight columns are a lot of bunk!"

Dr. Frank W. Barr, diplomate of the American Board of Bariatric Medicine, said, "If most people get right down to the Metropolitan figures, they would actually be underweight, unhealthy and more susceptible to illness and disease."

One Northwestern University survey of 1,233 people found that those with the lowest mortality rates were 25 to 35 percent overweight.

Brand-new evidence—look into it! Tell the doctors and the insurance companies that use the Metropolitan tables as an index to proper weight, that the authorities in the medical field have been debunking that ancient gauge.

ARE THOSE CHARTS REALLY ANCIENT AND REALLY NOT SO VALID?

But, I can hear you protesting, *I've been hearing all my life that those charts were perfect guides!* Well, the charts in question were prepared in *1959.* In spite of the changes in the American body itself in the last two decades, and in spite of the world of new research on the subject, we still hark back to that study as the final word on proper weight advice. Dr. Ancel Keys, the noted psychologist from the University of Minnesota, long ago questioned the validity of the outdated charts' assertion that obesity is a health hazard. He correctly judged that the insurance statistics represented such a small portion of *only those people who buy life insurance,* that it was unfair to judge the modern health standards of the entire populace by the data obtained on only one small segment of the then fat population.

A Harvard University researcher, Dr. Carl C. Seltzer, concluded that the data on which the Metropolitan Charts are based is totally off base. "The insurance companies claim that your mortality rate increases proportionately to how much overweight you are," states Selzer. "I analyzed the Society of Actuaries' [the group which compiled the data for the charts] own figures and showed that this isn't true!"

And a Mayo Clinic Study in 1952 stated that the obese actually had a better coronary survival rate than the nonobese.

So much for the "untouchable" charts that have been plaguing overweight people for years. They are wrong and outdated. Simple as that.

BUT DOESN'T EVERYBODY SAY THAT WEIGHT IS A KILLER?

More people than you would dream of are beginning to say no. New evidence is coming out which suggests that excess weight, by itself, is not the significant factor in heart disease and premature death it's been made out to be.

Dr. Ancel Keys says, "Apart from the insurance data, all of the published information is in agreement that coronary heart disease is not related to overweight." The famed researcher found that body build is more significant than overweight in determining factors of heart disease.

The prestigious and famous Framingham studies concur. In 1967, one study concluded, "While the belief that obesity and cardiovascular mortality are related is widely held, the exact nature of this relationship requires further clarification. Weight is only one parameter of body form and it is possible that body build is more closely related to development of CHD [coronary heart disease] than is adiposity."

In the Framingham report of 1972, sponsored by the National Heart, Lung and Blood Institute, 5,209 adults were studied for sixteen years. Obesity was *not* listed as a major risk factor in hardening of the arteries of the heart, head or legs. In 1973, another Framingham report said that it was still difficult to judge how or to what extent excess weight was involved in heart disease. In fact, the report says, the *lowest* death rates were among men and women aged forty to fifty-nine whose average weight was 15 to 20 percent *over* the Metropolitan "ideal" weight charts.

One heavy woman put it this way: "Many insensitive doctors blame everything on a person's excess weight, saying it causes everything from hangnails to cancer. If that were the case, no thin person should ever get sick!"

It is indeed becoming increasingly clear that if you are fat and if you are free of the risk factors of high blood sugar, blood pressure and blood fat, you are no more liable to heart disease than anyone else. *Obesity, by itself, does not mean a higher coronary risk factor!* Look, no fair-minded person can say that obesity cannot aggravate existing high blood pressure or diabetes—but thin people have these ailments as well. The stress of constant dieting can be as large a disease-causing factor as excess weight. In study after study, researchers have found that temperament, more than pounds, causes heart trouble. Other factors like metabolism, genetics, sugar and salt intakes and general environment play key roles in diseases that kill: but notice how all of these are played down by worried mothers and brainwashed and, yes, hostile-to-fat doctors who find it easier to pin the whole rap on weight.

Dieting and Diets

YO-YO'S ARE FUN, BUT NOT YO-YO DIETS

That kind of yo-yoing can kill you. Weight loss followed by weight gain and a quick weight loss and then another gain elevates serum-cholesterol levels and subjects women to more arterial fat-clogging than a weight that is high but consistent. Yo-yo diets also give you wrinkles and more sagging skin than you ever saw before.

Dr. Maria Simonson, a specialist at Johns Hopkins Obesity Clinic, has said, "It is worse to lose and gain, lose and gain. Many obese people will add more weight when they gain it back. . . . If you are comfortable with your weight, healthy physically and psychologically, I do not believe it is necessary to lose weight."

The yo-yo syndrome comes about because weight is so difficult to keep off. Dr. Norman Lindenmuth, director of the George Washington Hospital Health Plan, has been quoted in an article in *The Washington Post* as saying, "What is so depressing for the doctor about treating the obese is that the success rate, at the very best, is one in twenty. More often it is far less than that. And that's for keeping weight off for only one year."

HOW COME THERE'S NO WAY OUT OF THE DIET JUNGLE FOR MOST OF US?

There are, at last count, over 27,000 ways to diet. The diet business is a dense, dangerous jungle planted by fashion magazines, get-rich-quick quacks, health writers, well-meaning but uninformed doctors, and mothers. Some of the paths through this jungle *are* sound and responsibly laid out by knowledgeable experts, and *some* people do manage to hack through the underbrush and actually leave some of their pounds behind. Most don't. Why? Because a great preponderance of the diet advice that grows in the jungle is worse than useless—it is dangerous as snake-infested bush. People get sick, discouraged and self-hating when they can't hack the jungle. On the fad diets, which either limit calories for a prescribed period of time or allow you unlimited amounts of certain foods for a while, you are bound to fail because you have not changed your regular eating habits, permanently and for all time. And it is absolutely true that you may have a body build that will not allow for weight loss, short of starvation. The number of fat cells in your body have been determined at birth and through your early childhood. They cannot be reduced in number. It *is* possible to reduce the *size* of fat cells, but again, it's extremely difficult. Dr. John H. Karam, associate director of the Metabolic Research Unit of the University of California at San Francisco, says that if a person has normal levels of insulin, triglyceride and glucose, his fat cells are probably of normal size even though they may be too numerous. He is doomed to failure, no doubt, if he tries to reduce, and his obesity, says Dr. Karam, should not be considered a medical problem that demands treatment.

If no diet has ever worked for you, it may be that you are beating your head against a stone wall. If you're healthy, relax, expand your psyche, learn to like yourself the way you are. You really have no choice. In a recent *New York Magazine* article, author Toby Cohen tells why diets don't work. "We spend about $10 billion a year trying to lose weight, but the stark fact is that 95 percent of those who do lose it gain right back," says Cohen. Some of the reasons may be, he says:

1. According to Susan Wooley at the Cincinnati Medical School Clinic for Eating Disorders, severe dieting may cause some (not all) people to actually *gain* weight. They "develop unusually thrifty metabolism: they become more efficient at storing calories as fat than at burning them up." This tendency may have come from prehistoric times when the ability to carry fat on one's back or in one's belly made the difference between survival and death during famine times. "In our clinic," says Wooley, "we work with many patients whose metabolism appears to have become much thriftier with years of dieting."

2. You may be born to fatness. Researchers Richard Keesey of the University of Wisconsin and Peter Herman of the University of Toronto feel, along with myriads of other scientists, that each individual has a *biologically controlled* ideal weight that is right and normal for that person; it is very difficult to alter this weight by dieting.

3. Because of your genes, you may get excessively nervous and tense when you diet, unlike others who diet easily. Toby Cohen says, "Overweight is not always due to lack of discipline, greed, or a Jewish mother, but can be the effect of machinery that's been programed unusually. It may be much harder for your fat friend to curb his appetite than it is for you."

4. Many people find the side effects of dieting extremely debilitating. These side effects include the monotony of dieting and a condition called ketosis, which is acidosis associated with the abnormal breakdown of fat tissue.

DOES EVERYBODY LOSE WEIGHT AT THE SAME RATE IF THEY JUST STOP EATING SO MUCH?

Dr. Barbara Edelstein, in her book *The Woman Doctor's Diet for Women* (Prentice-Hall, Inc.), says no. "It is much, much harder for an overweight woman to lose weight than it is for a naturally thin woman or for any man. Men lose weight almost twice as fast as women do. It is not superior willpower or self-discipline that keeps a person thin, but simply the luck of the draw when metabolisms were being passed out."

WHAT CAN ANTI-FAT CAMPAIGNS DO TO PSYCHES?

Plenty. Overweight is neither immoral nor ignoble, but we start to hate ourselves if we're heavy. Researcher Dr. Hilde Bruch says, "There is no doubt about the damaging effect on mental health of the current campaign against overweight." Self-hate leads to depression and inactivity. Being constantly aware of a struggle not to eat can drive you crazy. Theodore Van Itallie, a noted expert on weight, said, "The price of leanness, like liberty, is eternal vigilance."

Liberty is worth eternal vigilance, I guess. But leanness?

ARE PEOPLE AUTOMATICALLY HAPPY WHEN THEY LOSE WEIGHT?

People who feel shame and sadness that they don't fit into the size 8s of their neighbors have been nothing less than brainwashed into thinking they would be better off thin. In fact, studies have shown that the pot at the end of the rainbow doesn't miraculously appear to those who have lost weight. Their problems and their fears, their liabilities and disabilities, remain remarkably the same. All that is different is that their bodies are smaller. Their heads still tell them that they are the same people they were fifty pounds ago. They didn't miraculously become the self-assured, successful, marvelous persons they expected to be from a weight loss. And they're confused.

Expecting to find successful dieters happy with their "new lease on life," Dr. Sandra Haber, a psychologist, discovered that "life was not a bed of roses" for many. New anxieties arose including confusion in marriage, relationships, work habits and worry about one's self-image. One of the formerly big women I spoke with corroborated Dr. Haber's view. "I am so nervous I'll gain it back!"

she lamented. "And I feel such anger at the guys who wouldn't look at me when I was forty pounds heavier. I'm the same me. What happens if I form a relationship with someone and then put the weight back? Will I be dropped like a hot potato?" Another woman complained, "I don't know. I look in the mirror and I see the same me, weight loss or not. But everyone else says I've changed—that I'm not as giving and warm. What the hell do they want from me? Fat or thin, they criticize."

There's one thing on which these rare, successful losers never plan but which happens, according to a *New York Times* article, 97 percent of the time:

DIETERS WILL PROBABLY GAIN THEIR WEIGHT BACK

Despite your perseverance (most dieters *never* give up), the odds are greatly against your losing weight permanently. Indeed, to lose weight forever, plan to spend a lot of time—the rest of your life—working on it *constantly*. In 1966, J. A. Glennon, after thoroughly reviewing available studies to that date, concluded that only 10 percent of patients in a scientifically controlled weight-reduction program maintained their weight loss after one year. After two years, it dwindled to only 6 percent. Imagine the statistics of those who are not buoyed by a controlled and supportive program. They're even dramatically lower! Albert Stunkard of the University of Pennsylvania tested ninety-seven patients at the Nutrition Clinic of New York Hospital and found that after a two-year follow-up, only two losers had managed to keep the lost weight off. The studies and the casebooks are solid with evidence that losing weight permanently is hardly ever done. Even the first recorded diet in 1873, which was the painstaking work of a mortician named William Banting, failed miserably. Banting, five foot five and 202 pounds, lost thirty-eight jubilant pounds in thirty-five weeks. A new fad was started: "banting," or dieting as it came to be known. When Banting died—at eighty, it was recorded—he was just as fat as he was when he started the misery that was to plague otherwise healthy and happy women up to 1980, at the current writing, anyway.

Why is this so? Well, for one reason among many, eating less, despite what the million-dollar weight-reducing plans will tell you, is only one part of losing weight. Your own genes may be working against you in preventing a slim body no matter how little you eat. Probably because it is thought that would-be dieters would throw up their hands in despair, the myth is retained that heredity has nothing to do with heaviness. Tell that to any farmer, says Harvard's expert Jean Mayer, and he'll look at you in disbelief. Traditionally, the fattest hogs and cattle are used when the farmer wishes to breed a fat strain of animal. Different breeds of the same species of animal (and that includes humans) definitely have different abilities to store fat, to gain weight. Some strains won't gain weight no matter what you stuff them with. Some strains, apart from near-starvation, can't lose weight. Still, the myth persists that your lineage has nothing to do with body weight—although no one tries to push the theory that lineage has nothing to do with blue eyes or red hair. We are what we eat, yes, certainly. But we also are what the genetic strains have preordained we will be, and sometimes fatness, barring starvation, may be as irreversible as blue eyes.

Being a baby girl, in the very first place, has given you a good deal more fat tissue than if you were a baby boy: the adipose tissue deposits were almost twice those of your brother's by the time you were adolescents.

What's Good About Being Heavy?

Although it is surely true that being heavy creates some medical problems, no one ever tells you the good parts. For instance, have you heard that according to a Metropolitan Life Insurance study, fat women have a much lower rate of breast cancer than thin women? Have you heard that fat people have less tuberculosis? Have you heard that they are less suicide prone? Have *less* schizophrenia and *no more* neuroses than anyone else? And furthermore, according to Dr. Mayer, "There are a few conditions in which weight reduction is not only unwise but actually dangerous. . . . Weight reduction is definitely contraindicated in regional ileitis, ulcerative colitis, and Addison's disease." Mayer also tells us that on the average, obese individuals have healthier skeletons than the average population as a whole.

Dr. James S. Arnold of the Veterans Administration Hospital in Hines, Illinois, agrees. After having examined the bones of more than 1,000 individuals, he found that the overweight have stronger, heavier bones than thinner people, making fat people lose less bone tissue as they age.

Fat people also seem to get fewer colds because they are better insulated against chill by their fat.

Ms. magazine, *Moneysworth* magazine and *The New York Daily News* all reported a study of DePauw University coeds that related hips to grades: according to a computer research study in that school, the bigger the hips, the better the grades.

The British Medical Journal says that underweight women are far more likely to suffer the side effects of The Pill than overweight women. And fat insulates to make winters easier, which is why Channel swimmers have to be fat-padded to endure seven or eight hours in cold water.

We could go on and on . . .

Help—Where Is It?

In the fat self-pride organizations. They are not diet clubs and they are not exclusively limited to heavy people. They are organizations open to anyone who is interested in helping heavy people fight the good fight—both socially and politically. Socially? You bet! The organizations hold dances, picnics, conventions and theater trips. The best-known of the organizations, National Association to Aid Fat Americans (NAAFA), has a monthly newsletter which is sent out to a growing national membership. Recently, NAAFAns have had television coverage on *60 Minutes* and the *Phil Donahue Show.* The president and founder, brilliant and articulate (and thin) engineer Bill Fabrey, feels that the thrust of the organization is to make members feel that they are not alone with their problems and that they should not let inhibitions stemming from pounds weigh down their lives.

Politically? For sure! Enlightened big women are changing the way they think. They will not be victims of discrimination any longer. Pride movements all over the country are attacking the terrible prejudice that sees excess pounds as being something sinful. And there are many areas of discrimination to be fought in the political arena. NAAFA and other Fat Pride groups have taken up the cudgel to help in cases like the following:

- Oral Roberts University in Tulsa, Oklahoma, evidently sees it as being democratic to expel students who have gained more weight than the university thinks appropriate. In fact they ask students to sign a pledge that they will maintain weight requirements.
- In the news recently a couple was denied a chance to adopt a baby *only because* they were heavier than the adoption agency thought pleasing or healthy.
- A woman was denied a job with a big electronics company because the company doctor thought she was too fat. She had a Masters in Business, was pronounced perfectly healthy by two impartial doctors outside the company and was requested by the division head for whom she'd been working. Still, the company doctor refused to pass her because she was "unpleasantly fat."
- Seven stewardesses were suspended by their employer, Ozark Airlines, for being overweight.
- National Airlines jumped on the bandwagon and fired twenty-three-year-old Ingrid Fee. The five-foot-seven woman was 138 pounds and too fat for them! Fat? She's almost skinny! But the airlines has a pound limit of 134. Wild.
- Joyce English is currently suing the Philadelphia Electric Company. Joyce passed all the preemployment tests except a company physical. On the basis of weight alone, she was found "unsuitable for employment." Dr. Anna-Marie Chirico, an internist for the University of Pennsylvania Medical Group, found her to be in good health with *none* of the complications so frequently (and often erroneously) associated with obesity.
- Five crew members of the nuclear submarine *Los Angeles* were asked to remain in the anonymous background when the President of the United States came to review his troops: the sailors, who were presentable enough to fight and maybe even

die for their country, were just not thought presentable enough, because of their girth, to greet their commander-in-chief.

NAAFA and the other organizations fight battles for people like this. Have you been a victim of prejudice? Write to a group which does not maintain that fat is best, but only that fat is a possible option and as worthy of respect and legal rights as thin. Here are some of the addresses of those groups if you should wish some information and literature on their activities:

National Association to Aid Fat
Americans, Inc.
P.O. Box 745
Westbury, NY 11590

Fat Underground
Box 5621
Santa Monica, CA 90405

Fat Liberator Publications
Box 342
New Haven, CT 06513

The Nasty Myths, Here Debunked!

MYTH #1: HIGH BLOOD PRESSURE IS ALWAYS CONNECTED TO FATNESS

Wrong.
More and more doctors are beginning to distrust our measurement systems. Sometimes, small blood pressure cuffs act like tourniquets and subsequently make blood pressure readings higher than they really are. Too often, heavy people have been told that they have hypertension because the small cuffs on their heavy arms are inaccurate. Dr. Hilde Bruch tells of the woman who had a blood-pressure reading of 280/140 when she was put on a strict diet. Finally, in despair and defeat, after a long while, she dropped the diet at the same weight she was upon beginning it, and her pressure, reevaluated, dropped to 200/110. Her weight was the same, but during the diet she had felt nervous, pressured and un-

gainly. When the diet was dropped, her spirits improved and, with a new reading, her pressure also "magically" improved.

Dr. Abraham I. Friedman, a specialist in weight, says that a study which appeared in *The American Heart Journal* in July 1978, indicates that the width of the arm cuff used for blood-pressure readings also has a bearing on the accuracy of the pressure measurements: "Ideally, the width should be as close to 40 percent of the arm circumference as possible. The inflatable bladder inside the cuff should also be longer so it can surround the arm. The cuffs usually used are too small. Therefore, a thigh cuff on an obese person's arm will give a more accurate and truer blood-pressure reading than the usual smaller cuff."

So if you are not certain that your doctor is getting an accurate reading on your blood pressure, and you think that diets and pills have been prescribed to service a "high" blood pressure that is actually a misread blood pressure, have your doctor either measure your pressure with a thigh cuff or some other more accurate gauge.

MYTH #2: DIETING MAKES YOU FEEL GOOD

Not always.

Robert Olson and Marvin Plessett have evaluated the effects on mental health of dieting. They note that dieting has often been fraught with serious emotional consequences, such as depression, suicide or psychosis. Albert Stunkard has said that "for a large number of overweight persons, the mechanical prescription of reducing diets has had unfortunate consequences; for a smaller number it has been disastrous." Hilde Bruch has said that great danger awaits the obese person who looks forward to slimming as a panacea for all ills. Diet if you want to. But be sure it's the right thing for you in terms of psyche and physical status.

Sheri Fram, a member of the Fat Underground, expresses fury at systems that force people into diets, pills and feeling crummy. "It isn't clear that being fat in itself is a health hazard, but it's very clear that diets can be. If your body is naturally fat, it shouldn't be forced into an unnatural, thin existence."

Even Dr. Theodore Rubin, who keeps changing his mind as to whether fat is good or bad, now says that fat people who decide to get thin should make the choice from accurate self-knowledge and not from a thin-obsessed society which fosters the decision on them. They will not feel good unless *they've* decided to lose the weight. He urges them to "refrain from sacrificing their characteristic personality traits like zest, enthusiasm and responsiveness to the tyrannical regime of keeping a new figure." Ah, Doctor Rubin, at last you're thinking properly!

MYTH #3: LOSING WEIGHT IS PERMANENT

Wrong.
The late Doctor Norman Joliffe of the New York City Department of Health said unequivocally, "At least 90 percent of all the people who lose weight on a diet gain back more than they have lost." Other doctors have put the failure rate even higher.

MYTH #4: IF YOU DON'T WATCH YOUR WEIGHT BY DIETING, YOU WILL JUST GET FATTER AND FATTER

Wrong again.
Llewellyn Louderback in his book *Fat Power* (Hawthorn Books, Inc.) says, "I have received any number of letters from women who were afraid that they would never stop eating if they didn't watch their diets. Instead, nearly all discovered that they leveled off at a certain weight (anywhere from ten to forty pounds over their artificially maintained one) and their weight has never varied more than a pound or so from the 'natural weight.' "

MYTH #5: NOBODY DIES FROM DIETING

False.
There is a dangerous and literal "die" in dieting. One coroner of a rural county in Illinois told a Senate subcommittee, "I see about one case in every six weeks in which I suspect the death was due to diet pills." Multiplied, that's a death rate of about fourteen people per 100,000 population—*just from pills.* The disease anor-

exia nervosa, which is a particular problem in the teenage girl population, is one where adolescents continue to see themselves as obese (and ugly) even when they are pitifully thin. We have been hearing more and more about such teenagers who die when they lose more than 50 percent of their normal weight. They literally starve themselves to death.

Recently many people have died while following a liquid protein diet, and as a result Senator Charles Percy requested the U.S. Food and Drug Administration to order liquid protein off the shelves immediately. This has not hurt the sales of *The Last Chance Diet*, a book that popularized liquid dieting—which only goes to show how desperate for a "fat cure" American women have become.

MYTH #6: YOUNG PEOPLE ARE THE BEST CANDIDATES FOR STRINGENT DIETS

Wrong.

Because children do not stop growing until their early twenties, drastic dieting is a very real danger. New growth requires new protein, and "fasting" diets tend to inhibit growth and body functions. Some starches and sugars *must* be included in a young person's diet. According to Dr. Abraham Friedman, "Strange as it may seem, most adolescents who are obese actually eat less food than their thinner counterparts. But they are much more inactive. Inactivity and lack of exercise is the most frequent cause of adolescent obesity." Jean Mayer tells us that using a moral approach to fatness ("You're a piggy eater," "You're a glutton") is particularly dangerous in adolescents, who may gain an unfavorable self-image that will haunt them all their lives. "They have a deep sense of isolation from other teenagers. They tend to withdraw, to be more dependent on their families than other girls, yet they are not happy even in their family relationships. They are obsessively concerned with food. If you ask them to list their bad habits, they put down 'eating.' Not *over*eating, just eating, as if all food intake were sinful." The *U.S. Public Health Report* of 1966 pointed out that fat youngsters lack both an "in group" and family support. And the worst thing is that the fat children tend to become antiobese themselves. They tend to identify with the ones who are oppressing them. Their lives become miserable and intolerable.

Like your teenager, fat or thin. Love her. Teach her about proper nutritional food needs but don't be a nag. Don't be a *nudge*. Don't be a fat-hater. It is as bad as being a Jew-hater, a black-hater, a gay-hater. It is prejudice of the worst sort and it hits adolescents particularly hard. As one nutritionist put it, "Don't make your teenager lead a life of diet desperation."

MYTH #7: YOUR PARENTS HAVE NOTHING TO DO WITH YOUR WEIGHT

Oh, really?

In the 1968–1970 *Ten State Nutrition Survey,* it was found that by age seventeen, the children of obese parents are actually three times as fat as the children of lean parents. (Obesity was defined by the famous skin-fold test every single diet book touts: if you can grasp more than one inch of fat in your thumb and forefinger by taking a pinch of skin from the back of the upper arm, they say you are obese.)

MYTH #8: AMERICANS ARE GETTING THINNER BECAUSE OF THEIR PREOCCUPATION WITH JOGGING, SWIMMING AND TENNIS

Wrong.

Despite their preoccupations with fast physical sports, Americans are getting heavier. According to *U.S. News and World Report,* a federal government survey showed the average American woman is three pounds heavier today than she was in the early 1960s. The average male is six pounds heavier. And a report from *The National Center of Health Statistics* says the average male is twenty to thirty pounds overweight. The average female is fifteen to thirty pounds overweight. Once-a-week athletics neither wards off fat nor improves muscle tone.

MYTH #9: BEING HEAVY IS DANGEROUS

Again wrong.

As Louderback points out in *Fat Power,* it is the *gaining* of the weight, not the already accomplished fact of fatness, that is dangerous. The Harvard nutritionist Dr. Frederick J. Stare, has pointed out that it is during the weight-*gaining* process that the most damage is done to the blood vessels. Louderback says that the best advice is, "If you are presently thin, do not get fat. If you are fat, try not to get fatter. But if you are not absolutely certain that you can sustain a lower weight for the rest of your life, do *not* attempt to lose weight."

"New and expanding evidence reveals that moderate obesity sustained for a lifetime poses no problems for your health or longevity if you don't have high blood pressure, diabetes and cholesterol problems." This statement comes from the prestigious Framingham International Cooperative Study.

And finally, Dr. Hilde Bruch says, "The optimal weight for any person is the weight at which they feel the best and their health is maintained in the very best manner. I just don't think we should be a nation of Twiggys."

MYTH #10: YOU CAN REDUCE THE NUMBER OF FAT CELLS IN YOUR BODY BY DIETING

Wrong.

Fat cells are constant. Continuous, close-to-starvation dieting can diminish the amount of fat within the cells, but the number of cells never changes. The number of cells you have is determined genetically and hormonally, and cannot be changed by exercise or diet.

MYTH #11: IF YOU GO ON AN EATING BINGE, IT IS BEST TO DIET FOR TWO DAYS AFTERWARD

Wrong.

Recent studies done by George Cahill and G. Hollifield show that it is best, for avoiding weight gain, to go on a diet *before* your eating binge, instead of the usual morning-after guilt-abstinence. Your weight will stay more stable if you diet *before* the party rather than after it.

MYTH #12: JUNK FOOD WILL KILL YOU

Nonsense!

That's the reaction of Gilbert A. Leveille, nutritionist and chairman of the Department of Food Science and Human Nutrition at Michigan State University. Leveille's studies have showed him that "there are no good or bad foods—it's the combination that counts in nutrition. It's not difficult to construct a good meal containing potato chips, a soft drink and a candy bar as long as you add foods that complement them." Leveille adds, "Managed snacking around the clock is better than eating three squares a day." A foe of the long-held belief that a preventive diet aborts heart disease and cancer, Leveille feels that the statistical rise of heart disease and cancer in the past half century is just the result of conquering infectious diseases. Although he says that junk foods are not sophisticated in a culinary sense, Leveille feels that limiting processed sugar, fats, cholesterol and salt will never solve the heart disease and cancer problem.

This researcher is one of the growing number of nutritionists who maintain that eating a lot does not mean gluttony. Working with laboratory mice, he discovered that the fat ones are not necessarily the gluttons. It is the animals that show lower enzyme activity that put out the least energy and are therefore the ones most likely to store fat. Again, genes, not diet, are often responsible for weight.

MYTH #13: FAT-PRONE WOMEN DEVELOP WONDROUSLY LARGE BREASTS

Not true.
Studies show that women gaining weight don't develop significantly larger bosoms. Buxom grandmothers or mothers are the only true influence on your bust size.

MYTH #14: VERY FEW AMERICANS ARE OVERWEIGHT

Incorrect.
The Food and Drug Administration estimates that, as a whole, over one-third of the nation's population is overweight. Perhaps we ought to reconstruct our concept of a "proper" weight if so many exceed it. Some more statistics? Across ages, income levels and races, a greater percentage of women than men are obese. Poorer women are more obese than richer ones. Dr. Stunkard has shown by his studies, however, that the richer women were more likely to be emotionally disturbed by the weight; it is more of a stigma in the upper classes.

MYTH #15: YOU GET FAT ONLY WHEN YOU'RE UNHAPPY, FRUSTRATED OR DISTURBED

Wrong, Wrong, Wrong.
According to the latest studies by Yale researcher Judith Rodin, "There is no single kind of obesity and no one obese personality." In fact, in many cases, many fat people were perfectly steady and happy before they gained weight. It is only *after* the weight gain, when society began to ostracize and browbeat them, that they became disturbed. Which goes to show that it's mostly society's problems causing the unhappiness, not ours. Said one patient at the University of Michigan's obesity program, "Look at Elvis Presley—he was a star. A great sex symbol. After he's dead, what do they talk about? How fat he was, how many rolls and bulges he

had. It's terrible." Rodin's study, while it shows that obesity can cause mistrust, low self-regard, anxiety and hypochondria, shows also that most overweight people are psychologically normal, at least to begin with.

Rodin also suggests that it is the constant vigilance required by dieters that often spells unhappiness. Continual restraint leads them to feel compelled and obsessed by food until their restraint weakens and then they feel guilty. She advises the healthy overweight to "get off diets as such and learn to live more normally with food."

MYTH #16: THE MORE EDUCATED YOU ARE, THE MORE YOU CAN FIGURE OUT HOW TO BE THIN

Untrue.
One off-the-cuff estimate by responsible researchers says that as many as one-quarter of the freshman college women in this country are victims of a syndrome that two Cornell University professors have named *bulimarexia*—being caught, according to Jane Brody of *The New York Times*, "in a physically and psychologically damaging cycle of starvation, binge eating and punishing urges." This syndrome often gives way to anorexia nervosa, the disease in which one literally starves herself—often to death. Book learning does not make for rational thinking about weight and proper nutrition.

MYTH #17: OBESITY AND "OVERWEIGHT" ARE THE SAME THING

Nope!
Weight is the added-up sum of pounds that the muscles, body fluids, bones and fat come to. The term *overweight* comes from outdated insurance charts, which tell what weight they'd like you to be, and the fashion and diet industries, which proclaim their ideas of proper weight. Obesity is no more than an excessive amount of fat tissue. To show how foolish the term *overweight* is, athletes can easily weigh sixty pounds or more over the so-called

normal weight for their height and age. But are they overweight? Are they obese?

MYTH #18: WHEN YOUR DOCTOR TELLS YOU YOU'RE OBESE OR OVERWEIGHT, DO WHAT HE TELLS YOU WITHOUT FURTHER INVESTIGATION

Don't!

At an October 1977 conference of The National Institutes of Health, an international panel acknowledged its "ignorance about what causes obesity and how best to treat it." This was reported in *Science Magazine* on December 2, 1977. Ten years earlier, another study reported the same thing despite an imposing body of information derived from research. "Our information concerning the etiology, pathogenesis and treatment of obesity is remarkable," said the doctors in an article in *Pediatrics* (1967).

If your doctor is so sure he can recognize "overweight" and cure it, perhaps he'd want to tell The National Institutes of Health his secret.

MYTH #19: GOING THROUGH A REAL DIETING PERIOD WILL ALWAYS MAKE YOU THINNER

It won't.

In a recent issue of the *Journal of Nutrition,* rats put on calorie-reduced diets gained more weight when the diet ended than non-dieting rats. The temporary diet caused the rats to be more efficient at turning less food into more fat. We *know* rats aren't people, but there's still food for thought here.

MYTH #20: FAT PEOPLE EAT MORE THAN THIN PEOPLE

The most insidious myth of all.

It simply isn't true. Sure, there are *some* fat people who eat more than thin people—and some thin people who eat more than fat people—but three decades of nutritional studies have proven that *all* fat people do not eat more than thin people. When fat peoples' caloric intakes are measured, they prove to be within ranges defined as "normal." J. S. Garrow, analyzing the literature from 1936 to 1972, found that in thirteen studies, all but one showed the mean caloric intake of fat people to be comparable to that of nonfat people. Garrow concluded, "The literature gives no evidence of any relationship between [caloric] intake and body weight in man."

MYTH #21: FAT-CAT INSTITUTIONS DELIVER WHAT THEY PROMISE

Oh no, they don't!
We spend millions of dollars a year at "spas" where we're wrapped in mud, pounded by mechanical devices, starved, submerged in ice packs, stifled in hot packs, fed laxatives, diuretics, wheat germ and propaganda. We dutifully attend meetings of Weight Watchers, Fat Anonymous, TOPS (Take Off Pounds Sensibly) and a hundred other groups which try to coerce, embarrass, tease, and bribe us into losing weight. (At one organization's meetings, we are made to sing, "We are plump little pigs, who eat too much, *fat, fat, fat!*") We plunk down many dollars to be told we're ungainly, unglamorous and sick in the head. We *actually pay* people to tell us that life must be an unending cycle of weighing mouthfuls, wiring jaws shut and listening to little refrigerator boxes screech, "No wonder you're so ugly!"

And what's the result? Less than 3 percent of us actually lose weight and *keep it off.*

Something's funny about that. We overweight people number one-third of the nation. Would anyone dare to tell one-third of the nation to be accountants? Or ambidextrous? How in the world, then, has the think-thin faction been getting away with telling one-third of the nation that we should weigh what they weigh?

To Sum Up

Dr. Hilde Bruch, a most respected authority in the field of obesity, says, "It may be too early to expect a change in taste that praises near-emaciation as beauty, but there is beginning to be a greater awareness and respect for the rights of minorities. Even fat people may come into their own."

If you suffer from an inferiority complex because of a million myths about overweight, if you have *had it* from do-gooders who tell you that you will die tomorrow if you don't diet, don't just sit there and absorb misinformation. Do your own reading and research on the subject. It has taken a long time to get the facts, but modern science is coming up with a picture of the big woman that contradicts all the easy myths about a "fat personality," all the quick and wrong medical knowledge about fat that has been with us too long.

Far from being the jolly, easygoing, dim-witted and sexless person who is sitting on a dangerous fuse of death from pounds, the image that is starting to emerge from the new data is one of a complicated and sensual and intelligent woman who is not so prone to physical risk from her pounds as *they* would have you believe. She is a woman who will not be put down anymore.

But don't believe me—or anybody else. You owe it to yourself to find out the truth—and then to do something about it.

And keep in mind one observation made by a gentleman who admires *zaftig* women: *"People who think thin have to have exceptionally narrow minds."*

We began this chapter with the saga of Jody White who was a victim of misguided family, of myths and of a think-thin society. Her story could end badly, if you, when you write the ending, decide to accept the myths without question. But if, after finding out the facts of fat, you decide to choose the upbeat ending, Jody will persevere and learn to be a big woman afraid of nothing. She will probably enjoy big fat career successes, big fat love affairs, big fat fun and very big fat dreams. She will use her weight to her advantage by giving herself dignity, class and poise. She will wear fabulous (and not necessarily expensive) clothing, be alert, alive and open to new experiences, and she will never, never be coerced into going on a trail of useless diets.

Give it some thought. Choose the right ending for Jody—and choose the right beginning for yourself.

Appendix: Large-Size Stores

The large woman who wants to shop at her local department store will be pleasantly surprised at the many changes in selection and depth of stock.

Starting with the northern part of the East Coast, there is *Porteous*, which has been busy opening well-stocked branches in addition to its main store in Portland, Maine. One of the largest stores is *Jordan Marsh*, which sports a young and enthusiastic group of professionals that are really gung-ho for their Women's World. Their branches are all over Boston, Cape Cod, New Hampshire and Rhode Island. In Providence, Rhode Island, you can also find the *Outlet Store.* If you live near Springfield, Massachusetts, check out the good stock at *Steiger's.* In New Haven, Connecticut, there's *Malley's.*

In and around New York City, of course, there's a glut of stores and if you haven't found chic large-size outfits, you just aren't looking. *Gimbel's* is dedicated to our size and if it's new, it's there! Ditto *Saks Fifth Avenue* and *Lord & Taylor. Macy's* has incredible depth and variety, and much of its stock is elegant and imported goods which you can find nowhere else. The best-known specialty shop in New York is *The Forgotten Woman,* run by a woman who has left a strong personal imprint on her shop. Many things are made just for her and are really individual.

In Upstate New York, there's *McCurdy's* in Rochester. Pennsylvania is a state with some great stores: *Gimbel's* in Philadelphia,

413

The Globe in Scranton and another great *Gimbel's* in Pittsburgh. *Hutzler's in* Baltimore is only one of many department stores that are concerned with large sizes; its management has been vitally interested in promoting good fashion.

In Washington, D.C., there's *Woodward and Lothrop*. Richmond, Virginia, has *Miller and Rhoads*, where the large-size buyer's enthusiasm is contagious.

There are a great group of buyers who carefully stock *O'Neills*, in Akron. Still in the Midwest, *McKelvey's* in Youngstown, Ohio, is marvelous, and there is a really dedicated buyer at *Lazarus*, in Columbus, Ohio. (This store has a load of branches including one in Indianapolis, Indiana.) In Chicago, there's *Charles A. Stevens* and *Carson's*. Milwaukee, Wisconsin has *The Boston Store* and a marvelous specialty store called *Fashions At Large*. Minneapolis, Minnesota has two large department stores. *ZCMI* in Salt Lake City, Utah, also believes in large sizes.

On the West coast, *The Bon* in Seattle, Washington, has been a leader in fashion for the large-size woman. Updated fashion is the byword at *Macy's San Francisco* as well as *Emporium-Capwell*. In Los Angeles, there's the *May Company*, whose fashion shows are the wildest and best in the country. *The Broadway* has well-stocked departments. Up and down the West Coast there are many specialty chains, the foremost being Women's World.

In the Rocky Mountain area, *Denver Dry* in Denver, Colorado, is notable for its large-size department.

Texas also has its share of department stores featuring well-stocked large-size departments as well as the *Women's Shops*, whose main store is in Houston.

Throughout the South can be found the *Catherine Stout Shops*. Their name is anything but up to date and fashionable, but the merchandise inside these stores is beautiful. Florida has a constantly growing selection of department stores, but they love biggies best at *Ivey's* and *Maas Brothers*.

Department stores, as a general rule, try to have the merchandise fit the ambience of the store, so the price range in Women's World departments will match the price range in the rest of the store.

Lane Bryant, *Roaman's* and *Catherine* stores always carry a good selection, no matter where they're located.